Applying Pathophysiological Concepts for the NCLEX-RN®: Through an Inclusive Lens

Applying Pathophysiological Concepts for the NCLEX-RN®: Through an Inclusive Lens

Kaveri M. Roy, DNP, RN, CNE

Assistant Professor
School of Nursing
MGH Institute of Health Professions
Boston, Massachusetts

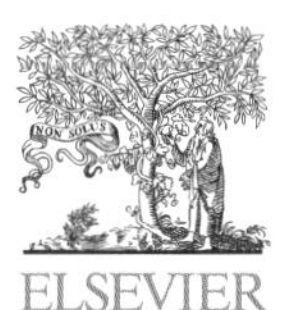

Elsevier
3251 Riverport Lane
St. Louis, Missouri 63043

APPLYING PATHOPHYSIOLOGICAL CONCEPTS FOR THE NCLEX-RN®:
THROUGH AN INCLUSIVE LENS ISBN: 978-0-323-93608-8

Content Strategist: Heather D. Bays-Petrovic
Senior Content Development Specialist: Sneha Kashyap
Publishing Services Manager: Deepthi Unni
Project Manager: Nandhini Thanga Alagu
Senior Book Designer: Amy L. Buxton

Printed in India

Last digit is the print number: 9 8 7 6 5 4 3 2 1

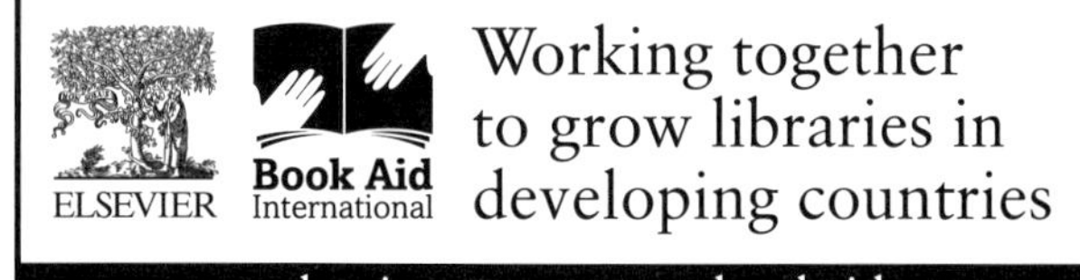

Dedication

I would like to dedicate this book to my late father, Dr. Kalyan K. Roy, my husband Dave, my cats, and all of my pathophysiology students. I could not have written this book without all of you. For my students, I hope that this book makes you proud of all you have achieved.

Preface

I started teaching pathophysiology pretty early in my academic career. While I was teaching medical/surgical nursing I noticed that students were often weak in the subject, often asking me to review "the patho." I realized that they needed a more rigorous experience and was allowed to take over the class with my colleague at the time, Dr. Eileen Searle. When designing the class, we knew that we had to integrate case studies into the classroom. However, when I looked for case studies to use in class, there were few resources. The ones I found were often long and cumbersome, with information that they did not know or perhaps did not need at the time. We started writing our own, which were shorter, and more focused on their class and clinical topics. This way, we hoped to give them a strong foundation in the science so that they could apply it as they progressed.

I ended up taking over the class and continued to make changes. The biggest issue I faced was integrating diversity, race-based medicine, climate change, and social determinants of health into every aspect of pathophysiology—the lectures, the exams, and the case studies. It was a time of change, and the students were hungry for this type of material. I also realized that students of color need to be reflected in the material, so that they can relate and incorporate their own culture and values into their practice. Slowly, I began to learn more about these subjects and to integrate them fully into my lectures and case studies. Surprisingly, pathophysiology is a terrific conduit to these subjects! One of the first pieces of feedback that I received on the class was from a student of color who told me that she felt that she "belonged" in the class and that it was the first time that she saw herself reflected in the class material. Over the years, there have been many comments like this and many students who were grateful to learn about race-based medicine so that they could better advocate for their patients. Students have also remarked on how applicable these case studies are to their clinicals.

By writing this book, I hope to provide another resource for you to test yourself and apply your knowledge, as well as to provide material in a more current context. In utilizing these case studies, please know that conditions can overlap and sometimes there is more than one answer to a case study. I always tell my students that if they can justify their answer, they will get credit. I hope that you benefit from these case studies as much as my students have. Think of it as a puzzle or a mystery and enjoy the process!

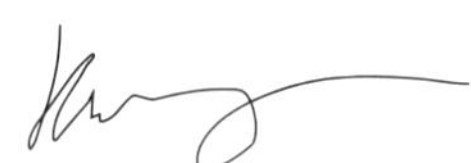

Acknowledgments

I would like to thank and acknowledge Dr. Rebecca Hill for all the support she has given me throughout the years. Thank you to Dr. Eileen Searle, with whom I started this pathophysiology journey; it was a daunting task, and I could not have done it without you. To Professor Julika Wocial, you have gone from being my student, to becoming an RN, to co-teaching with me, and your help and support are invaluable. To my parents, thank you for instilling the love of education and learning in me. I hope this makes you proud! Thanks to my sister, Soma, who is the real writer in the family. Love and thanks to my husband, Dave, for always encouraging me and believing in me and to all my animals at home, for loving me no matter what. And finally, thank you to all my students—I learned more from all of you than you did from me.

Contents

Introduction

Pathophysiology is a class that nursing students often fear. The comments I hear from my pathophysiology students every semester are things like—"I'm so stressed about this class!" or "Everyone talks about how tough this class is." Pathophysiology may be difficult at first, but all of you can succeed! Many students wonder why they need to learn pathophysiology in such detail. Learning about disease process is the key to assessing, diagnosing, planning, intervening, and evaluating clients. It is a language that you are learning as your first step to becoming a nurse and becoming a peer with the team treating your future clients. Most importantly, it is the key to advocating for and educating your clients and families on disease process and why certain interventions are important. This book is meant to supplement the textbook(s) that you are using in your class and to help provide an overview of the material.

One of the important things to realize about pathophysiology is that many diseases are epigenetic, which means that both environment and genetics play a role in disease expression and manifestations. Understanding epigenetic variables is important, as we will be looking at risk factors for diseases. Although your text may include race as a risk factor, race/skin color is no longer considered a biological risk factor by the scientific community. In actuality, disease often has its roots in genetics or familial clusters. When we talk about environment, we must also consider the social determinants of health (access to health care, education, green spaces, good jobs, healthy food, and safe housing) and equity. These determinants are not always considered. However, they can complicate or alleviate many diseases and can sometimes be the difference between life and death for the client. Clients also identify in many ways. Asking clients how they identify can aid in breaking down barriers of mistrust and increasing access for all populations. Addressing gender openly can also help you provide client-centered care and help with specific health issues a client may have.

Learning in Nursing School

Nursing school is going to change the way you work and think. However, before that happens, you need to understand that many of your old ways of learning will not work in a clinical discipline such as nursing. One of the first things that you need to modify is how you learn. Think back to your prerequisite or undergraduate courses. Do you remember sitting in large lecture halls, memorizing information, regurgitating it for the exam, and then forgetting most of what you learned? That method may have served you well then, but it will not work in nursing school!

Nursing school is about active learning. What is active learning? I'll tell you what it is not. Reading, memorizing, highlighting, notecards, and filling out study guides are all forms of passive learning. Active learning is really any method that helps you take the next step to understand and be able to apply, analyze, and evaluate the client and disease processes. Here are some active learning tips that I share with students:

- Use critical thinking strategies. With each disease, picture a client scenario. Think to yourself:
  - D: What do I *d*iscern about the client?
  - I: How would I *i*nterpret my findings?
  - R: How would I *r*espond to these findings?
  - E: How would I *e*valuate my response?

  Here's an example: A client comes to the emergency room. They are pale, sweating, clutching their chest, and short of breath.

  D: Client is pale, sweating, appears to have chest pain, and is short of breath.

  I: This client may be having a myocardial infarction (heart attack).

  R: This is an emergency. This client needs to be brought back to a bed and a provider needs to see the client immediately. An ECG, labs, and an IV need to be ordered STAT.

  E: The patient is stable, has tolerable pain, is getting ordered medications, and is being transported to the cardiac catheterization lab.

  If you think about each scenario this way, you will have the background to answer almost any question!
- Think about how you learn best. Are you a visual, auditory, or kinesthetic learner? Utilize the methods that suit you. There are lots of videos, cartoons, and pictures online to help you. Don't be afraid to Google!
- If you have or make a study guide/disease template, do not fill it out like a book. Going back and having to wade through 30 pages will not help come exam time. Study guides should test your knowledge. After your lecture, try to answer the study guide questions, or even formulate questions about each disease process and answer them on your own. By "on your own", I mean no notes! Once you've done this, go back, look at your book and notes, and fill in the gaps. This way you can separate concepts that you understand from the concepts that you need to work on.

  Write three or four bullet points, draw a picture, or make a chart. That is much more helpful than repeating words on a slide. Study guides should be prompts to help you remember concepts, not books repeating the material.

- Invest in a dry-erase board or large pads of paper. Test your knowledge on disease by drawing the disease process out on the dry-erase board or writing it out on a large piece of paper. Reasoning out each pathophysiological process this way will help you ingrain the concepts in your mind.
- Say it out loud. If you can't explain the disease process to yourself, chances are that you don't fully understand it. You don't need to memorize the book or the PowerPoint. What you do need to do is put the concept into your own words. That is the best way to understand and explain it to someone else, like your clients!
- Teach someone. Remember the saying, "See one, do one, teach one"? Teaching is by far the best way to learn a topic. Yes, I know, you are on the spot. But having to explain it to someone else is harder to do, because you need to make the connections and then explain your thoughts coherently. There is no better way to solidify your learning. Also, teaching someone does not only mean your fellow students. Professors, teaching assistants, parents, siblings, cats, dogs, other pets, stuffed animals, significant others, other family members, are all fair game when it comes to your learning!
- Look for connections. The body makes sense. This is something that my students hear me say all the time. So often I see students reaching for a complex answer when the correct answer is in front of them the whole time. When I ask why they do this, they tell me that they didn't think the answer was that simple! It can be that simple if you break down what you are learning and say it in your own words. When you are looking at the systems, such as cardiac, pulmonary, renal, and hepatic, all of them connect to each other. If you figure out how they connect, it makes the learning much easier.

Hint: Don't memorize the clinical manifestations unless your instructor emphasizes certain hallmark symptoms or lab values that you need to know. Again, the body makes sense. If you are going over a gastrointestinal disorder, the client is going to have abdominal pain, maybe a change in stool (diarrhea), or nausea and vomiting. If the client has a cardiac disorder, they will likely have chest pain, palpitations, and shortness of breath. Learn to understand the pathophysiology, then think logically about what the clinical manifestations would be.

- Test yourself. The one thing that we are all (myself included) afraid to do is to test ourselves. This means putting away your notes, PowerPoints, and books and seeing what you know. After a lecture, use a study guide or objectives as a tool to test yourself with. How many of the study guide questions or objectives can you answer on your own? This tells you how much you have retained. After doing that, go back to the notes and fill in what you missed.
- You need to synthesize the information. This means that you cannot just copy what you missed from your notes or the book. You need to work out how you are going to put concepts into your own words, so that you truly understand. This means talking out loud, drawing it out on a dry-erase board, or teaching someone the content. Once you synthesize the information, you will be able to retain the knowledge.

The last thing we need to talk about is your study habits. I'm just going to say it, and some of you may not believe me, but cramming doesn't work! There is so much information coming at you so fast that you need to keep up every week. Not only do you need to keep up, but you also need to test yourself on the concepts covered every week. What I suggest is that you slot out defined study periods each week. Most pathophysiology courses are three or four credits. You should be studying for 3 hours per credit hour. For pathophysiology, you should be studying 9 to 12 hours a week. It sounds like a lot, doesn't it? But the truth of the matter is, you are probably already studying close to this many hours, but it is not focused studying. Here's how I tell my students to lay out their weekly calendars:

Day1 (2-3 hours)
Prework
- Skim/read over chapters
- Look over PowerPoint
- Read over objectives for the week

Day 2 (2-3 hours)
Lecture
- Listen actively
- Ask questions
- Record the lecture if possible so that you can actively listen
- Mark notes or slides where you missed information so that you can go back and listen to that section again

Day 3 (2-3 hours)
Synthesis
- Test yourself
- Use the study guide from class, this book, or the objectives
- Answer the questions and see how much you have retained
- Then go back and look at what you missed
- Synthesize the information into your own words, a picture, or a chart and put it on the study guide

Day 4 (2-3 hours)
Practice questions/case studies/synthesis
- Act as if you are going to take an exam on the week's material
- Complete any practice questions that you have access to; your textbooks often have questions you can complete
- Complete the case studies in this book that apply to the week's material

Now, you do not have to use this way of organization. But you will need some form of organization to direct your studying and get the most out of it. You can also use your method of organization for your other nursing classes.

A method students find helpful is to break down and compare similar disease processes with T-charts. Below is modified version of the pathophysiology template.

	Cobalamin (B_{12}) deficiency	Folic acid deficiency
Cause?		
Pathophysiology?		
Symptoms?		

An example would be the B_{12} and folic acid deficiencies. These deficiencies both cause anemia, but the mechanisms of disease as well as the symptoms are very different. By looking at these diseases side by side, you can clearly see the similarities and differences.

Another way to organize your thoughts is by using a disease template. Here is an example:

Pathophysiology	
Causes and risk factors	
Clinical manifestations	
Diagnostic studies	
Treatments/interventions	
Complications	

This template can help you organize information as you take notes. You can also use it to test yourself on different diseases. Hopefully, some of these tips have helped.

Each chapter in this book consists of an overview, a study guide, and multiple case studies. A study guide is in every chapter to help you guide your studying for class. But the primary learning method is using case studies. Case studies are one of the best ways to apply your pathophysiology knowledge and make it stick. Please use the study guides and case studies with your textbook and class notes. Feel free to use reputable websites and research studies to supplement your learning. Now, let's get started on the pathophysiology case studies. A note of caution: Do not look at the answers before you have finished answering the case studies. I know it's tempting, but you will not gain as much by doing this. And if you get an answer wrong, make sure you understand the rationale for the correct answer.

1 Inflammation and Immunity

Inflammation and immunity are typically one of the first topics in a pathophysiology class. Why? Because inflammation and immunity are the basis for all disease. Most of the manifestations of disease process come from the reaction of the body to the injury, whether it is from pathogens, the environment, or a direct physical insult. The body's first line of defense includes the skin, mucous membranes, and epithelial cells. Once the body's first line of defense has been breached, the second line of defense, inflammation, quickly goes into effect to control the injury.

Inflammation consists of redness from vasodilation and slower blood flow, isolation of the affected area through clotting, swelling from the formation of exudate, mast cell degranulation and secretion of chemical mediators and cytokines, activation of complement proteins to lyse and kill pathogens, and migration of phagocytes to the area of injury to aid in pathogen destruction and wound healing. If it is a minor injury, sometimes inflammation and wound healing are enough. However, if it is a more involved injury or infection, systemic inflammation and the adaptive immune systems come into play (Figs. 1.1 and 1.2).

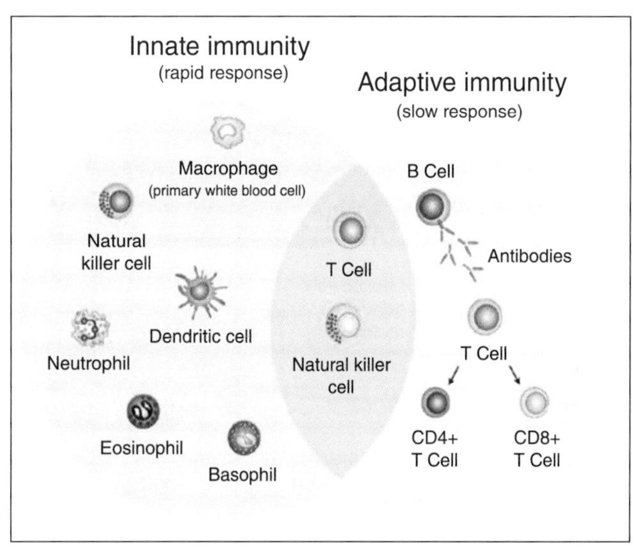

• **Fig. 1.1** Cells of the innate and adaptive immune system. (Used with permission from Dranoff, G. Cytokines in cancer pathogenesis and cancer therapy. Nat Rev Cancer 4, 11–22 (2004). https://doi.org/10.1038/nrc1252)

A few key points when looking at innate and adaptive immunity:

- Inflammation is nonspecific. Think of the five cardinal signs: redness, swelling, pain, heat, and loss of function.
- Mast cells degranulate and secrete chemical mediators and cytokine. They also synthesize prostaglandins and leukotrienes. They are significant in innate immunity (Fig. 1.3).
- You will always see clotting with inflammation.
  - Disorders such as atherosclerosis and myocardial infarctions are due to inflammation.
- Systemic inflammation typically means:
  - Fever
  - Increased white blood cells (leukocytosis)
  - Increased C-reactive proteins (CRP)
  - Increased erythrocyte sedimentation rates (ESR)
- Bradykinin and prostaglandin are chemical mediators that cause pain.
- Tumor necrosis factor and interleukins are cytokines that cause fever.
- Macrophages and dendritic cells are antigen-presenting cells that help bridge the innate immune response and the adaptive immune response.
- The adaptive immune system can take a few days to a week to mount a response, as it is specific to the antigen and the T helper cells need to recognize the antigen first.
- Repeated exposures create more memory T and B cells, which helps the adaptive immune system respond faster.

Passive and active immunity are ways that the body deals with infection. Acquired passive immunity is transfer of antibodies from parent to fetus or by injection/infusion. Active immunity is the body's response to infection—antibodies, T cells, and B cells. Acquired active immunity occurs when you contract a disease or when you are vaccinated, and the body is prompted to make antibodies and memory T and B cells.

If a component of the innate and immune system is deficient or absent, it can lead to serious consequences in the body's immune surveillance system. This can happen because of genetics (severe combined immunodeficiency—T and B cells absent) or it can be acquired (HIV/AIDS—destruction of T helper cells by virus).

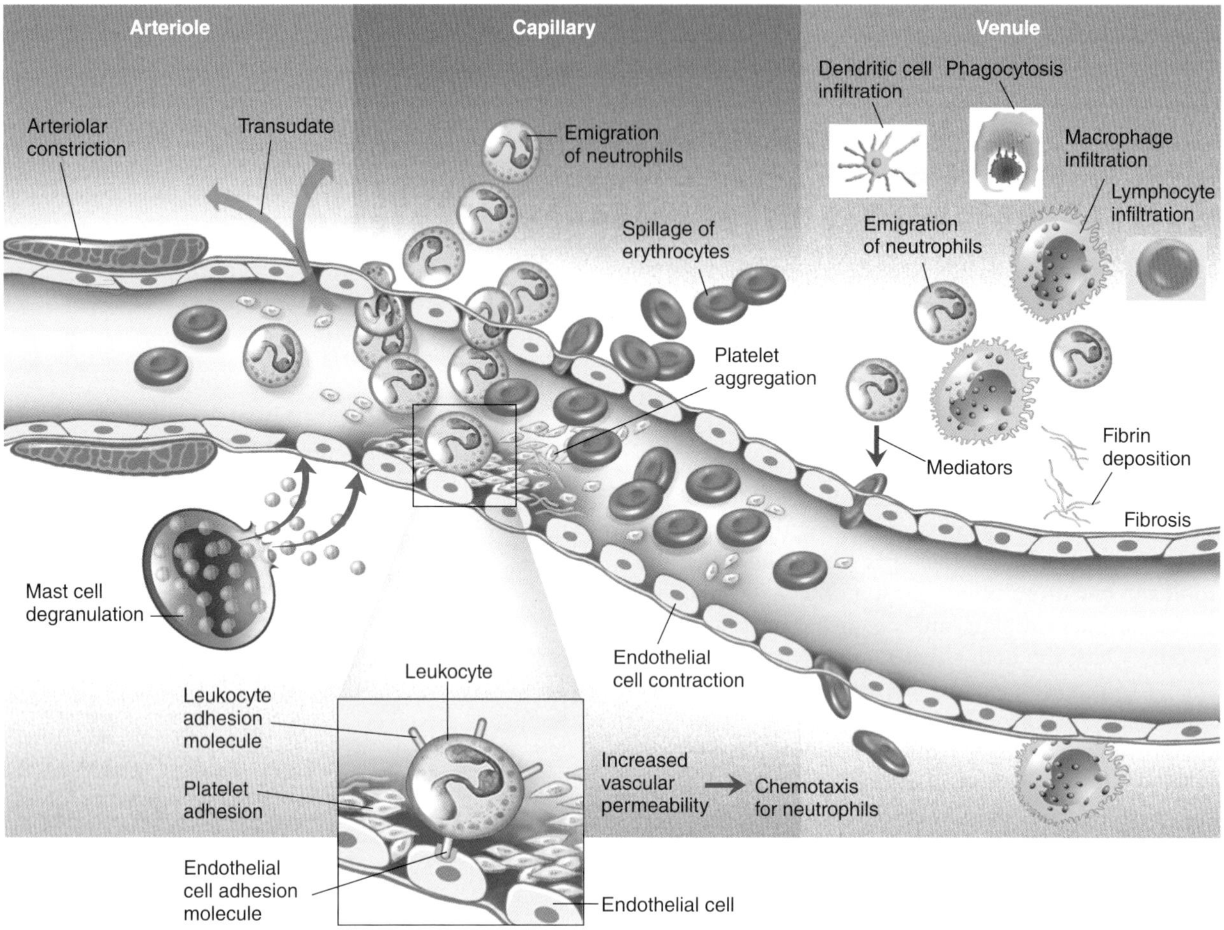

• **Fig. 1.2** Acute inflammatory response. (From Huether, S. E., & McCance, K. L. (2019). *Understanding pathophysiology* (7th ed.). Mosby.)

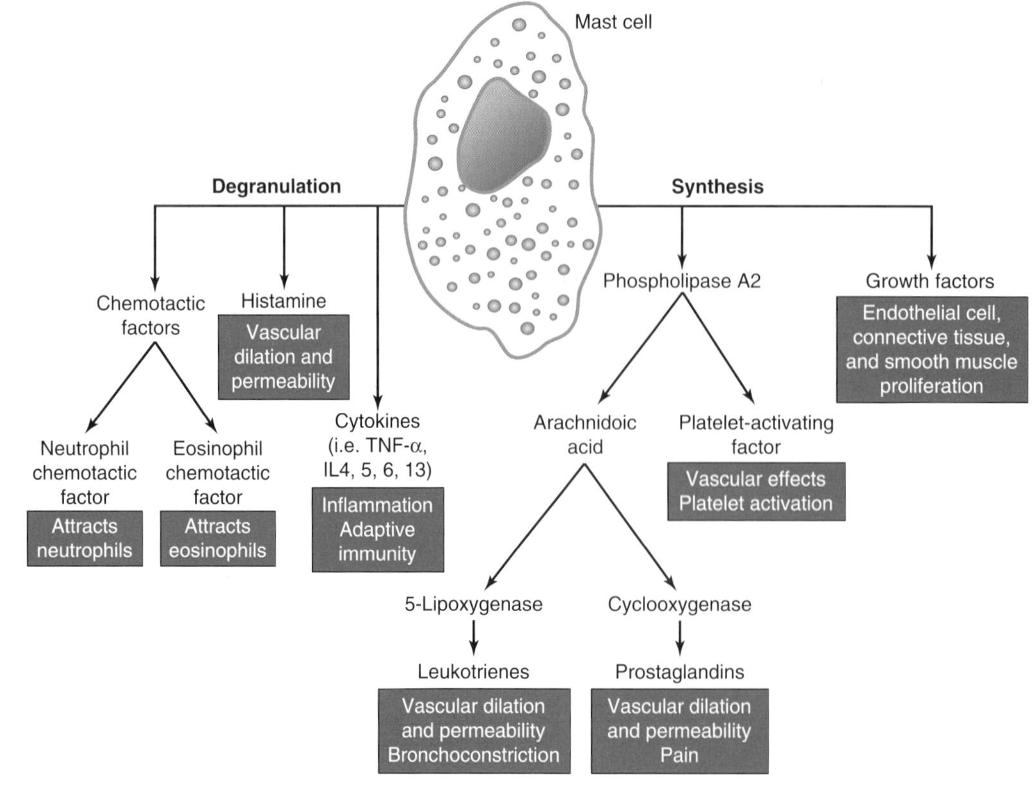

• **Fig. 1.3** Mast cell functions. *IL,* Interleukin; TNF-α, tumor necrosis factor alpha.

Study Suggestions

- To understand the roles of the different types of cells, draw them out—innate, antigen-presenting, and adaptive immune cells and look at how they work together in mounting immune response.
- Remember—synthesize information, don't write a book!

Study Guide for Chapter 1

Make sure that you have your class notes and textbooks on hand to answer these questions.

1. What are the ways that the body protects us? What is the difference between innate and immune response?

Innate (Inflammation) Response

2. When do you have an innate inflammatory response? What is the purpose of this response?

3. What is exudate? What are the different types?

4. What are the functions of interleukins, tumor necrosis factor, and interferons?

5. What are the functions of mast cells? What clinical manifestations would you expect to see with histamine release and with prostaglandin and leukotriene release?

6. What is a chemokine?

7. What do neutrophils, macrophages, and dendritic cells do?

8. What happens in the vascular stage of inflammation? What happens in the cellular stage of inflammation?

9. How does the body mount a systemic inflammatory response? When does a systemic response happen? What do you see when there is a systemic response?

10. What is the difference between acute inflammation and chronic inflammation? When would you see an abscess? When would you see a granuloma?

11. What is an antigen-presenting cell and what function does it serve in adaptive immunity?

Adaptive Immune Response

12. When does adaptive immunity start? What is adaptive immunity? What cells take part in it?

13. What function do the T helper cells play? How do they identify antigens and activate the immune system?

14. How does the major histocompatibility complex (MHC1 and MHC2) play a role in adaptive immunity? How do they interact with T helper cells and cytotoxic T cells?

15. What is an epitope? How do antibodies and antigens bind to each other?

16. How does an antibody function? (opsonization, neutralization, agglutination, complement proteins)

17. Differentiate between antibody primary response and secondary response.

18. What are the different classes of antibodies?

19. What role do complement proteins play in innate (inflammatory) and immune (antibody) reactions?

Immunity and Immune Deficiency

20. What are some examples of active and passive immunity? Why do you need a booster shot with active immunity?

21. How is HIV diagnosed? What are the different stages?

22. What are the most common opportunistic infections seen with HIV?

23. What do the HIV/AIDS therapies accomplish?

Get to Know Your Cells!

Use this cell map to link each cell to its role in inflammation and immunity. This way you will be able to see not just what the cells do, but how inflammation and immunity connect. Fill in the innate and immune cells and their functions. How do they connect?

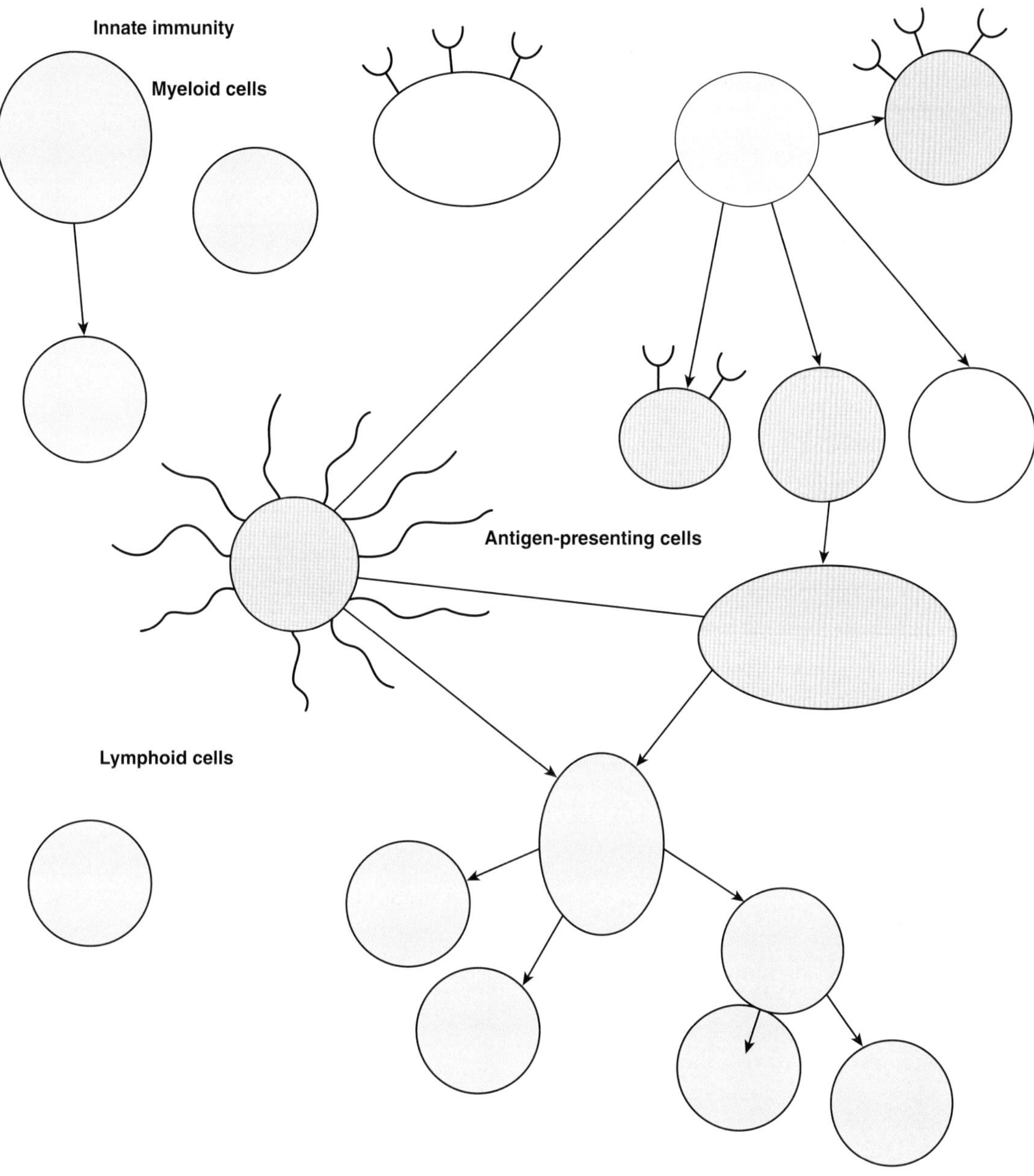

Case Studies for Chapter 1

Make sure that you have your class notes and textbooks on hand to answer these questions.

Case Study 1.1

Leah, a 45-year-old Black cis-female (she/her/hers), fell while hiking in Yosemite National Park. She sustained a laceration on her left forearm with some bruising. She cleaned up the laceration, put an antibiotic ointment on it, and bandaged it up. Two days later, she was changing her bandage and noticed that the area around the laceration was red, painful, and swollen. She observed thick yellow discharge on the bandage.

1. In terms of inflammatory response, describe the vascular and cellular events.

____

____

____

____

2. Is this an acute or chronic inflammation? Is it systemic? Explain your answers.

____

____

____

____

Leah went to the urgent care center near her home and received oral antibiotics. A week later, she noticed that her entire left arm was swollen and painful. There was a red line going from the laceration on her forearm to her upper arm. She felt fatigue and muscle aches. When she went back to the urgent care center, staff took her vital signs and found that Leah had a fever of 101°F.

3. What has caused Leah's worsening symptoms?

4. What lab work would you expect?

5. How would you treat Leah's symptoms?

Case Study 1.2

Matt is a 34-year-old White cis-male (he/him/his) with a history of inflammatory bowel disease, which was diagnosed 10 years ago. On a recent colonoscopy, a lesion was found in his small bowel. A biopsy showed that the lesion contained giant cells, macrophages, and lymphocytes.

1. What is the biopsy indicative of? Explain.

2. Is this an acute inflammation or a chronic inflammation? Why?

When Matt met with the provider to go over the colonoscopy results, the provider told him that Matt has a high risk of gastrointestinal cancer because of his inflammatory bowel disease. Matt became very upset, stating, "It's bad enough that I have this disease. Now you are telling me that I will get cancer too?"

3. Explain why Matt is at a higher risk for cancer.

4. What would you say to Matt about his risk of getting cancer?

Case Study 1.3

Kasey, a 35-year-old Latinx trans-male (they/them/their), has had a sore throat and myalgias for the last 3 weeks. They went to see their provider because they were worried that they had mononucleosis. The provider ordered lab work and asked to add an HIV test as well. Kasey agreed to this. When the lab work came back, the provider told Kasey that they were tested negative for mononucleosis, but positive for HIV.

1. What stage of HIV infection is Kasey in? Describe the stage.

2. Do their symptoms fit with the HIV diagnosis?

3. What kind of HIV testing is done initially? Is just having one of those tests enough to confirm the diagnosis? Explain.

After the provider shares the lab results, Kasey becomes tearful. They ask, "Is this a death sentence?"

4. How would you answer Kasey?

Kasey is put on highly active antiretroviral therapy (HAART) and their viral load becomes negligible. They and their spouse want to have a child. Kasey's partner is a cis-male (he/him/his) who is HIV negative. When they go in for a regular checkup, they ask if it would be possible for them to have a child if they have HIV.

5. What would you tell them?

6. How can they prevent the child from having HIV?

Kasey gets pregnant and has an uneventful pregnancy and delivery. When the baby has blood tests taken, the baby is found to have HIV antibodies.

7. Does this mean that the baby has HIV? Explain your answer.

8. What would be the most definitive HIV test for a newborn?

2 Genetic Disorders and Cancer

Genetics and Cancer Overview

Genetics and cancer are often paired together as the subjects immediately following inflammation and immunity. Why? Genetics and familial clustering are major causes and risk factors for disease. When we are talking about genetic diseases, we are talking about autosomal dominant, autosomal recessive, sex-linked traits, and multifactorial inheritance diseases. We are also talking about epigenetic issues such as toxins, viruses, and bacterial illnesses that can cause significant mutations and congenital defects. Cancer is a response to chronic inflammation and the increased chance of genetic mutation. Cancer can also be caused by genetic traits passed on by family members.

Autosomal Dominant and Recessive Traits

Think back to genetics and Punnett squares. The following table shows a Punnett square that is a cross between a brown-eyed parent (BB) and blue-eyed parent (bb). The "B" signifies the dominant trait and "b" signifies the recessive trait.

BB	Bb
Bb	bb

An autosomal dominant trait is expressed whenever there is a dominant allele, in this case "B," in one of the two alleles for the genotype, regardless of whether the other allele is dominant (B) or recessive (b). So, looking at the Punnett square, there is a 75% probability that the parents will have a child with brown eyes. An autosomal recessive trait is only expressed when both alleles have the recessive gene. In this case, blue eyes (bb) are recessive and there is a 25% chance that the parents will have a blue-eyed child. Examples of autosomal dominant disorder would be neurofibromatosis. An example of an autosomal recessive disorder would be phenylketonuria.

Sex-Linked Traits

Sex-linked characteristics are typically carried on the X chromosome. This means that if an assigned female at birth (AFAB) with the gene mutation for hemophilia X^HX is crossed with an assigned male at birth (AMAB), the female children have a 50% chance of being carriers (X^HX) and a 50% chance of having a normal phenotype. The AFAB children are only carriers because they have two X chromosomes, and the healthy X chromosome can mask the effects of the mutation. However, because AMAB children only have one X chromosome, if they have an X chromosome with a gene mutation, they will show the effects of the mutation. In this case, the AMAB children have a 50% chance of having hemophilia (X^HY) and a 50% chance of having a normal phenotype.

X^HX	XX
X^HY	XY

Aneuploidy

Aneuploidy is when there are an abnormal number of chromosomes. This is seen in Turner syndrome, where AFABs have one X chromosome paired with an incomplete or absent second X chromosome. Klinefelter syndrome is when AMAB have multiple X chromosomes along with a Y chromosome (Fig. 2.1). Another well-known example is Down syndrome, or trisomy 21. This is when there are three chromosomes instead of two for chromosome 21.

Multifactorial Inheritance Disorders

As is probably evident by the name, multifactorial inheritance disorders, many factors figure into these disorders, not only genetic but also environmental factors. Examples of these diseases include congenital issues, such as cleft lip and palate, clubfoot, and heart defects. However, diseases such as diabetes, Alzheimer disease, schizophrenia, depression, heart disease, and obesity are also classified as multifactorial inheritance disorders. Individuals with these diseases may be predisposed genetically, but environmental factors such as stress, diet, exercise, and determinants of health and equity also play a role in whether the genetic traits are actually expressed.

Cancer

Cancer is the rapid, uncontrolled proliferation of abnormal cells. This can be in response to genetic or epigenetic factors,

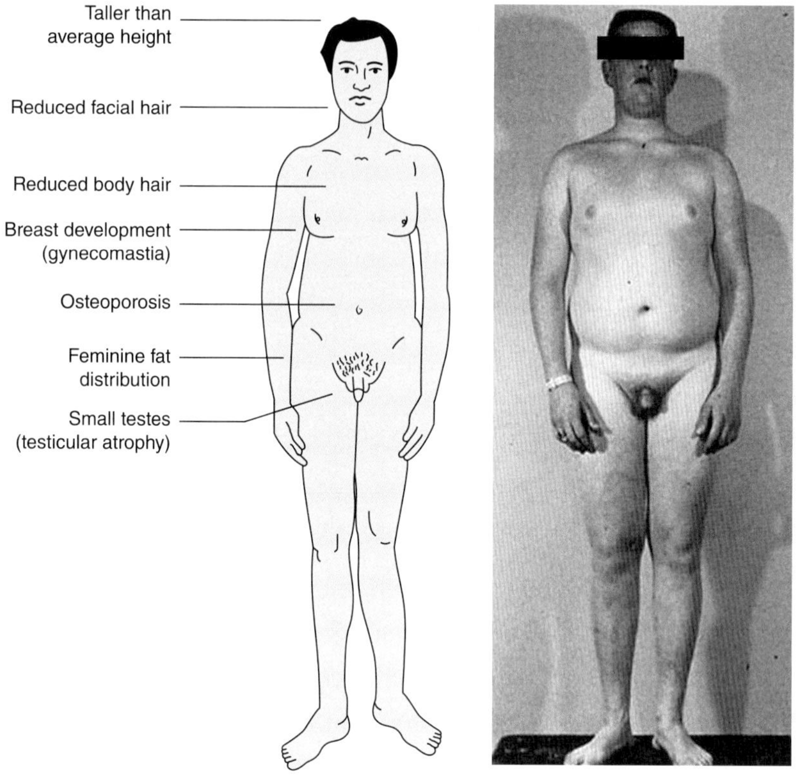

Taller than average height
Reduced facial hair
Reduced body hair
Breast development (gynecomastia)
Osteoporosis
Feminine fat distribution
Small testes (testicular atrophy)

• **Fig. 2.1** Klinefelter syndrome. (From Matsumoto, A.A., & Anawalt, B.D. (2020). Testicular Disorders. Williams Textbook of Endocrinology (14th ed.). Elsevier.)

exposure to carcinogens, or chronic inflammation (Fig. 2.2). The first step in developing cancer is having a genetic mutation. Let's look at an example of a client who sunbathes frequently. The ultraviolet radiation from the sun may cause mutations of the DNA in the client's skin cells. These mutations initiate cells that can go on to become cancerous. However, that does not mean that the client has cancer. We have a myriad of defenses within our body to deal with mutated cells, such as our innate and adaptive immune system. We also have protective mechanisms within our genes, such as the tumor suppressor genes and apoptosis genes (cause cellular death). It takes a failure of these protective mechanisms for cancer to develop.

After cellular mutations have occurred, promotion needs to occur. This is the stage where normal growth genes called proto-oncogenes mutate to become oncogenes. This causes mutated cells to proliferate. Tumor suppressor genes inhibit the proliferation of mutated cells. However, if there is a mutation in the tumor suppressor genes, they may no longer protect against the proliferation of these abnormal cells. Apoptosis genes are also a layer of protection, as these genes cause cellular death if there is a mutation or damage to the cells. If there is a mutation in the apoptosis genes, it could "shut off" apoptosis, causing these cells to proliferate indefinitely. That's why cancer cells are said to be immortal. For cancer to develop, rapid, aggressive proliferation must occur due to a great number of these mutations. Cell division needs to be promoted or occur in a hospitable environment. If the client sunbathes for 4 hours daily, they would be in an environment where mutations would be promoted.

Cancer cells also must be nourished to proliferate. The cells utilize angiogenesis for this purpose. Angiogenesis is the growth and development of new blood vessels. Cancer cells secrete chemical mediators, such as vascular endothelial growth factor, to cause blood vessel growth into the tumor (Fig. 2.3). The blood flow into the tumor allows cancer progression. Blood and lymph vessels are also important in metastasis, as they both allow cancer cells to escape and colonize other areas of the body. Cancer cells proliferate more and more aggressively and become anaplastic. Anaplasia means that the cancer cells mutate and no longer look or function like the parent cell. There is a loss of differentiation between these cancer cells and the original parent cell (Fig. 2.4).

Cancer can be diagnosed in many ways: tumor marker cells found in the blood (e.g., prostate-specific antigen), cytology studies, biopsy, monoclonal antibodies (specific to cancer cell antigens), and genetic analysis. Cancers are graded and staged to track progression. When a tumor is graded, you are looking at how differentiated a cancer cell is. If the cell is well differentiated, then it is a low-grade cancer. If a cell is poorly differentiated, it is a high-grade cancer. Staging looks at the size and spread of the cancer. The TNM (tumor, node, metastasis) system looks at how big the tumor is, if it has spread to the lymph nodes, and if there is distant metastasis. Tumors can compress organs and impede vital

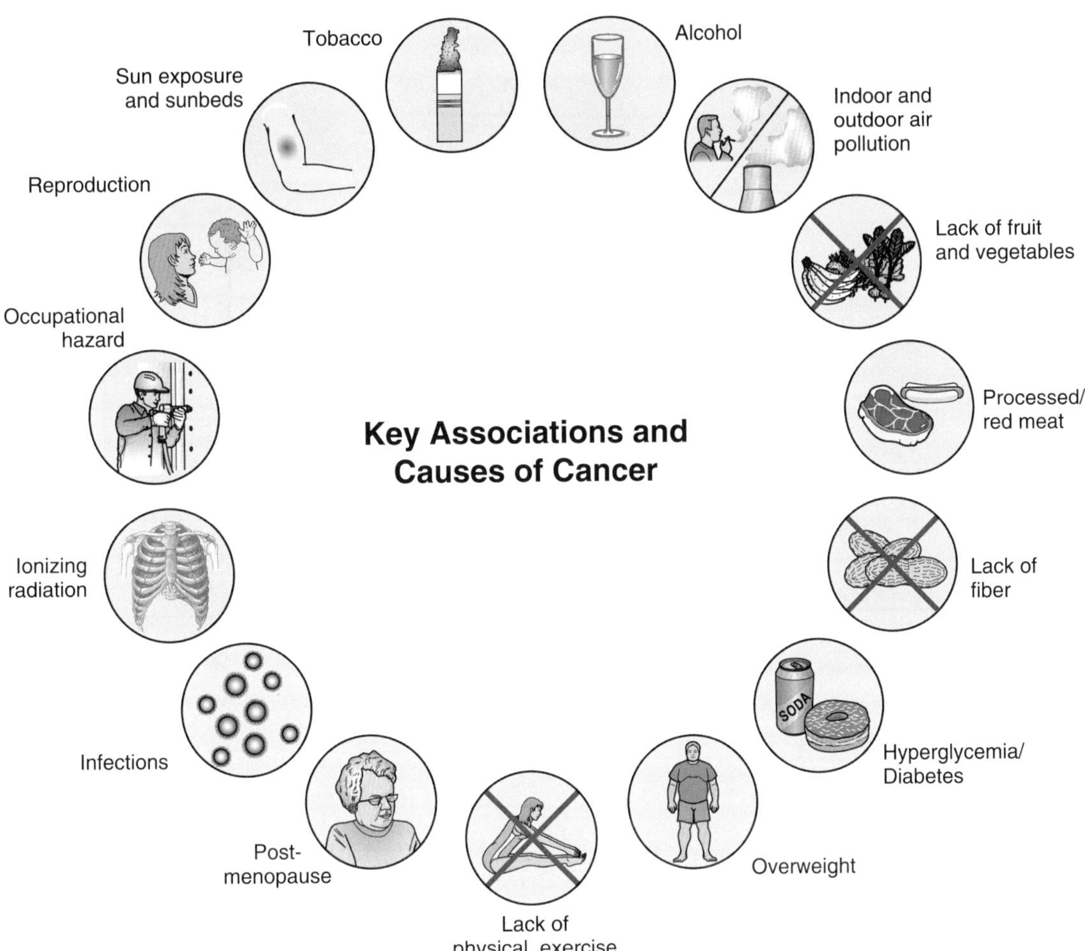

• **Fig. 2.2** Risk factors for cancer. (From Power-Kean, K., Zettel, S., El-Hussein, M. T., Huether, S. E., & McCance, K. L. (2022). *Huether and McCance's understanding pathophysiology, Canadian edition* (2nd ed.). Elsevier. Fig. 11.1.)

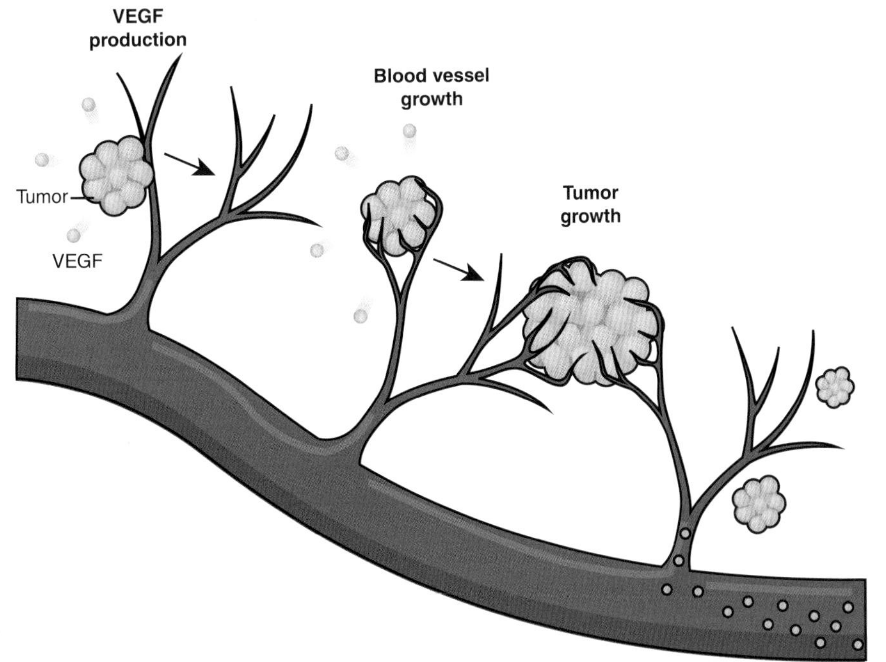

• **Fig. 2.3** Angiogenesis. *VEGF,* Vascular endothelial growth factor. (From Mohammed, H. H. (2015). Angiogenesis and cancer. *Int J Sci Eng Technol Res*, 4(41), 9089–9096. Fig. 2.)

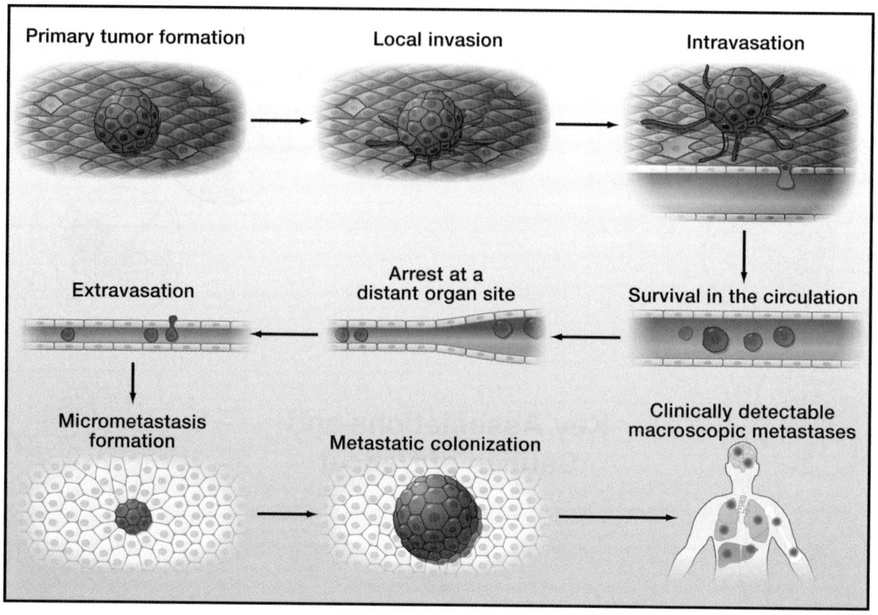

• **Fig. 2.4** Invasion and metastasis. (From Valastyan, S., & Weinberg, R. A. (2011). Tumor metastasis: Molecular insights and evolving paradigms. *Cell*, 147(2), 275–292. https://doi.org/10.1016/j.cell.2011.09.024. https://www.sciencedirect.com/science/article/pii/S0092867411010853.)

functions. Metastasis is typically to nearby organs and lymph nodes initially. Common areas for metastasis are lymph, bone, brain, lungs, and liver.

Benign tumor cells also proliferate at a higher rate than normal. However, the rate of proliferation is slower than that of cancer cells and the cells are well differentiated and continue to function the same way as the parent cells. The danger with a benign tumor is when it runs out of space and causes compression (brain) or when it impedes a vital function (lung, heart).

There are many ways to treat cancer—surgery, chemotherapy, radiation, immunotherapy, and hormone therapy being among them. Most of the time, two therapies are paired together, such as surgery to remove the tumor and adjuvant chemotherapy to kill off cancer cells that have metastasized. No treatment is meant to kill 100% of the cancer cells; instead, the treatments are meant to destroy enough cancer cells that the body's immune system can then take over and get rid of the rest. Treatments such as chemotherapy and radiation are targeted to rapidly dividing cells but can damage healthy cells and tissue as well.

Study Suggestions

- When learning the genetic diseases, classify them by type: autosomal dominant, autosomal recessive, multifactorial inherited, etc. Compare and contrast them to help remember details.
- Utilize the disease template. Separate the etiology, pathophysiology, manifestations, and complications. Use the template to test yourself!
- With cancer, divide up the topic into parts; for example, cancer formation, diagnosis, treatments, complications.

Study Guide for Chapter 2

Make sure that you have your class notes and textbooks on hand to answer these questions. A concept map is included to help you to diagram and link disease concepts together.

Genetic Disorders

1. Describe the etiology (genetics, incidence), clinical manifestations, and risk factors of Klinefelter syndrome, Turner syndrome, and Down syndrome.

2. Describe the etiology and manifestations of Marfan syndrome and neurofibromatosis and compare the differences between the two.

3. Discuss the genetics and manifestations of Tay-Sachs disease.

4. How does phenylketonuria occur? What are the manifestations and long-term complications?

5. What is a multifactorial genetic disorder?

6. What causes cleft palate/cleft lip?

7. Describe the prenatal testing that can be done for fetal genetic defects.

Cancer

8. What are the differences between benign and cancerous cells?

9. How do you classify tumors? (grading, staging, TNM)

10. How do you diagnose cancer?

11. What is the role of oncogenes and tumor suppressor cells in causing cancer cells to proliferate?

12. How does angiogenesis occur? What role does angiogenesis play in metastasis?

13. How do cancer cells metastasize? Where are the most common areas of metastasis?

14. How do risk factors such as obesity, age, genetics, and immune system function increase/affect risk of cancer?

15. What are some of the side effects of cancer?

16. What is paraneoplastic syndrome?

17. What are the side effects of chemotherapy and radiation? What tissues are most susceptible? Why?

18. How does radiation work to destroy cancer cells? Is it a local or systemic treatment?

19. How does chemotherapy work? Is it a local or systemic treatment?

20. Why is immunotherapy used to treat cancer? In what cases would hormone therapy be used for cancer?

Concept Map

Use this concept map to link each disease to its pathophysiology, diagnostics, causes, risk factors, complications, and clinical manifestations together. This way, you will be able to see the whole picture of the disease.

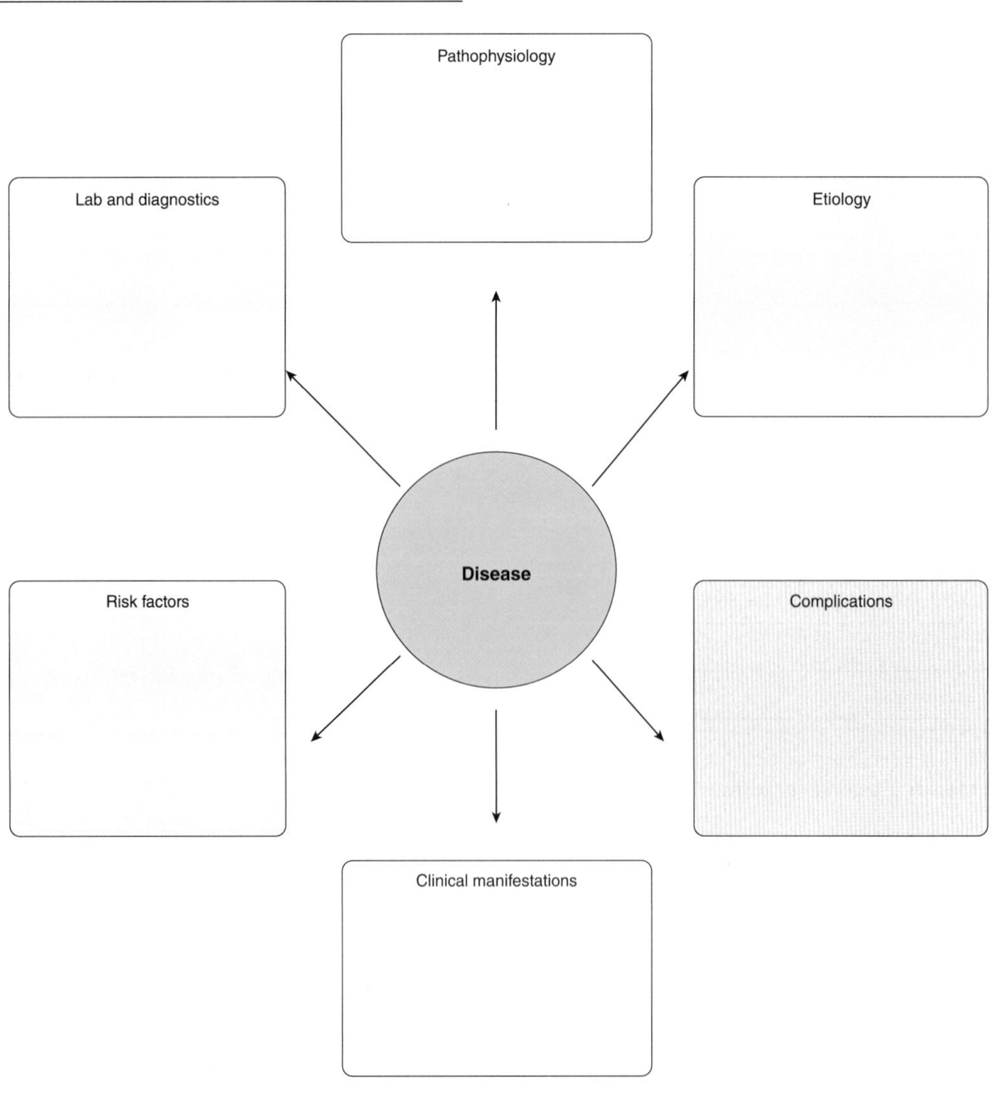

Case Studies for Chapter 2

Make sure that you have your class notes and textbooks on hand to answer these questions.

Case Study 2.1

Mateo is an 18-year-old Brazilian cis-male (he/him/his). He is a varsity soccer player and an avid runner. During his last soccer game, Mateo collapsed and was rushed to the emergency room. In the emergency room, Mateo was assessed and found to be short of breath and tachycardic.

Vital signs: BP 88/60, pulse 136 beats/minute, respiratory rate 28 breaths/minute. Height: 6′5″, weight 180 pounds.

Assessment: Client is pale, using accessory muscles to breathe. Chest is noted to be concave. Electrocardiogram (ECG): ventricular tachycardia.

1. What disorder do you think that Mateo has? Why?

2. Explain the reason why Mateo may be short of breath and tachycardic.

With supportive care, Mateo's vital signs are back to baseline, and he can breathe normally. He tells the nurse, "I can't wait to go back and play in the championship game!"

3. What would you say to Mateo about continuing his athletic activities?

4. What complications are associated with this disease and how can they be monitored?

Case Study 2.2

Mia is a White cis-gender female (she/her/hers) who has a 5-month-old daughter, Lana. She and her wife have noticed that Lana has stopped meeting the growth milestones. At 4 months, Lana was able to roll over and was starting to crawl. Over the last few weeks, they have noticed that Lana has stopped rolling over and crawling and seems to be much weaker. They are concerned that Lana may be ill. After examining Lana, the pediatric provider lets Mia and her wife know that she may have Tay-Sachs disease.

Mia's wife asks, "What is Tay-Sachs disease? Can it be cured?"

1. How would you answer Mia's spouse?

Mia starts to cry, asking if it is her fault that her child has Tay-Sachs disease. "Did I give this to my baby? I'm healthy and I made sure that the sperm donor was healthy too!"

2. Explain how Mia could have a child with Tay-Sachs disease.

3. What is the prognosis for children with Tay-Sachs disease? Is there a way to find out if a child will be born with the disease? How?

Case Study 2.3

Patrick is a 40-year-old Asian cis-male (he/him/his). He has a history of type 2 diabetes mellitus, hypertension, depression, and is mildly overweight. He has been prescribed medications for his diabetes, hypertension, and depression. He goes to the health clinic to see his health care provider for a follow-up visit. He says to his provider, "I don't know how I got all of these conditions. I live a pretty healthy lifestyle. My mom and brother have some of these problems too."

1. Discuss any risk factors, including epigenetic risk factors, Patrick may have. What would be the next step in the assessment?

When looking at Patrick's lab results and vital signs, the provider notices that Patrick's blood sugar is elevated, and his blood pressure is high. The provider asks Patrick if he is taking medications and exercising. Patrick appears embarrassed and says, "I went to the drug store, but I couldn't afford the medications. My insurance does not cover it. I tried to exercise, but the gym is too expensive. I live in an apartment building in the city and there aren't any places close by to run or exercise. The big chain grocery store near my house just closed, so I have to buy all my food at the corner store. I really want to be healthy, but I don't know how I can do more."

2. How do the social determinants of health and health equity play a role in Patrick's health?

3. How can the health clinic team help Patrick achieve his goal to become healthier?

Case Study 2.4

Leticia is a 52-year-old Latinx cis-female (she/her/hers). She has a past medical history of atherosclerosis, hypertension, and is overweight. She has recently emigrated to the United States and is living with her daughter, son-in-law, and grandchildren. Leticia has temporary resident status but does not have health insurance yet. Three months ago, while showering, Leticia noticed a small nodule near her right armpit. Leticia did not pay much attention to it at that time. A week ago, she noticed that the nodule was bigger and told her daughter. She also told her daughter that breast nodules run in the family. Her daughter made an appointment at a free clinic nearby and has accompanied her mother on the visit. The provider finds the nodule suspicious and helps Leticia and her daughter schedule an appointment for a free/low-cost mammogram. The mammogram shows a suspicious right breast lesion.

1. What would be the next step in properly diagnosing Leticia's condition?

2. How would the social determinants of health and equity impact her diagnosis and treatment?

3. What risk factors does Leticia have for breast cancer?

The clinic social worker is able to help Leticia obtain Medicaid coverage. She is diagnosed with breast cancer, which is staged as T3N1M2. She is scheduled for surgery and adjuvant chemotherapy.

4. How advanced is Leticia's cancer?

5. Why is she scheduled for chemotherapy? Will surgery and chemotherapy get rid of all of the cancer cells? Why or why not?

6. What are three common side effects of chemotherapy? Explain the pathophysiology behind why these side effects occur.

Leticia's treatment regimen is effective. Five years later, Leticia notices that her skin has a yellow tinge, and her abdomen is distended. Her daughter notices that Leticia is more confused than usual and becomes agitated easily.

7. What could these symptoms be a result of?

3

Fluid, Electrolytes, and Arterial Blood Gases

Fluid, electrolytes, and arterial blood gas (ABG) disorders can be quite overwhelming for the new nursing student. While I don't usually recommend memorizing for pathophysiology as a rule, for this chapter you will need to memorize the normal lab ranges of serum osmolality (275–295 mOsm/kg), electrolytes, and ABGs. Flashcards can help with this. A method that helps in learning the electrolytes is to compare the disorders in a table. For example, compare fluid volume deficit and fluid volume excess, or hypocalcemia and hypercalcemia. Typically, the causes and clinical manifestations are opposite, so if you know one, you know the other!

Fluids

A common mistake students make is to try to memorize everything—lab values, causes of the disorders, clinical manifestations, everything! This is not the way to go if you want to be successful. While there are some things you need to memorize, if you understand the pathophysiology, there is a lot that you can figure out without memorizing. Clinical manifestations are a perfect example. Let's take fluid volume deficit and fluid volume excess. Fluid volume deficit happens when you lose blood volume. This can happen through third spacing (ascites), hemorrhaging, or dehydration. So, think about what this will look like (Fig. 3.1):

The client will look dry, sunken in, be thirsty, confused, and produce less urine. With less blood volume, the client's blood pressure will go down. This will make the heart work harder, increasing heart rate and respiration. Capillary refill will be longer than 2 seconds. You all know what dehydration looks like. Use what you know! Don't just throw your knowledge out the window. Remember, the body makes sense (Fig. 3.2).

Now, think about fluid volume excess. Common sense would tell you that the manifestations would be just the opposite, right? Well, that's exactly right!

Increased fluids due to heart failure (blood backs up because the heart can't pump), renal failure (the kidneys can't filter out fluid and electrolytes), and liver failure (edema due to lack of protein and increased pressure in liver circulation) are some of the common causes. The client with fluid volume excess would look bloated and edematous. Blood volume will increase, which increases blood pressure and causes bounding pulses.

This leads us to the question → What controls our fluid balance? Three body systems figure prominently in this process—the central nervous system, kidneys, and heart.

Central Nervous System

Our brain has osmoreceptors within and around the hypothalamus. These receptors measure the concentration of the blood. When the blood volume rises, the osmoreceptors swell up, signifying fluid volume excess. When the blood volume falls, the osmoreceptors shrink, signifying fluid volume deficit. If there is fluid volume deficit, the osmoreceptors signal the brain to cause thirst. They also signal release of antidiuretic hormone (ADH), a hormone that is produced in the hypothalamus and stored in the posterior pituitary gland. ADH causes the kidneys to retain water. When there is fluid volume excess, the osmoreceptors stop signaling thirst and stop the release of ADH (Fig. 3.3).

Baroreceptors are located within our great vessels: our carotid arteries, large lung vessels, and aortic arch. These receptors sense pressure changes in our blood vessels. When blood volume increases, blood pressure increases. The baroreceptors signal to the brain, which then causes neurons to secrete acetylcholine. This activates the parasympathetic nervous system (PNS), our "rest and digest" system, causing vasodilation, decreased blood pressure, and decreased heart rate. When there is a drop in blood pressure, the baroreceptors signal the brain, which then activates the adrenal medulla to secrete epinephrine and norepinephrine. This activates the sympathetic nervous system (SNS), our "fight or flight" system, to increase vasoconstriction, heart rate, force of contraction, and blood pressure. The SNS also decreases the amount of urine produced and causes ADH to be secreted so that fluid is retained.

Kidneys

The kidneys are extremely important, as they filter out excess fluid or retain fluid during fluid deficits. When the

BACKGROUND

* LOW EXTRACELLULAR VOLUME
  ~ OFTEN INVOLVES ↓↓ in SODIUM & WATER

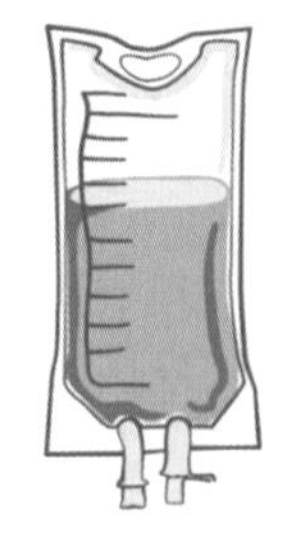

TREATMENT

* ORAL HYDRATION & DIET MAINTENANCE
* IV FLUIDS
* BLOOD TRANSFUSION

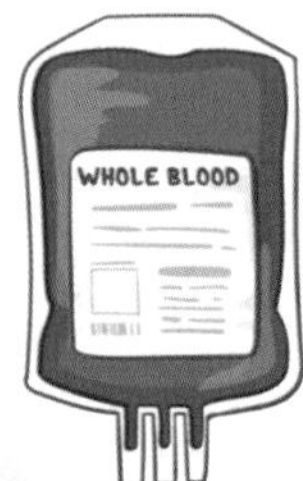

SIGNS & SYMPTOMS

* WEAKNESS
* FATIGUE
* DIZZINESS
* ↑↑ THIRST

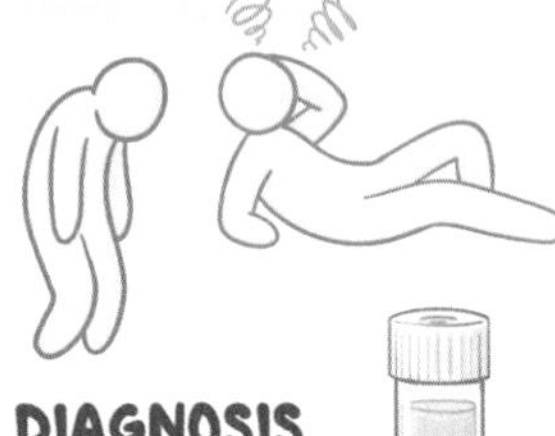

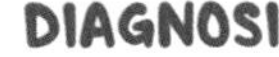

CAUSES

* DEHYDRATION
* TRAUMA
* EXCESSIVE FLUID ACCUMULATION between CELLS
* MEDICAL CONDITIONS:
  ~ RENAL DISEASE
  ~ CONGESTIVE HEART FAILURE

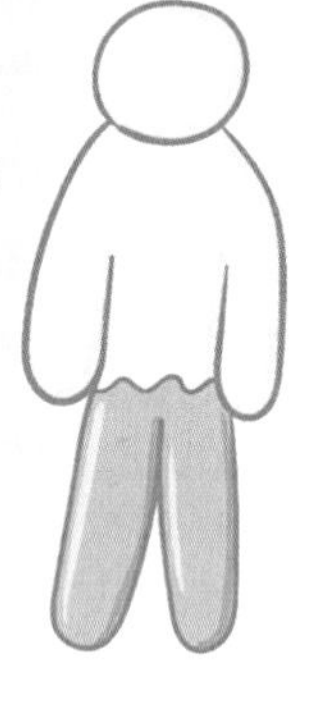

DIAGNOSIS

* BLOOD TEST
  ~ CBC
  ~ CHEMISTRY PANELS
* URINE TEST
  ~ ↑↑ BUN, CREATININE, URINE SODIUM CONCENTRATION, URINE pH
* X-RAY or MRI

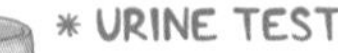

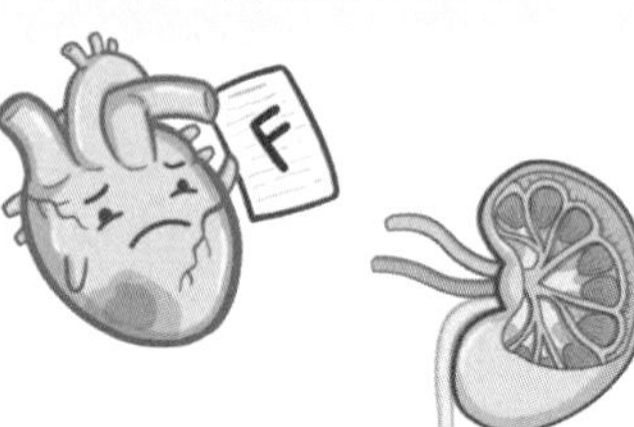

• **Fig. 3.1** Fluid volume deficit. *CBC,* Complete blood count; *IV,* intravenous; *MRI,* magnetic resonance imaging. (From https://www.osmosis.org/answers/hypovolemia.)

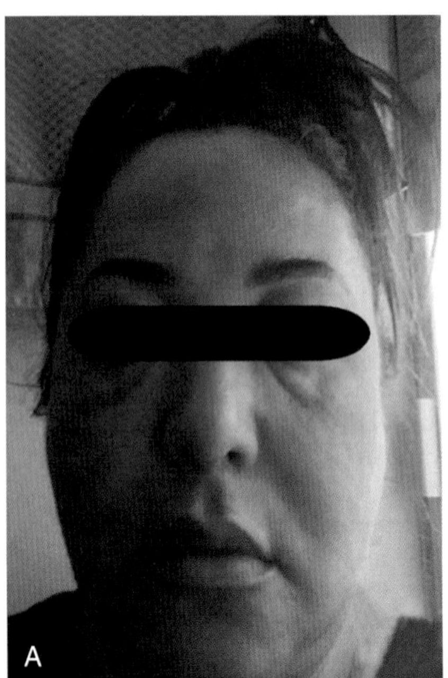

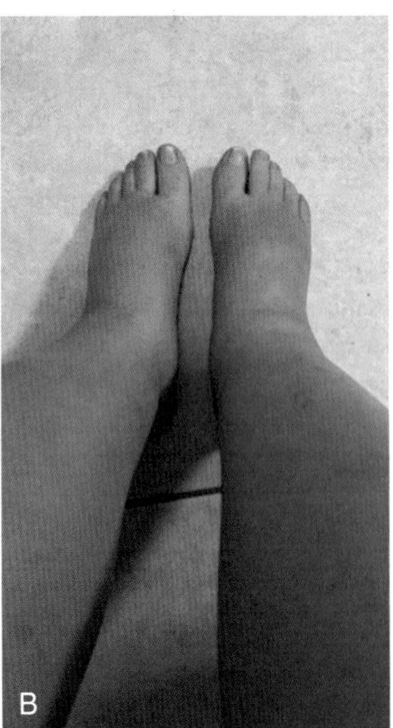

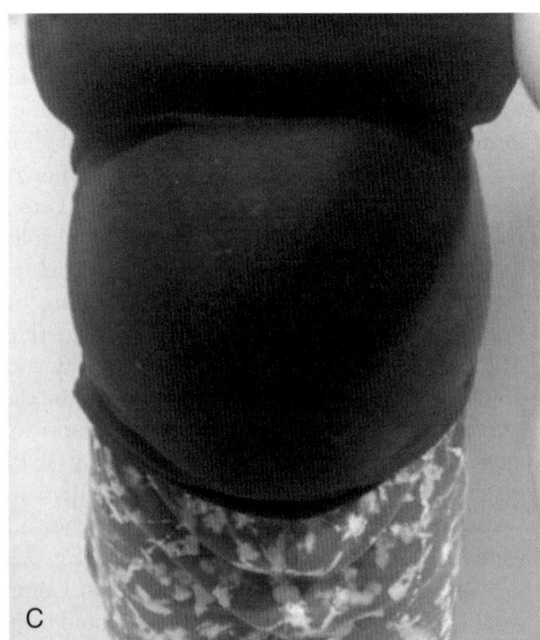

• **Fig. 3.2** Fluid volume overload. (From Martínez, H. R., Figueroa-Sanchez, J. A., Rodriguez-Gonzalez, I., Rodriguez-Gomez, G. P. (2023). Generalized edema with pregabalin in a patient with fibromyalgia. *Neurologia (Engl Ed).*, 38(3):218–219. doi: 10.1016/j.nrleng.2022.04.001.)

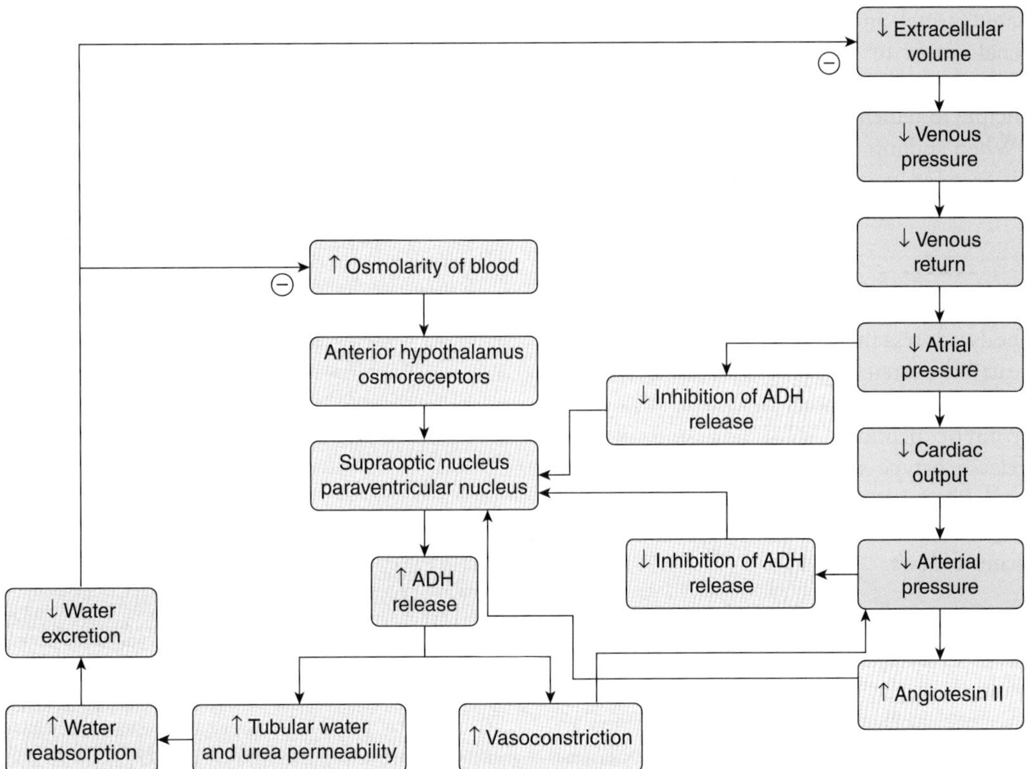

• **Fig. 3.3** Mechanisms for fluid balance. *ADH,* Antidiuretic hormone. (From Feher, J. (2017). Hypothalamus and pituitary gland. In J. Feher (ed.). *Quantitative human physiology* (2nd ed., pp. 870–882). Academic Press. https://doi.org/10.1016/B978-0-12-800883-6.00085-9; https://www.sciencedirect.com/science/article/pii/B9780128008836000859.)

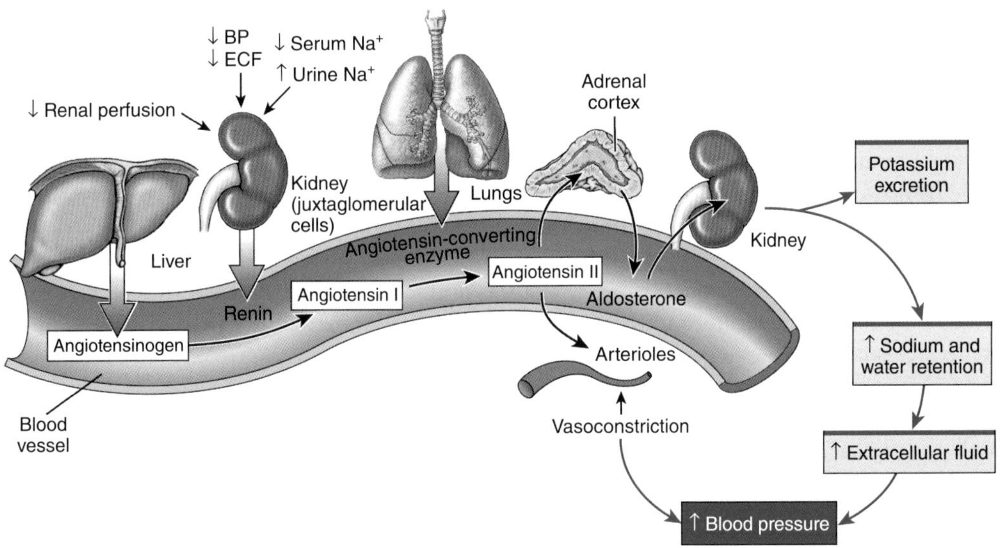

• **Fig. 3.4** Renin-angiotensin-aldosterone system. *BP,* Blood pressure; *ECF,* extracellular fluid. (Modified from Herlihy, B., & Maebius, N. (2011). The human body in health and disease (4th ed.). Saunders. Borrowed from. Roberts L.D., et al. (2014). Medical-surgical nursing: Assessment and management of clinical problems (9th ed.). Mosby.)

SNS goes into effect, it causes vasoconstriction of peripheral blood vessels, to perfuse the heart, lungs, and brain, considered the vital organs. The kidneys, though incredibly important, are not considered vital, so blood flow to the kidneys will drop with SNS activation. The kidneys respond by secreting a peptide hormone called renin. Renin causes a chain reaction, called the renin-angiotensin-aldosterone system (RAAS) (Fig. 3.4). Renin triggers the activation of angiotensin 2, a potent vasoconstrictor. Angiotensin 2 also causes the kidneys decrease glomerular filtration rate (less, more concentrated urine) and retain sodium. RAAS also causes the adrenal cortex to release aldosterone, a steroid hormone. Aldosterone causes the kidneys to retain sodium. Now, a key principle to remember is ≥Where sodium goes, water follows. When sodium is retained, water is retained. When sodium is excreted, water is excreted. So, both angiotensin 2 and aldosterone cause sodium and water retention.

Heart

How does the body address fluid excess? The atria and ventricles of the heart have stretch receptors that detect an excess volume of fluid. These receptors signal the atria to release atrial natriuretic peptide (ANP) hormone and the ventricles to release b-type natriuretic peptide hormone (BNP). ANP and BNP cause the kidney to excrete more sodium, therefore excreting more water. Remember, where sodium goes, water follows.

Edema

Edema, excess fluid that is trapped in the tissues, is a concept that seems simple, but it often confuses students. Edema affects fluid equilibrium between the blood vessels (capillaries) and the tissues (interstitium). In a capillary, there is an arterial end and a venous end. Hydrostatic pressure, or capillary filtration pressure, is high on the arterial end. This makes sense because the capillary needs to push oxygenated blood out to the tissues. The tissues also exert hydrostatic pressure, but the pressure is very weak on the arterial end, so the net result is that the capillaries can push out large amounts of oxygenated blood into the tissues, but the tissues are not able to push any deoxygenated blood back. However, edema can develop if the arterial pressure increases above normal levels. This causes increased hydrostatic pressure, with increased fluid being pushed out into the tissues, causing edema. This is why your feet swell when you have been standing for a long time. The increased arterial pressure leads to edema.

Capillary colloidal osmotic pressure, or oncotic pressure, is exerted by proteins in the blood serum and interstitial fluid. These proteins are usually too big to go through capillary pores and the pressure they exert causes fluid to stay in the vessel and bound to blood proteins, such as albumin. On the arterial end, the capillary colloidal pressure is weaker than the capillary filtration pressure and there is net filtration to the tissues.

At the venous end of the capillary, the capillary filtration pressure drops. The capillary colloidal osmotic pressure is greater than the capillary filtration pressure, causing deoxygenated blood to be reabsorbed, bind to albumin, and eventually circulate back to the heart. Note that the interstitium also has colloidal osmotic pressures, but these pressures are normally quite weak. If a client is malnourished (not eating enough protein) or has liver failure (the liver makes most blood proteins), it will result in a loss of serum protein. Question: If there is no serum protein, what is exerting the capillary colloidal osmotic pressure? Answer: Nothing! That is why you will see these clients have a large amount of generalized body edema, called anasarca.

TABLE 3.1 Electrolyte Disorders

Electrolytes	Extracellular (Serum Blood)	Neuromuscular Excitability
Sodium	135–145 mEq/L	Increased
Potassium	3.5–5.0 mEq/L	Increased
Calcium	8.5–10.5 mg/dL	Cardiac—Increased Neuromuscular—Decreased
Phosphorus	2.5–4.5 mg/dL	Cardiac—Decreased Neuromuscular—Increased
Magnesium	1.8–2.6 mg/dL	Decreased

Inflammation and immune responses can also cause a loss of serum proteins due to increased capillary permeability. This means that the capillary pores become larger so that the serum proteins can escape into the tissues. With the larger pores and the loss of proteins, fluid also escapes into the tissues causing edema. Anaphylaxis, allergic reactions, inflammatory disorders, and severe burns may all lead to edema due to increased capillary permeability.

All the fluid that is not reabsorbed is trapped by the lymph nodes and vessels and returned to the heart. However, if the lymph nodes and vessels are removed, destroyed, or blocked, fluid will collect in that area, causing lymphedema. This is often seen in cancer treatment when lymph nodes are removed.

Electrolytes

Electrolyte disorders can be caused by disease process, chemical/medication reactions, and over-/under- ingestion of the electrolyte (Table 3.1). You will need to memorize the normal ranges for these electrolytes and their effect on neuromuscular excitability (flashcards).

Sodium (Na)

Sodium is the major cation in the bloodstream (extracellular fluid) that maintains extracellular osmolality. It is regulated by the kidneys and adrenal glands. Hormones regulating sodium levels are aldosterone, angiotensin 2, ANP, and BNP. It is important in the function of sodium-potassium pumps and acid-base equilibrium. Sodium helps to initiate action potentials from neurons to muscle fibers, and so causes increased neuromuscular excitability.

Hyponatremia, or low sodium levels in the blood (<135 mg dL), can be caused by sudden large increases in water intake. Athletes are particularly prone to this after extreme activities such as running a marathon. If an athlete runs a marathon and then drinks 2 to 3 L of water, they will dilute the electrolytes in their blood. This will cause hyponatremia.

Therefore, electrolyte drinks, such as Gatorade or Pedialyte, are needed to maintain electrolyte balance. Another disorder that causes hyponatremia is the syndrome of inappropriate antidiuretic hormone (SIADH). This disorder can be due to issues, such as brain tumors or medications. Basically, the body secretes too much ADH, causing the body to retain water. Remember, ADH causes the kidneys to retain only water. The client will look swollen and edematous. Severe hyponatremia is sodium levels below 120 mg/dL. Treatment can be fluid restriction, increased sodium intake, or hypertonic intravenous (IV) infusions. Hypertonic IV infusions must be run in slowly to not cause a sudden shift in fluids in the brain, which may result in seizures and brain death.

Hypernatremia, or too much sodium in the serum blood levels (>145 mg/dL), typically results from dehydration or very high intake of sodium. However, disease process can also cause hypernatremia. One example of this is diabetes insipidus (DI). With DI, ADH is either deficient or the kidneys aren't responding to it. What happens next? If ADH is not there, water is not being retained by the kidney, so large amounts of water are being excreted. Remember that ADH causes only water retention, not sodium retention. The result is that the client has large amounts of extremely diluted urine and becomes extremely dehydrated and hypernatremic. All the symptoms of dehydration are clinical manifestations of hypernatremia. Hypernatremia is treated with fluids, orally or IV, and electrolyte balance must be maintained. Mild hypernatremia can be treated with oral fluids of normal saline infusions. Severe hypernatremia is seen at levels greater than 160 mg/dL and may require hyponatremic fluid infusion. Infusing fluids too fast or fluids that are too diluted may cause hypotonicity. Fluid will rush into the cells in the brain, and lead to cerebral edema.

Now we get to neuromuscular excitability and clinical manifestations. In the electrolytes chart, you can see that sodium helps to generate action potentials. Thinking logically, if the sodium level drops, it won't be as easy to generate an action potential, so you would have decreased neuromuscular excitability. This means a decrease in neuromuscular function. What does that mean for your client? It means that the client will look confused and disoriented. They will also have headaches, decreased deep tendon reflexes, and muscle weakness. The increased fluid will cause the pressure in the brain to increase. This may trigger the chemoreceptor trigger zone and cause nausea and vomiting. All of these are neuromuscular symptoms. Ultimately, if severe hyponatremia is not treated, the client will become lethargic, develop seizures, and go into a coma.

Hypernatremia has the opposite effect. The excess sodium will lead to more action potentials being generated, so you would have increased neuromuscular activity. Picture what increased neuromuscular function will look like. Agitation, increased deep tendon reflexes, muscle cramping, and headaches are all common neuromuscular symptoms of hypernatremia. The client will also look dehydrated, and may have fever, tachycardia, and dry mucous membranes. Ultimately, if you don't treat hypernatremia, the client will develop seizures and go into a coma. Now, you are probably asking—How are the some of the symptoms of hypo- and hypernatremia the same? Think about the effect on brain cells. Whether the cells are inundated with fluid from the blood vessels, or the fluid is being pulled out of the cells and into the blood in extreme hypernatremia, the brain cells are irritated and damaged. This is what causes the headaches, seizures, coma, and finally, brain death (Fig. 3.5).

Now let's put everything together. If you know whether the electrolyte disorder increases or decreases neuromuscular excitability, you can reason out the clinical manifestations without having to memorize. Also, if you know the excitability and manifestations of one disorder (hypo-), you will automatically know the excitability and manifestations of the other (hyper-). They are opposites. Hallmark symptoms, or important distinguishing symptoms, are clinical manifestations that you may need to memorize. But the good news is that there aren't many of them! The best way to attack electrolytes is to pair disorders in a table. Table 3.2 may be helpful.

Does this seem more manageable? Table 3.3 has been completed for sodium as an example.

Potassium (K^+)

Potassium is the major cation inside the cells (intracellular fluid). Potassium is critical for neuromuscular excitability, acid-base balance, and maintaining intracellular osmolality. It is the electrolyte that you will look at first when you look at labs. This is because potassium has such a huge impact on cardiac function. Potassium is regulated by the kidneys and the transcellular buffer system. The kidneys secrete renin, which causes the activation of the RAAS system and aldosterone secretion. Aldosterone can cause fluid retention by retaining sodium. But the electrolyte balance needs to be maintained. So, for every sodium ion retained, a potassium ion is excreted. When there is fluid excess, potassium ions are retained, and sodium is excreted. The kidneys also have a potassium (K^+)/acid (H^+) exchange mechanism that helps retain and excrete potassium. The transcellular buffer system is a mechanism that exchanges H^+/K^+ ions from the blood to bone, muscle, red blood cells, or hepatic cells temporarily. If the blood is too acidic (H^+), the hydrogen ion will be shifted into the cells and K^+ ions will be shifted into the blood. If there is too much potassium in the blood, the K^+ ions will be shifted into the cells and the H^+ ions will be shifted into the blood.

Hypokalemia, or low serum potassium levels (<3.5 mg/dL), can be caused by low intake, diuretic use, and eating disorders. Severe hypokalemia is at levels below 2.5 mg/dL and can cause cardiac arrest. Hypokalemia is extremely dangerous because it affects cardiac function. Potassium is very important in the conduction of action potentials. The stimulus to generate action potentials must reach the threshold potential to cause the action potential. When potassium levels are low, the stimulus is not able to reach the threshold and cells don't fire as easily.

PATHOPHYSIOLOGY

The Opposing Syndrome to Diabetes Insipidus

- Presents as a dilutional hyponatremia.
- Excess ADH secreted into the bloodstream.
- Excessive water resorbed at the kidney tubule, → dilutional hyponatremia.
- Because minimal sodium is present in this fluid, edema usually does not result.
- Without ADH and aldosterone, water is retained, ↓ U/O, ↑ sodium excreted in urine.
- ↑ urine osmolality → ↓ water excretion.
- Malignant bronchogenic small cell carcinoma causes production and release of ADH regardless of the body's needs.

ASSESSMENT & DIAGNOSIS

Clinical Manifestations

- Early clinical manifestations of dilutional hyponatremia include lethargy, anorexia, & N/V.
- Edema usually not present, slight weight gain from ↑ fluid.
- Severe neurologic symptoms usually occur when serum sodium < 120 mEq/L.
- S/S of severe hyponatremia → inability to concentrate, mental confusion, apprehension, seizures, ↓ LOC, coma, & death.

Early recognition of neurologic or hemodynamic deterioration

Laboratory Values

- ↓ Plasma osmolality
- ↑ Urine osmolality
- ↓ Serum sodium
- ↑ Urine sodium
- Measurement of serum ADH levels not recommended for diagnosis.

NURSING DIAGNOSES

- ↓ Cardiac Output R/T alterations in preload.
- ↓ Fluid Volume R/T absolute loss.
- Anxiety R/T threat to biologic, psychologic, & social integrity.
- ↓ Knowledge RT previous lack of exposure to information.

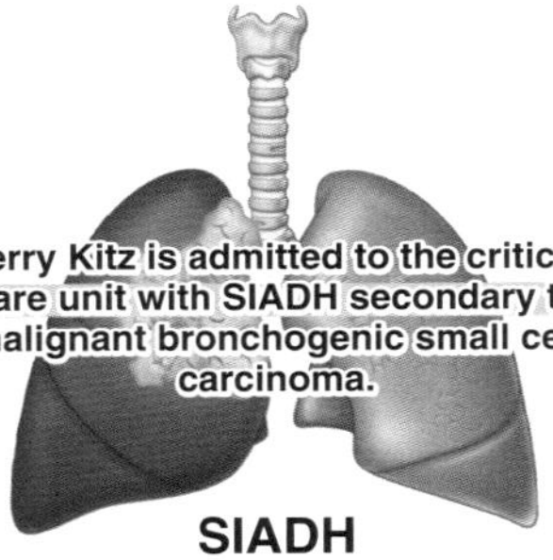

Jerry Kitz is admitted to the critical care unit with SIADH secondary to malignant bronchogenic small cell carcinoma.

SIADH

Syndrome of Inappropriate Secretion of Antidiuretic Hormone

Results in

Dilutional Hyponatremia
↑ Blood Volume
↓ Serum Osmolality

GOALS OF MEDICAL MANAGEMENT

RESTORE FLUID AND SODIUM BALANCE

The patient will demonstrate adequate fluid and sodium balance by

PATIENT OUTCOMES

- Hemodynamic values within normal (CO, BP, HR, CVP, PAP, PAOP)
- Sodium within normal range
- Maintain O_2 Saturation of 90% or greater
- Mental clarity, skin warm/dry
- Urine output ~ 60 mL/hr.
- RR within normal, clear breath sounds

Nursing Care Includes

MEDICATIONS TO CORRECT SIADH

When Water Restriction is Ineffective - Medications

- Indicated for SIADH secondary to a small cell lung carcinoma, the vasopressin receptor antagonists "vaptans" will ↑ water excretion while conserving sodium (aquadiuresis).
- Administer IV infusion of Conivaptan (Vaprisol) or Tolvaptan (Samsca) administered orally.
- Monitor serum sodium levels carefully.
- Monitor for hypotension.
- Astute clinical judgment warranted when using these medications.

NURSING INTERVENTIONS

Patient & Family Health Education

- Show sensitivity to family's fears by using words indicating empathy.
- Teach about SIADH & its effect on water balance, & reasons for fluid restrictions.
- Provide time for the patient & family to ask questions & express their concerns.

Frequent Assessment of Patient's Hydration Status

- Fluids restricted to 500 - 1000 mL per day.
- Slow infusion of 3% saline to replenish sodium without adding extra volume.
- Slowly ↑ serum sodium (10 mEq/L in 24 hrs).
- Evaluate sodium at least every 4 hours during acute phase of sodium replacement.
- Extreme caution is warranted when infusing hypertonic saline solution.
- Calculation of hourly sodium amount and over 24 hours.
- Serial measurements of urine output, serum sodium levels, & serum osmolality.
- Frequent mouth care.
- Daily weight.

A

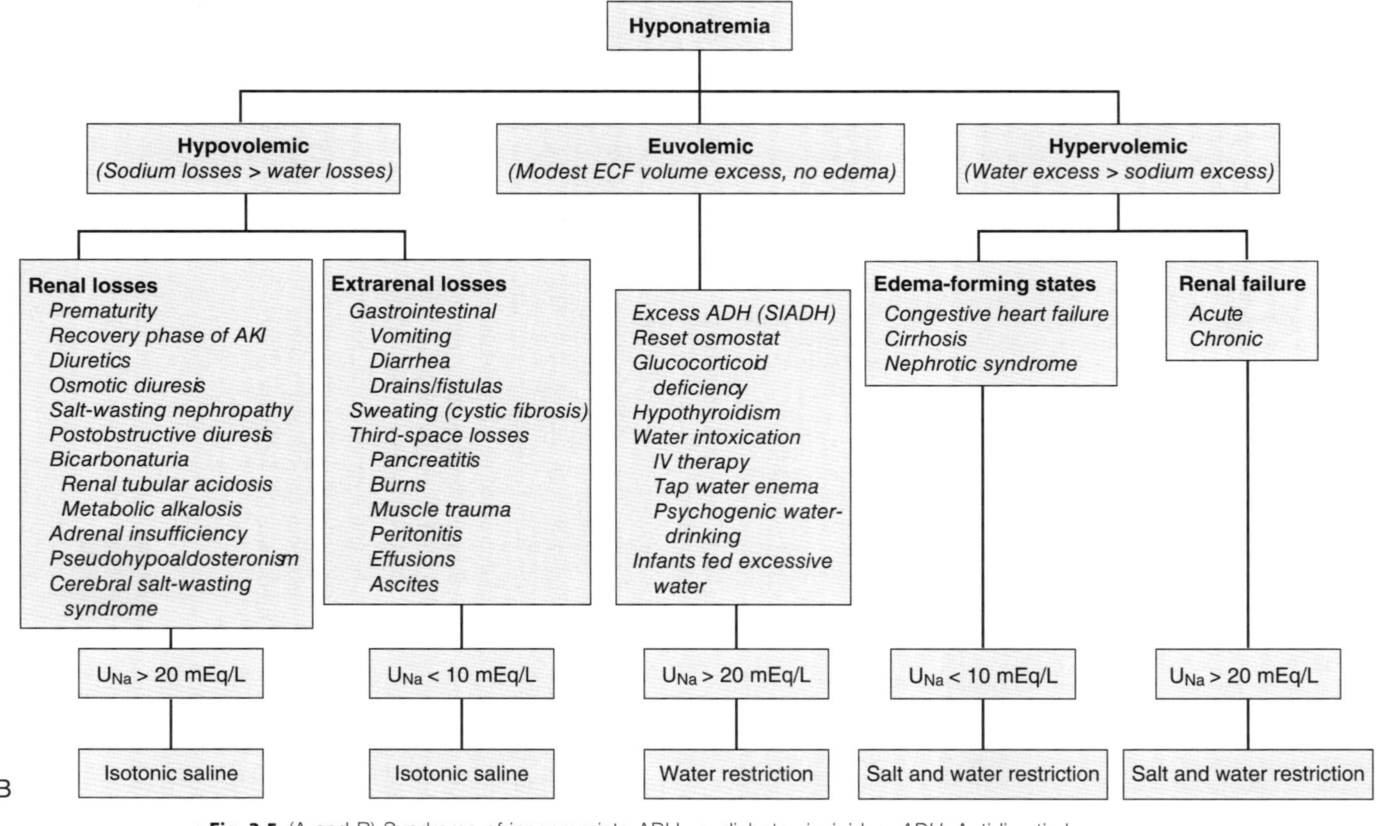

• **Fig. 3.5** (A and B) Syndrome of inappropriate ADH vs. diabetes insipidus. *ADH,* Antidiuretic hormone; *ECF,* extracellular fluid; *IV,* intravenous; *LOC,* level of consciousness; *SIADH,* syndrome of inappropriate antidiuretic hormone. (Modified from Berl, T., Anderson, R.J., McDonald, K.M., et al. (1976). Clinical disorders of water metabolism. Kidney Int, 10:117–132 (Figure 2).)

TABLE 3.2 Electrolyte T charts

Hypo-	Hyper-
Increased or decreased neuromuscular excitability?	Increased or decreased neuromuscular excitability?
Under what conditions do you see this disorder? (i.e., alcoholism, diuretic use, starvation, etc.)	Under what conditions do you see this disorder?
What are the hallmark symptoms? (i.e., cardiac arrest, tetany, etc.)	What are the hallmark symptoms?

TABLE 3.3 Sodium (Na) T chart

Hyponatremia	Hypernatremia
Decreased neuromuscular excitability	Increased neuromuscular excitability
SIADH, water intoxication, diuretics, diarrhea, vomiting, low salt intake	Dehydration, diabetes insipidus, high salt intake
Confusion, edema, nausea/vomiting, headache	Fever, tachycardia, dry mucous membranes, agitation

SIADH, Syndrome of inappropriate antidiuretic hormone.

What does this mean as far as clinical manifestations of hypokalemia? Hypokalemia causes a decrease in action potentials, so it leads to decreased neuromuscular excitability. Now, we talked about the clinical manifestations of decreased neuromuscular activity with sodium. Here, you see the same kinds of symptoms, only with pronounced cardiac symptoms. With decreased neuromuscular activity, there are electrocardiogram (ECG) changes, decreased heart rate (bradycardia), cardiac arrhythmias, and cardiac arrest. A hallmark symptom is the presence of a U wave on the ECG. Anything that interferes with the electrical activity of the heart will cause arrhythmias. Confusion, muscle weakness, a decrease in smooth muscle tone (leading to constipation) are all symptoms of hypokalemia. All these symptoms should make sense when you think in terms of decreased neuromuscular excitability.

Hyperkalemia, or high potassium levels (>5 mg/dL), is commonly caused by renal failure. It can also be caused by potassium infusions that are too fast or at too high a dose. Hyperkalemia is also extremely dangerous. Hyperkalemia increases the resting membrane potential so that initially, action potentials are generated and cells fire more easily. This means that neuromuscular excitability increases. Again, anything that affects cardiac conduction and contraction may lead to lethal cardiac arrhythmias. With

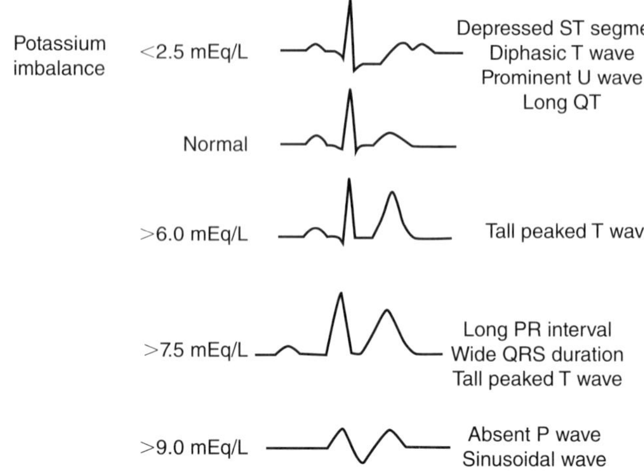

• **Fig. 3.6** Electrocardiogram changes with potassium abnormalities. (From Polin, R. A., & Ditmar, M. F. (2017). *Pediatric Secrets: First South Asia Edition*. Elsevier.)

increased excitability, arrhythmias such as ventricular tachycardias and fibrillation may occur. A hallmark sign is peaked T waves on an ECG (Fig. 3.6). Numbness and tingling (paresthesias), muscle twitching, irritability, abdominal cramping, and diarrhea are all manifestations of increased excitability.

However, this changes with severe hyperkalemia (>6.5 mg/dL). The resting membrane potential decreases less than the threshold potential, and repolarization cannot occur. So that means that the cell membrane is "stuck" in a depolarized state. The cell membrane needs to repolarize before it can depolarize again. Because action potentials cannot be generated, cells cannot fire. The clinical manifestations of severe hyperkalemia are the same as those of hypokalemia and decreased neuromuscular excitability, such as cardiac arrhythmias, bradycardia, cardiac arrest, decreased muscle tone, and decreased reflexes.

Now, using this information, try to fill out the chart for hypo- and hyperkalemia. Remember, if you know if there is increased and decreased neuromuscular excitability, you can reason out the clinical manifestations. You will only need to memorize the hallmark clinical signs (Table 3.4).

TABLE 3.4 Potassium (K) T chart

Hypokalemia	Hyperkalemia (Mild and Severe)
Increased or decreased neuromuscular excitability?	Increased or decreased neuromuscular excitability?
Under what conditions do you see this disorder?	Under what conditions do you see this disorder?
What are the hallmark symptoms?	What are the hallmark symptoms?

Calcium

Calcium is important for bone formation, clotting, strengthening cardiac contractions, and stabilizing neuromuscular cell resting potentials. Most calcium is bound to proteins, or contained in complexes, such as calcium carbonate ($CaCO_3$) or calcium phosphate ($Ca_3(PO_4)_2$). Ionized calcium, or free calcium, is the second most common cation in blood serum. Calcium and phosphorus (phosphate) are inversely related. When serum calcium levels are high, serum phosphate levels are low. When serum phosphate levels are high, serum calcium levels are low. Serum calcium and phosphate are regulated by two hormones, parathyroid hormone (PTH) and calcitonin. PTH is produced and secreted by the parathyroid gland and is released when serum calcium levels are low and/or serum phosphate levels are high. PTH causes bone to release calcium and the kidneys to retain calcium and activate vitamin D. Vitamin D is essential for calcium to be absorbed from the gut. PTH also causes increased secretion of phosphate.

When serum calcium is high and/or serum phosphate is low, PTH secretion stops, and calcitonin secretion starts. Calcitonin, produced and secreted from the follicular cells of the thyroid gland, causes reabsorption (bone) and excretion (kidneys) of calcium. Calcitonin also regulates high levels of phosphate, causing phosphate reabsorption and excretion. PTH and calcitonin act in tandem to ensure equilibrium of serum calcium and phosphate.

Note that calcium has a different effect on cardiac cells and neuromuscular cells. For cardiac muscle cells to contract, calcium ion channels open and allow calcium into the cells, which is crucial for muscle contraction, increasing cardiac excitability. However, for neuromuscular cells, calcium acts as a stabilizer, stabilizing cell membranes so that they are less likely to react and depolarize, decreasing neuromuscular excitability.

Hypocalcemia

Hypocalcemia ($<$8.5 mg/dL) occurs most with renal failure (kidneys cannot retain calcium or activate vitamin D), PTH deficiency (hypoparathyroidism), vitamin D deficiency, and hyperphosphatemia (when serum phosphate levels go up, serum calcium levels go down). Low levels of calcium affect the heart and neuromuscular cells differently. Hypocalcemia decreases excitability of the heart, causing decreased contractile strength, arrhythmias, and hypotension. Severe hypocalcemia ($<$7.6 mg/dL) may cause heart failure and cardiac arrest. However, with neuromuscular cells, calcium acts as a cell membrane stabilizer. Low levels of calcium will cause the cell membrane to become less stabilized, leading to more action potentials. This will lead to clinical manifestations such as tetany, twitching, and muscle spasms. Low levels of calcium also lead to bone breakdown and osteoporosis. Hallmarks of hypocalcemia are Chvostek sign and Trousseau sign (Fig. 3.7 and Fig. 3.8).

Hypercalcemia

Hypercalcemia ($>$10.5 mg/dL) can be caused by PTH excess (hyperparathyroidism), prolonged immobilization

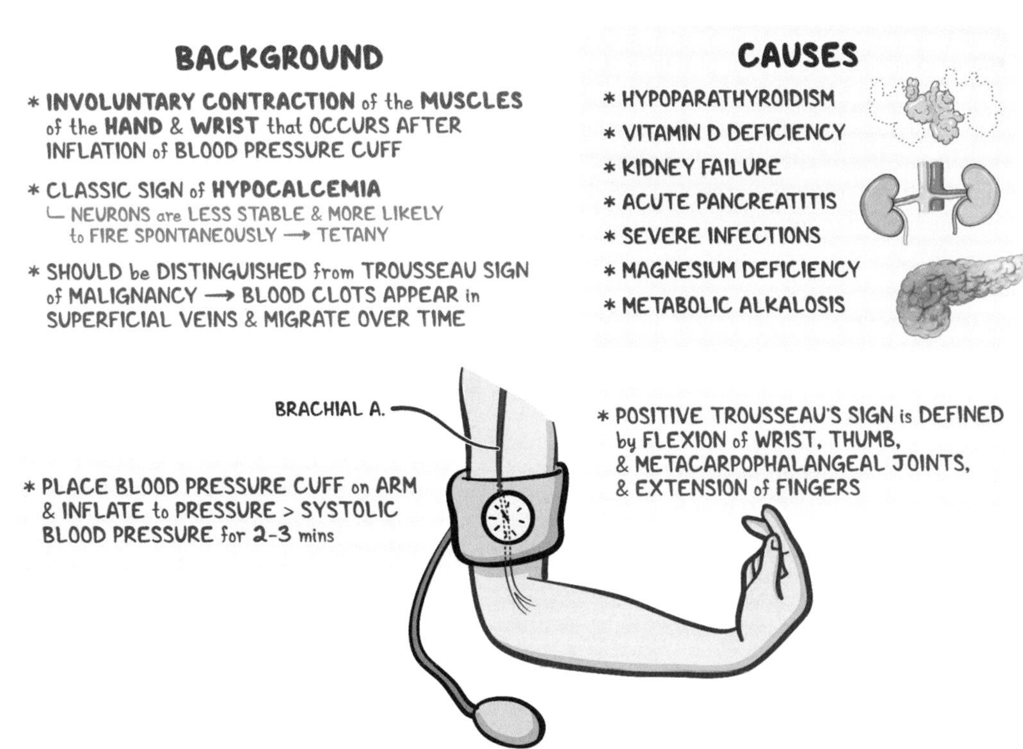

• **Fig. 3.7** Trousseau sign. (From https://www.osmosis.org/answers/trousseau-sign.)

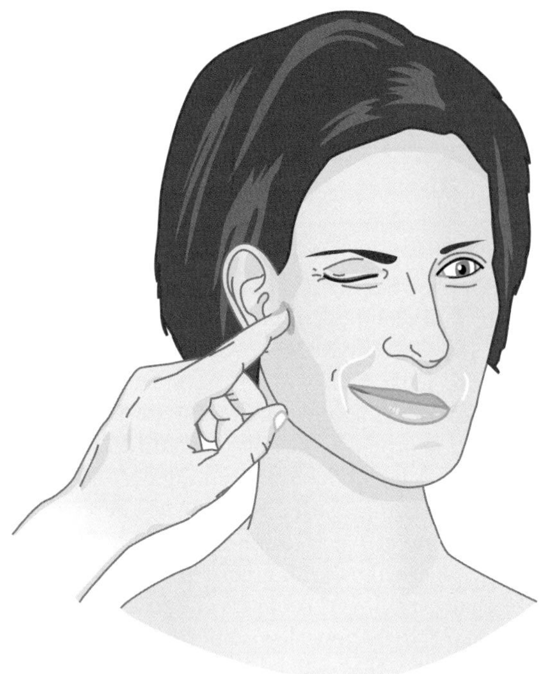

• **Fig. 3.8** Chvostek sign. (From Carlson K. (2009) AACN Advanced Critical Care Nursing. Elsevier. (pp. 841-864; Fig. 31.10.)

(causes bone breakdown), and cancer (paraneoplastic syndrome). Hypercalcemia causes increased cardiac excitability because the heart needs calcium to contract. This increased excitability leads to increased contractility, tachycardic arrhythmias, and hypertension. However, calcium stabilizes the neuromuscular cell membranes. Increased levels of calcium will cause decreased neuromuscular excitability. This will lead to lethargy, loss of smooth muscle tone, constipation, lethargy, and coma. A hallmark sign of hypercalcemia is behavioral change. Severe hypercalcemia (>15 mg/dL) may result in hypercalcemic crisis. Because the blood is so concentrated, the client will feel extremely thirsty and will experience polyuria. Altered mental status and psychosis may occur. Cardiac arrhythmias and arrest may also result.

Table 3.5 show how to set up your chart for hypo- and hypercalcemia.

Phosphorus (phosphate)

Phosphorus is important in many bodily functions. Bone formation, ATP, metabolism, DNA and RNA production, and acid-base balance all depend on adequate levels of phosphorus. Red blood cells, white blood cells, and platelet function also rely on phosphorus. Typically, phosphorus is found in the body as phosphate. Phosphate is regulated by PTH and calcitonin. Phosphate levels are inversely related to calcium levels. If there is an increase in phosphate, there is a decrease in calcium, and vice versa.

Hypophosphatemia (<2.5 mg/dL) can occur with intestinal malabsorption; increase use of antacids with magnesium, aluminum, or calcium (binds with phosphate); chronic alcohol use (alcohol interferes with absorption); and malnutrition (low intake of protein and dairy). Because phosphate has an inverse relationship with calcium, hypophosphatemia occurs when hypercalcemia is present (hyperparathyroidism). Therefore, the clinical manifestations of hypophosphatemia are the same as those of hypercalcemia. Like hypercalcemia, hypophosphatemia leads to increased cardiac excitability and decreased neuromuscular activity.

Hyperphosphatemia (>4.5 mg/dL) is most commonly by muscle breakdown and chronic renal failure. It can also be caused by low calcium levels (hypoparathyroidism) and use of antacids and laxatives that contain phosphate. The clinical manifestations of hyperphosphatemia are the same as those of hypocalcemia. Hyperphosphatemia leads to decreased cardiac excitability and increased neuromuscular activity (Table 3.6).

Magnesium

Magnesium is the second most abundant intracellular cation. I call magnesium the "Great Stabilizer." It is needed to stabilize both cardiac and neuromuscular cell membranes. It is essential in the function of the sodium/potassium pump, calcium transport, and parathyroid gland function. Magnesium relaxes neuromuscular and smooth muscle tissue. For this reason, magnesium is used to treat severe asthma exacerbation, preterm labor, pre-eclampsia, and a

TABLE 3.5 Calcium (Ca) T chart

Hypocalcemia	Hypercalcemia (Separate Mild and Severe!)
Increased or decreased neuromuscular excitability? Cardiac Neuromuscular	Increased or decreased neuromuscular excitability? Cardiac Neuromuscular
Under what conditions do you see this disorder?	Under what conditions do you see this disorder?
What are the hallmark symptoms?	What are the hallmark symptoms?

TABLE 3.6 Phosphorous (P) T chart

Hypophosphatemia (Hypercalcemia)	Hyperphosphatemia (Hypocalcemia)
Increased or decreased neuromuscular excitability? Cardiac Neuromuscular	Increased or decreased neuromuscular excitability? Cardiac Neuromuscular
Under what conditions do you see this disorder?	Under what conditions do you see this disorder?
What are the hallmark symptoms?	What are the hallmark symptoms?

ventricular tachycardia called *torsades de pointes*. Magnesium compounds can also act as laxatives.

Hypomagnesemia (<1.8 mg/dL) can be caused by alcoholism (malabsorption) and malnutrition. Diarrhea and diuretics can also reduce the amount of magnesium in the body. When magnesium levels are low, cell membranes are not stabilized, so there are increased numbers of action potentials, leading to increased neuromuscular activity. Tetany, personality changes, hyperactive reflexes, seizures, and coma can occur. Cardiac symptoms include ventricular arrhythmias (tachycardia), and hypertension. Hallmark signs include agitation, irritability, Chvostek sign, and Trousseau sign.

Hypermagnesemia (>2.6 mg/dL) is typically caused by renal failure (failure to filter magnesium) and overuse of antacids and laxatives containing magnesium. When magnesium levels are high, cell membranes are extremely stable and do not depolarize. The lack of action potentials causes decreased neuromuscular excitability. Clinical manifestations include confusion, decreased reflexes, weakness, lethargy, and coma. Cardiac manifestations include hypotension, cardiac, arrhythmias, and cardiac arrest (Fig. 3.9 and Tables 3.7 and 3.8).

Along with electrolytes and fluid balance, acid-base balance is key in balancing the body's equilibrium. While there are some strong acids in the body, like hydrochloric acid (HCl), most acid in the body is carbonic acid (H_2CO_3). Carbonic acid is a weak acid that is in dynamic equilibrium with H^+ (acid) and HCO_3^- (bicarbonate). Acidity and alkalinity, or pH, are closely monitored by the body's central and peripheral chemoreceptors. The central chemoreceptors are in the medulla and monitor levels of carbon dioxide in the blood. The peripheral chemoreceptors are in the carotid and aortic arteries and detect changes in the levels of oxygen in the blood.

The pH needs to be within a narrow range, between 7.35 and 7.45, which is considered neutral. If the pH is below 7.35, it is considered acidic. If the pH is above 7.45, it is considered alkaline. The pH must stay consistent because when the pH is too low (acidic), it causes denaturation of proteins, which are the "workhorses" of the body. If proteins do not function, body processes would shut down. When the pH is high (alkaline), it is extremely hospitable to proteins. High pH causes proteins to bind too tightly to substrates, such as oxygen. The proteins are not able to release their substrates to the tissues that need them.

The pH of the blood is constantly fluctuating. However, the body contains chemical buffers that respond instantly to pH changes to push the pH back to neutral range. Proteins and bones act as buffers by releasing H^+ ions when the pH is too alkaline or absorbing H^+ ions when the pH is too acidic. Aside from the chemical buffers, the pH is buffered by the respiratory system and kidneys. The respiratory system can act as a buffer within minutes of pH changes by releasing carbon dioxide (hyperventilation) and retaining carbon dioxide (hypoventilation). Hyperventilation releases CO_2, decreasing acidity. Hypoventilation increases acidity, as CO_2 is retained. The kidneys take the longest to respond, but they are the most efficient and long-acting buffers. This is because the kidneys can eliminate or retain H^+, as well as create and retain HCO_3^-. These buffers are important when talking about acid-base disorders. Note: Think of CO_2 as acid and HCO_3^- as base.

Acid-base disorders can occur from disease processes, trauma, ingestion, or anything that causes stress to the body. The two classes of disorders are respiratory and metabolic. Respiratory disorders are caused by breathing issues and lung diseases. Metabolic disorders are caused primarily by disease, trauma, or chemical ingestion, causing the body to go into acidosis or alkalosis. The four disorders are listed below:

- Metabolic acidosis: diabetic ketoacidosis, renal failure, ingestion of acids (salicylate), shock, diarrhea
- Respiratory acidosis: caused by hypoventilation due to airway obstruction, lung disease, neuromuscular disease, opioid overdose
- Metabolic alkalosis: caused by vomiting, nasogastric drainage, antacid overuse, diuretics
- Respiratory alkalosis: caused by hyperventilation, anxiety, fever, often seen with vented clients

With each disorder, the body typically tries to compensate by pushing the body in the opposite direction. For example, if a client has metabolic acidosis, the body will compensate with respiratory alkalosis. The chemical buffers start working instantly; a few minutes later the lungs start compensating through hyperventilation, called Kussmaul breathing. Later, the kidneys start compensating through bicarbonate production and retention.

However, if a client has respiratory acidosis, the body tries to compensate with metabolic alkalosis, by triggering the chemical buffer system first, then a day or two later, triggering the kidneys to retain and create more bicarbonate and excrete more acid. The lungs cannot compensate for respiratory disorders as they are the cause of the problem.

If the client has metabolic alkalosis, the body tries to compensate with the chemical buffer system first, then respiratory acidosis, triggering the lungs to hypoventilate and retain more acid. Later, the kidneys will start to compensate by excreting bicarbonate and retaining acid. If the client has end-stage renal failure, the kidneys may not be able to fully compensate.

With respiratory alkalosis, the body responds with metabolic acidosis. The chemical buffer system responds instantly; then the kidneys compensate hours to days later. However, respiratory alkalosis, or hyperventilation, can occur with anxiety, with no underlying lung disease. In that case slowing down the client's breathing will resolve the alkalosis.

Like electrolytes, acidosis and alkalosis can have severe effects on neuromuscular excitability. Remember, acidosis causes protein denaturation and decreased function. Therefore, it leads to decreased neuromuscular excitability. Cardiac manifestations such as vasodilation, decreased cardiac output, hypotension, decreased contractility, and arrhythmias may occur. Confusion, muscle weakness, lethargy, obtundation, seizures, and coma are all neuromuscular

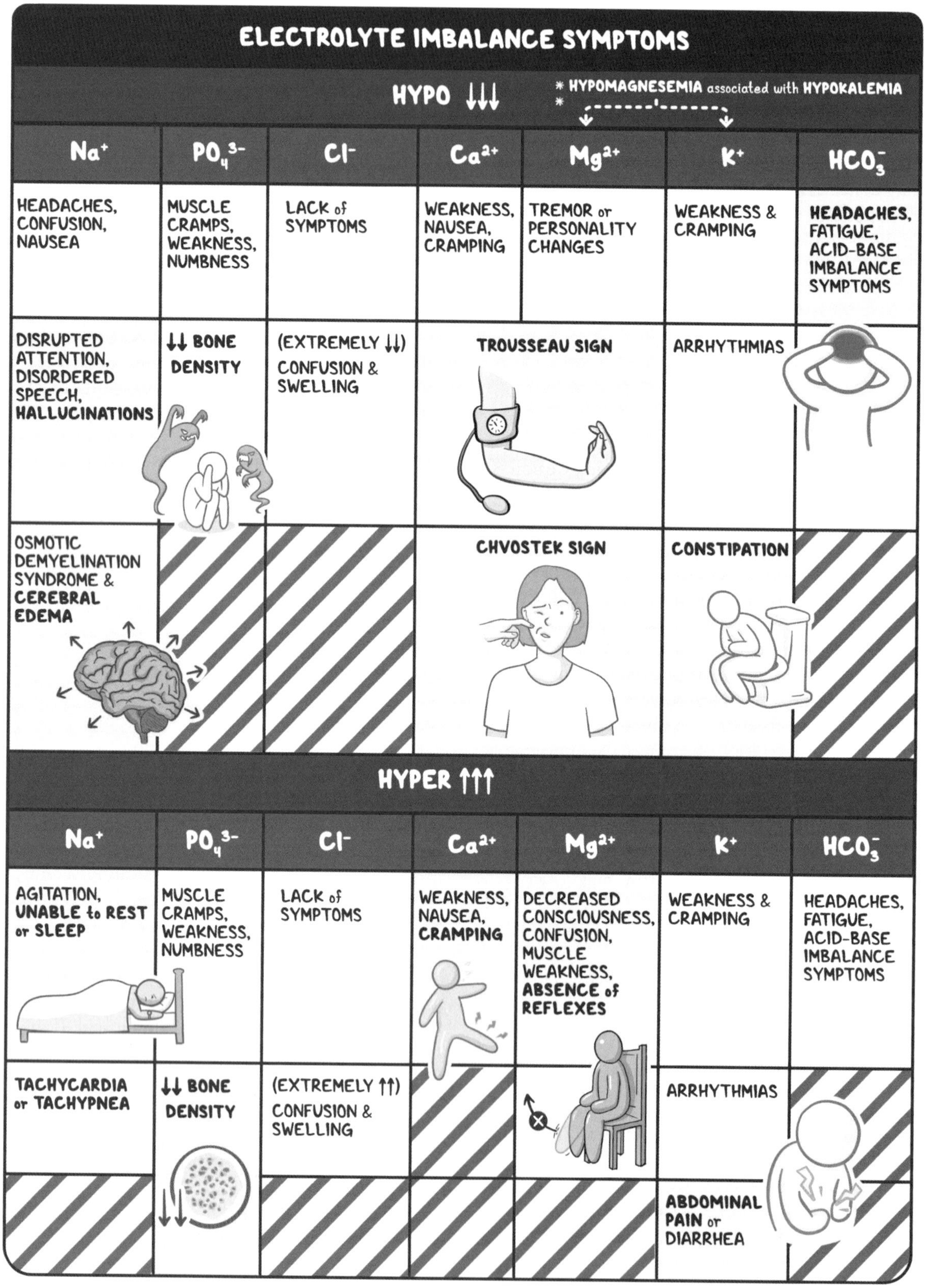

ELECTROLYTE IMBALANCE SYMPTOMS

HYPO ↓↓↓

* HYPOMAGNESEMIA associated with HYPOKALEMIA

Na^+	PO_4^{3-}	Cl^-	Ca^{2+}	Mg^{2+}	K^+	HCO_3^-
HEADACHES, CONFUSION, NAUSEA	MUSCLE CRAMPS, WEAKNESS, NUMBNESS	LACK of SYMPTOMS	WEAKNESS, NAUSEA, CRAMPING	TREMOR or PERSONALITY CHANGES	WEAKNESS & CRAMPING	**HEADACHES,** FATIGUE, ACID-BASE IMBALANCE SYMPTOMS
DISRUPTED ATTENTION, DISORDERED SPEECH, **HALLUCINATIONS**	**↓↓ BONE DENSITY**	(EXTREMELY ↓↓) CONFUSION & SWELLING	**TROUSSEAU SIGN**		ARRHYTHMIAS	
OSMOTIC DEMYELINATION SYNDROME & **CEREBRAL EDEMA**			**CHVOSTEK SIGN**		**CONSTIPATION**	

HYPER ↑↑↑

Na^+	PO_4^{3-}	Cl^-	Ca^{2+}	Mg^{2+}	K^+	HCO_3^-
AGITATION, **UNABLE to REST or SLEEP**	MUSCLE CRAMPS, WEAKNESS, NUMBNESS	LACK of SYMPTOMS	WEAKNESS, NAUSEA, **CRAMPING**	DECREASED CONSCIOUSNESS, CONFUSION, MUSCLE WEAKNESS, **ABSENCE of REFLEXES**	WEAKNESS & CRAMPING	HEADACHES, FATIGUE, ACID-BASE IMBALANCE SYMPTOMS
TACHYCARDIA or TACHYPNEA	**↓↓ BONE DENSITY**	(EXTREMELY ↑↑) CONFUSION & SWELLING			ARRHYTHMIAS	
					ABDOMINAL PAIN or DIARRHEA	

• **Fig. 3.9** Electrolyte disorders chart. (From https://www.osmosis.org/answers/electrolyte-imbalances.)

TABLE 3.7 Magnesium (Mg) T chart

Hypomagnesemia	Hypermagnesemia
Increased or decreased neuromuscular excitability?	Increased or decreased neuromuscular excitability?
Under what conditions do you see this disorder?	Under what conditions do you see this disorder?
What are the hallmark symptoms?	What are the hallmark symptoms?

TABLE 3.8 Arterial Blood Gases

What are we Measuring?	Normal Ranges
pH	7.35–7.45
pCO_2	35–45 mm Hg
pO_2	80–100 mm Hg
$HCO_3 2$	22–26 mEq/L

manifestations. Acidosis may also lead to hyperkalemia. When there is too much acid (H^+) in the blood, the transcellular buffer system shifts H^+ and K^+ temporarily. Acid (H^+) is pushed into bone, muscle, liver, and red blood cells. Potassium (K^+) is pushed into the blood serum, resulting in hyperkalemia. Hallmark signs are the relative hyperkalemia, increased oxyhemoglobin disassociation (proteins are denatured and release oxygen molecules too early), and increased concentrations of ionized calcium and magnesium (due to lack of protein binding affinity).

Alkalosis causes increased protein binding and, therefore, increased neuromuscular excitability. Cardiac manifestations include vasoconstriction, hypertension, and arrhythmias. Neuromuscular symptoms include twitching, tetany, irritability, anxiety, delirium, and seizures. The transcellular buffer system temporarily shifts H^+ back out to blood and K^+ back into the cells, leading to relative hypokalemia. Hallmark signs include hypokalemia, decreased oxyhemoglobin disassociation, and decreased levels of ionized calcium and magnesium (proteins have a strong binding affinity in alkaline solutions) (Table 3.9).

Figuring Out Arterial Blood Gases

In the last part of this chapter, I will explain how to figure out what an acid-base disorder is and whether the body is compensating or not. Important to remember:

CO_2 is an indicator of acidity. CO_2 and pH have an inverse relationship.

Low CO_2 levels (<35 mm Hg) $\rightarrow$ High pH levels (>7.45)
High CO_2 levels (>45 mm Hg) $\rightarrow$ Low pH levels (<7.35)

TABLE 3.9 Acidosis vs. Alkalosis T chart

Acidosis	Alkalosis
Increased or decreased neuromuscular excitability?	Increased or decreased neuromuscular excitability?
Under what conditions do you see this disorder?	Under what conditions do you see this disorder?
What are the hallmark symptoms?	What are the hallmark symptoms?

R Respiratory

O Opposite pH↓ pCO_2↑ Respiratory acidosis

pH↑ pCO_2↓ Respiratory alkalosis

M Metabolic

E Equal pH↓ $pHCO_3$↓

pH↑ $pHCO_3$↑

• **Fig. 3.10** ROME (respiratory opposite, metabolic equal) method.

HCO_3 is an indicator of alkalinity. HCO_3 and pH have a direct relationship.

Low HCO_3 levels (<22 mg/dL) $\rightarrow$ Low pH (<7.35)
High HCO_3 levels (>26 mg/dL) $\rightarrow$ High pH (>7.45)

Oxygen really is not a good indicator of the disorder, so it is often left out of these problems.

When I was in nursing school, the way I learned to do this was by using the ROME mnemonic (respiratory opposite, metabolic equal) (Fig. 3.10).

This method requires more memorization, as you need to remember which way the arrows go with each disorder. Looking at the pH, you must determine whether there is acidosis or alkalosis. Using the ROME mnemonic, determine the cause. Is it respiratory or metabolic? Finally, determine compensation. Is it uncompensated, partially compensated, or fully compensated?

The method that I teach students is the Tic-Tac-Toe method (Fig. 3.11).

Here, you assign the pH to be acidic, neutral, or basic. Then figure out whether the pCO_2 is acidic, neutral, or basic. Finally, place HCO_3 into the correct category, acidic, neutral, or basic. Depending on whether CO_2 or HCO_3 is under the pH, the disorder is respiratory (CO_2) or metabolic (HCO_3). There are many great videos on YouTube to help you understand how to work out acid-base problems. I learned how to figure out acid-base problems from videos too. Don't be afraid to Google resources for yourself. There is nothing wrong in finding effective learning tools for yourself!

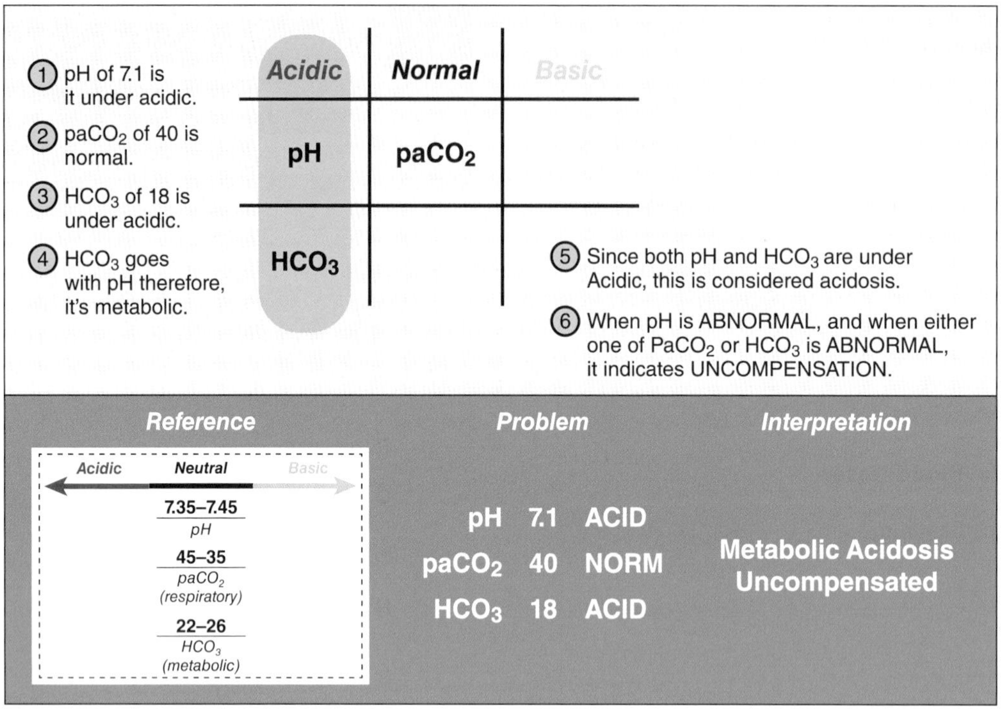

① pH of 7.1 is it under acidic.

② $paCO_2$ of 40 is normal.

③ HCO_3 of 18 is under acidic.

④ HCO_3 goes with pH therefore, it's metabolic.

Acidic	Normal	Basic
pH	$paCO_2$	
HCO_3		

⑤ Since both pH and HCO_3 are under Acidic, this is considered acidosis.

⑥ When pH is ABNORMAL, and when either one of $PaCO_2$ or HCO_3 is ABNORMAL, it indicates UNCOMPENSATION.

Reference	Problem			Interpretation
Acidic / Neutral / Basic: 7.35–7.45 pH	pH	7.1	ACID	Metabolic Acidosis Uncompensated
45–35 $paCO_2$ (respiratory)	$paCO_2$	40	NORM	
22–26 HCO_3 (metabolic)	HCO_3	18	ACID	

• **Fig. 3.11** Tic-Tac-Toe method.

Study Guide for Chapter 3

Make sure that you have your class notes and textbooks on hand to answer these questions. A concept map is included below for you to help you diagram and link disease concepts together.

Fluid

1. Define isotonic, hypertonic, and hypotonic fluid effects on the cell.

2. What happens in fluid volume deficit and fluid volume overload?

3. What is ADH? What role do renin and aldosterone play?

4. Describe the differences between SIADH and diabetes insipidus.

5. How do you develop edema? Describe the role of colloidal osmotic pressure and capillary filtration pressure in causing edema. How do you assess edema?

Electrolytes

(Hint: Compare and contrast hypo and hyper. Note hallmark characteristics of each electrolyte imbalance.)

6. Know the ranges of sodium, potassium, calcium, phosphorus, and magnesium.

7. What happens to cells in hypotonic hyponatremia?

8. What is hypertonic hyponatremia? When does it happen?

9. What are the causes and symptoms of hyponatremia?

10. What happens to cells in hypernatremia? What are the causes and symptoms of hypernatremia? Who is at risk?

11. When does hypokalemia develop? When does hyperkalemia develop? Who is at risk for each? What are the causes and manifestations of each?

12. What are the causes and manifestations of hypo- and hyperparathyroidism? What electrolyte(s) do they affect? How?

13. What are the causes and manifestations of hypo- and hypercalcemia? What is the function of calcium? What kinds of cells are affected?

14. What is vitamin D? How is it produced? What electrolyte does it affect? How?

15. What are the causes and manifestations of hypophosphatemia?

16. Why is magnesium important in cells? What electrolytes and functions does it affect?

17. What causes hypo- and hypermagnesemia? What are the manifestations of each?

Acid-base

18. Know the normal ranges of acid-base: pCO_2, pO_2, HCO_3^-, pH.

19. What are the causes and manifestations of acidemia and alkalemia?

20. Be able to identify primary ABG disorders and compensatory effects given pH, pCO_2, and HCO_3^- values.

21. Describe the compensatory mechanisms in acid-base regulation (chemical buffers, lungs, kidneys). When and how quickly does each work? How effective is each?

STUDY TIPS

Try these problems using ROME or Tic-Tac-Toe:

a. pH: 7.48; pCO_2: 25; HCO_3: 18
b. pH: 7.24; pCO_2: 35; HCO_3: 10
c. pH: 7.38; pCO_2: 40; HCO_3: 24
d. pH: 7.30; pCO_2: 50; HCO_3: 32
e. pH: 7.53; pCO_2: 48; HCO_3: 34
f. pH: 7.37; pCO_2: 60; HCO_3: 38

Answers:

a. Respiratory alkalosis partially compensated.

Acidic	Normal	Basic
		pH
HCO_3		CO_2

Compensation (→ HCO_3); Cause of pH (CO_2 → pH)

b. Metabolic acidosis, uncompensated. Let's try ROME.

pH↓ HCO_3↓

Now go back and look at the ROME method. The arrows both going down tell you that this is metabolic acidosis (metabolic equal). Remember, the body compensates for these disorders by causing the opposite disorder to occur. So, an increase in metabolic acid will be compensated with an increase in respiratory alkalosis. A decrease in CO_2 signifies an increase in pH (respiratory opposite). When you look at the CO_2 level, it is normal. Therefore, there is no compensation happening.

c. Normal. All values are within normal range.

Acidic	Normal	Basic
	pH	
	CO_2	
	HCO_3	

d. Respiratory acidosis, partially compensated.

pH↓ CO_2↑ HCO_3↑

Looking at the ROME diagram and the arrows, the only one that fits is respiratory acidosis. The pH is acidic and an increase in CO_2 is causing the acidity (respiratory opposite). To compensate, the bicarbonate would need to increase, becoming more alkalotic. Sure enough, the bicarbonate is increased indicating partial compensation.

Why is it partial compensation? Because the pH is still abnormal. To have full compensation, the pH must go back to normal.

e. Metabolic alkalosis partially compensated.

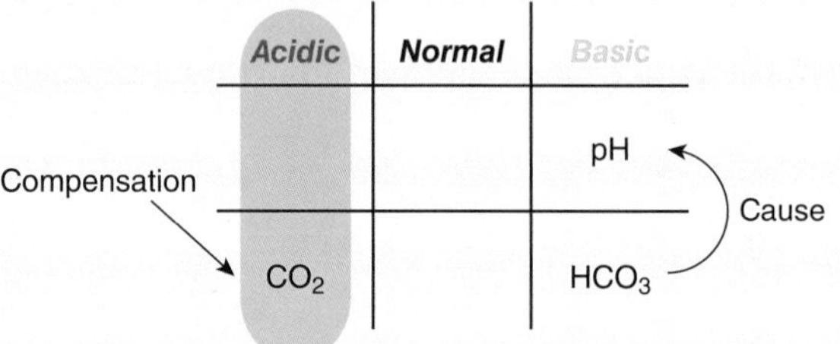

The pH is alkalotic, caused by an increase in bicarbonate, metabolic alkalosis. It is partially compensated by an increase in CO_2.

f. Respiratory acidosis, fully compensated.

Acidic	Normal	Basic
	pH	
CO_2		HCO_3

Oh no, now what?!!

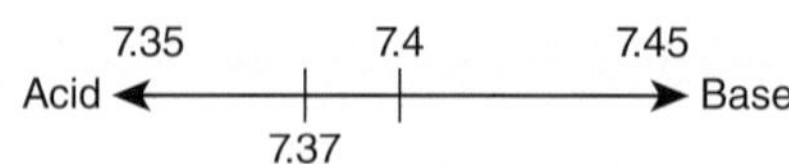

Even though the pH is normal, you can see that the acid-base balance is completely out of whack. The CO_2 and HCO_3 levels are both abnormal. This does not happen when the acid-base balance is normal. In this case, the CO_2 and HCO_3 levels have fully compensated for the acid-base disorder. So, is this acidosis or alkalosis? Look at where the pH value lies in the normal range. Is it more toward the acidic side or basic side? It is more toward the acidic side, acidosis. Once you figure that out, you can see that it is caused by the increase in CO_2, so it is respiratory acidosis, fully compensated (with a normal pH).

Acidic	Normal	Basic
pH ←	pH	
CO_2		HCO_3

Concept Map

Use this concept map to link each disease to its pathophysiology, diagnostics, causes, risk factors, complications, and clinical manifestations together. This way, you will be able to see the whole picture of the disease.

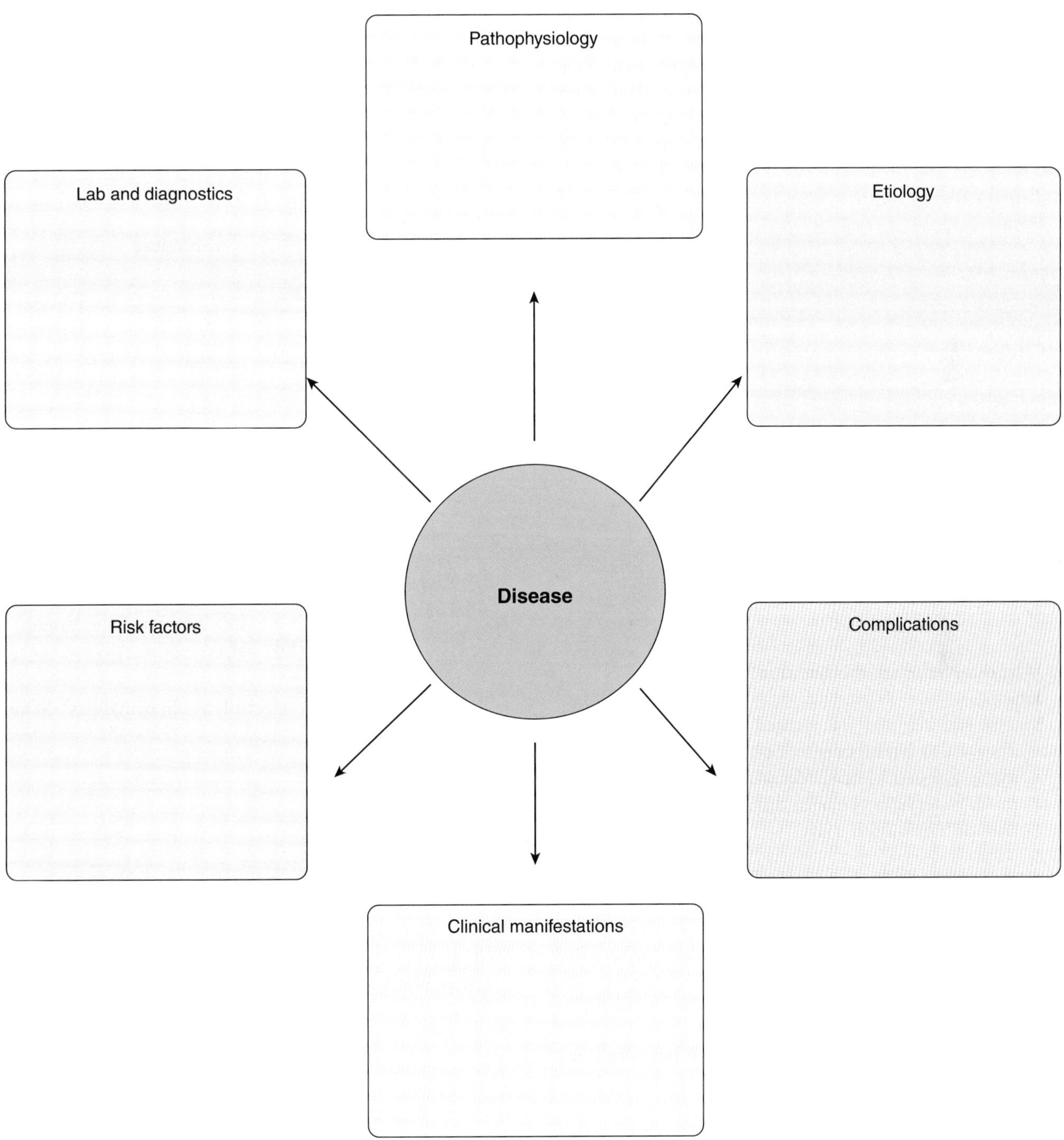

Case Studies for Chapter 3

Make sure that you have your class notes and textbooks on hand to answer these questions.

Case Study 3.1

Marcos, a Latinx nonbinary person (they/them), was traveling in South India with their husband, Nikhil (he/him). Despite the weather being extremely hot and humid, Marcos and Nikhil went out sightseeing on foot during the day. Marcos was very hot and was sweating copiously. They made sure to stay hydrated by having a water bottle on hand and making sure to refill it at water stations. After a few days of travel, Marcos woke up and was alarmed to find that their feet and lower legs were extremely swollen.

1. Explain the pathophysiology behind the swelling and edema.

2. What conditions may have led to this?

3. Why did Nikhil ask this question? Why did he assess the lungs?
   Marcos was alarmed and wanted to go to the hospital. They called Nikhil over to look at their feet. Nikhil, a nurse, assessed Marcos' feet and asked, "Marcos, how much water have you been drinking?" Marcos replied, "About 5 or 6 liters a day."

4. What does Marcos' response indicate? What condition do they have?

5. Does Marcos need to go to the hospital? How can their condition be treated?

Case Study 3.2

Sam, a 20-year-old client with a uterus (they/them), is brought into the emergency room (ER) confused and lethargic. They are put on oxygen, an IV is put in, and labs are drawn. The nurse assesses Sam's vital signs and labs.

Labs	Lab Values
Potassium (mg/dL)	6.5
Magnesium (mg/dL)	4
Calcium (mg/dL)	12
Sodium (mg/dL)	145
pH	7.28
HCO_3 (mg/dL)	16
pCO_2 (mm Hg)	35
Blood glucose	515 mg/dL

VITAL SIGNS AND ASSESSMENT	
Respiratory rate (breaths/minute)	30, deep and rapid
Pulse (beats/minute)	120, weak and thready
Blood pressure	90/50
Temperature (°F)	100, skin warm and flushed
Oxygen saturation (%)	97

1. Does Sam have any electrolyte abnormalities? Which electrolytes?

2. How would you interpret Sam's arterial blood gas? If there is a disorder, how would the body compensate?

3. Are there any electrolyte imbalances that are common with Sam's condition? Explain.

The emergency medical technicians (EMTs) tell the nurse that Sam was newly diagnosed with type 1 diabetes. The nurse realizes that Sam is likely in diabetic ketoacidosis. When the nurse goes in to check on Sam, they find that they are unconscious, breathing deeply and rapidly at 32 breaths/min.

4. How would you explain Sam's somnolence and respiratory rate? Explain the pathophysiology.

5. Why is Sam's face warm and flushed? What would cause their weak, rapid pulse?

Case Study 3.3

- Kal is a 75-year-old South Asian cis-male with a history of severe pulmonary disease. He has a wheezy, congested cough and needs to use oxygen at night.
- Lei is a 16-year-old Asian cis-female with a history of depression. She is brought to the emergency room (ER) after 24 hours of slurred speech, dizziness, nausea and vomiting, and abdominal pain.
- Jess is a 48-year-old White cis-female, brought into the ER after spending the day working in the sun. Jess is experiencing a severe headache, and she has a temperature of 101°F. She has not urinated in the past 4 hours.

	Kal	Lei	Jess
Na^+ (mEq/L)	138	132	150
K^+ (mEq/L)	5.6	2.0	4.8
Ca^+ (mg/dL)	11	6.6	10
Mg^+ (mg/dL)	4	0.7	2.0
pH	7.32	7.64	7.40
pCO_2 (mm Hg)	50	42	40
pO_2 (mm Hg)	78	80	86
HCO_3 (mmol/L)	30	46	26

1. Based on the above information, which patient needs to be assessed first? Why?

2. Kal is complaining of numbness and tingling, especially around the mouth. Identify the electrolyte imbalance(s) this patient has that could be causing these symptoms.

3. How would you interpret Kal's blood gas? What would cause this? What body system(s) will attempt to compensate?

4. Jess' blood pressure is 88/50 mm Hg and her heart rate is 116 beats/min when lying down. When she attempts to sit up, she feels faint. What could be causing her symptoms?

5. Would you treat Jess' sodium level? If yes, how?

The EMTs tell the nurse that Lei drank a bleach-based cleaner (pH of 11) in a suicide attempt. (Fact: Suicide is the leading cause of death among Asian-Americans, ages 15 to 24.) Her roommate found her and called 911. On emergency medical services (EMS) arrival, she was extremely anxious, complaining of numbness and tingling to her hands and feet. When the nurse goes in to assess Lei, they find that she is seizing. She has a decreased respiratory rate (10 breaths/min), and the cardiac monitor shows an irregular heart rate.

6. What do Lei's blood gas results indicate? What condition does she have? What is an electrolyte disorder that often accompanies this condition?

7. How would you account for her seizures and respiratory rate?

8. How would you explain Lei's heart rate and paresthesias?

4

Renal Diseases

After fluid and electrolytes, the renal system is the next logical topic to cover because the kidney has so much to do with maintaining fluid and electrolyte balance, as well as acid-base balance.

STUDY TIP

One big tip: Review your anatomy and physiology of the kidney before you start to work on renal disorders.

It is important to know how the kidneys work and how they function before you can understand what happens to them during a disease process (Figs. 4.1 and 4.2).

You need to know the normal ranges of important renal lab values (Table 4.1).

NOTE

It is important to realize that some facilities continue to use different equations to calculate the glomerular filtration rates from creatinine levels in melanated clients who are Black, resulting in readings that are falsely high.

- This has caused delayed diagnosis of renal disease and renal failure, as evidenced by the fact that individuals who are Black have the highest rates of end-stage renal disease and death from renal failure.
- This has also caused delayed referrals to specialists and for kidney transplants.
- Treatments and medications that may harm the kidneys would not be identified with falsely high values.
- Hospitals and labs have started removing these "race-corrected algorithms," but the practice persists in many facilities.

When looking at renal disorders, it's helpful to divide up the diseases into different categories and make T charts to compare.

Example:

	Cystitis	Pyelonephritis
Cause?		
Pathophysiology?		
Symptoms?		

- Lower urinary tract infections (UTIs)
  - Cystitis

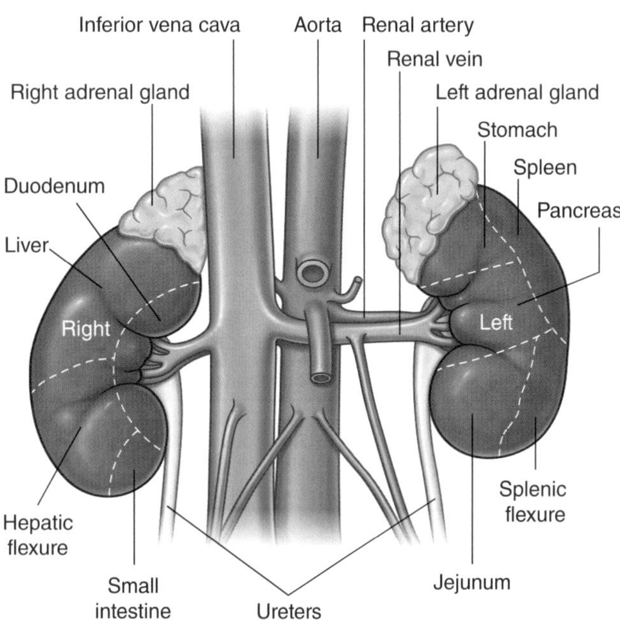

• **Fig. 4.1** Anatomy and physiology review of the kidney. (From Waugh, A., & Grant, A. (2022). *Ross & Wilson anatomy and physiology in health and illness* (14th ed.). Elsevier, Fig. 13.2.)

- Upper UTIs
  - Pyelonephritis
- Obstructive disorders
  - Benign prostatic hyperplasia (BPH)
  - Neurogenic bladder
  - Nephrolithiasis (kidney stones)
  - Hydronephrosis and hydroureter
- Glomerular disorders
  - Glomerulonephritis
  - Diabetic glomerulosclerosis
  - Nephritic syndrome
  - Nephrotic syndrome
- Acute kidney injury (AKI)
- Chronic renal failure (CRF)

Lower Versus Upper Urinary Tract Infections

Students often find it helpful to be able to compare different disorders. Let's start with urinary tract disorders. Cystitis, or

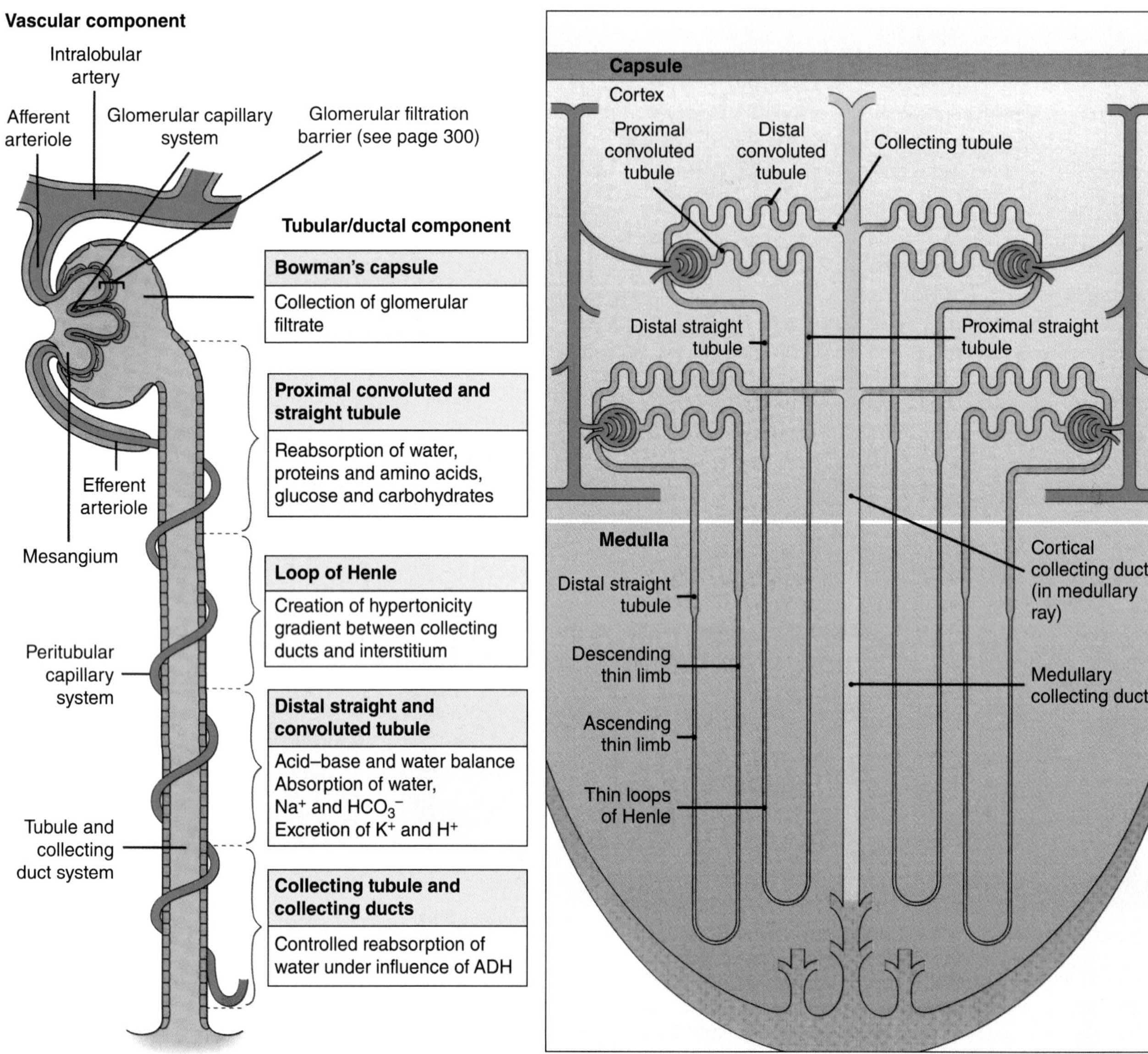

• **Fig. 4.2** Functions of nephrons. *ADH,* Antidiuretic hormone. (From Stevens, A., & Lowe, J. Human Histology (3rd ed.), Mosby/Elsevier. Copyright 2005, Elsevier.)

TABLE 4.1 Normal Ranges of Important Renal Lab Values

Kidney Function Test	Normal Values and Ranges
Glomerular filtration rate (GFR)[a]	>90 mL/minute/1.73m^2 <60 mL/minute/1.73m^2 signals kidney failure
Average urinary output	60 mL/hour[b]
Blood urea nitrogen (BUN)	8–20 mg/dL
Creatinine[a]	0.6–1.2 mg/dL
Urine analysis	
• **Specific gravity**	1.010–1.025
• **Protein**	Negative
• **Blood**	Negative

[a]Most important lab values for kidney function
[b]Concern if this drops below 30 mL/hour

a UTI, is a common infection, especially for assigned females at birth (AFAB) and trans-females who have undergone gender affirming surgery. This is because the urethra is much shorter than the urethras of assigned males at birth (AMAB). Bacteria enter through the urethra and ascend to the bladder, causing inflammation, urinary urgency and frequency, dysuria, and/or bleeding. Urine may be cloudy or foul smelling, though this is not always the case.

NOTE

Symptoms can be very different in the old individuals and individuals with diabetes. Infections in these populations can by asymptomatic or manifest as confusion and lethargy.

UTIs are most often caused by *Escherichia coli* bacteria from fecal matter. That's why AFABs are encouraged to wipe themselves front to back after urination. Another major cause of UTIs is catheter-associated UTIs (CAUTI). Other causes might be sexual intercourse, urinary reflux (backflow of urine), or urinary stasis (hospitable environment for bacteria). The urethra protects itself by having a slightly acidic pH, "good" bacteria (probiotics), and producing mucus to trap "bad" bacteria. A urine analysis and urine culture are done to confirm the infection and the UTI is treated with antibiotics.

Let's contrast a UTI with pyelonephritis. Pyelonephritis ("itis" = inflammation) is a kidney infection (sometimes called an "upper UTI") and usually stems from an untreated or undertreated lower UTI. It can also be caused by stents, trauma, or an obstruction, all of which can directly introduce bacteria into the kidney. The bacteria ascend the ureter and end up in either one or both kidneys, causing an infection. This is a much more serious infection and can progress to become a systemic infection, resulting in sepsis and acute renal failure.

Pyelonephritis starts suddenly with the common manifestations of fever, chills, flank/back pain, and nausea/vomiting. AFABs may present with hematuria or purulent urine. Tests to diagnose this may include a complete blood count, blood cultures, urine analysis, and urine culture. Treatment is typically intravenous antibiotics.

If pyelonephritis becomes recurrent or persistent, it can develop into chronic pyelonephritis. The ongoing inflammation and immune response cause scarring and necrosis within the kidney, ultimately leading to decreased glomerular filtration rate (GFR), increased creatinine, and increased BUN.

As you can see, there is a continuum:

UTI → acute pyelonephritis → chronic pyelonephritis → renal failure

Obstructive Disorders

Obstructive disorders are anything that blocks the passage and excretion of urine. This includes kidney stones, neurogenic bladder (nerve damage preventing voluntary urination), tumors, and enlarged prostate. These blockages can cause backflow of urine into the ureters and kidneys, which can lead to hydroureter and/or hydronephrosis (dilations of ureters/kidneys). When talking about obstructions, it is important to look at where blockage is, whether it is partial or complete, and whether it is acute or chronic.

If the blockage is below the uterovesical junction (neurogenic bladder, bladder cancer, or BPH) it will have a bilateral effect, causing urine to back up into both ureters and both kidneys. If the blockage is above the junction, the effect will be unilateral, causing urine to back up on one side only. The most common blockages are due to BPH and kidney stones. As AMABs age, their prostates enlarge. This is a normal development with age but can impede urine flow and lead to complications. With a unilateral obstruction, the unobstructed kidney will continue to function and can take over for the obstructed kidney for a time, so renal failure does not occur. The obstructed kidney and unobstructed kidney may be damaged if the obstruction is not resolved. If there is a bilateral obstruction that is not resolved, it can lead to bladder rupture and renal failure.

Kidney stones are typically composed of calcium salt, and less commonly, struvite. Hypercalcemia, or increased blood levels in blood and urine, can cause crystal formation in the urine, which continues to increase in size and may eventually create a blockage. Dehydration can also cause relative hypercalcemia and lead to kidney stones.

NOTE

Kidney stones are common issues. If the stones are stuck in the renal calyces, renal pelvis, or the ureter, they can cause severe pain, hematuria, nausea and vomiting, and chills. Smaller kidney stones can pass on their own. However, larger stones may get stuck and may need lithotripsy (ultrasonic waves) to break apart the stones or removal of the stones using ureteroscopy. Pain relief, fluid, and antiemetics may be needed.

Think of renal diseases on a continuum:

Obstruction → urinary stasis → hydroureter/hydronephrosis → renal failure

Glomerular Disorders

Acute glomerulonephritis is commonly caused by immunoglobulin A (IgA) nephropathy (autoimmune) and infections, such as *Streptococcus* (strep throat). Antibody-antigen complexes accumulate and damage the glomeruli. Cell-mediated immune reactions cause T lymphocytes and macrophages to flood the kidneys and cause damage. Glomerulonephritis can also be caused by glomerular injury caused by diabetes mellitus, hypertension, and nephrotoxic drugs. Diabetic glomerulosclerosis is caused by hyperglycemia, which leads to thickening of the glomerular basement membrane and damage to the glomerular capillaries. This cuts down on the surface area needed for filtration, which decreases GFR (Fig. 4.3).

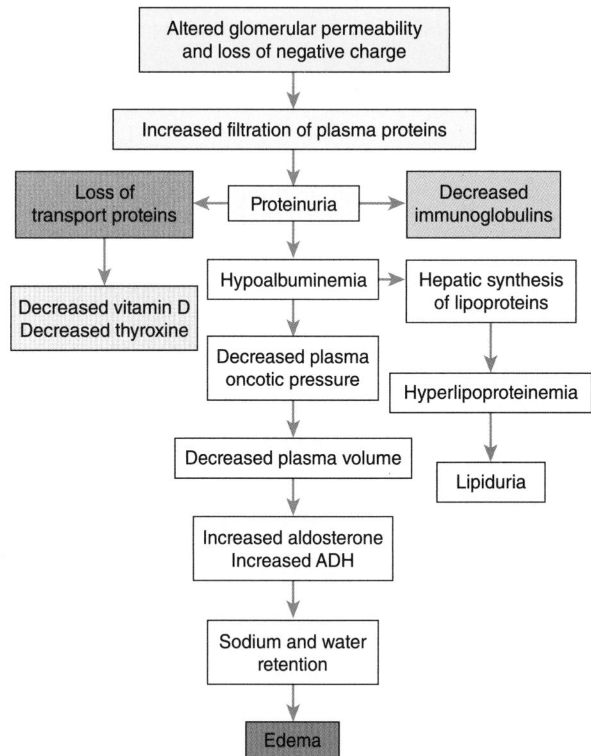

• **Fig. 4.3** Acute glomerulonephritis. *ADH,* Antidiuretic hormone. (McCance, K. L. (2019). Cancer Epidemiology. In K. L. McCance, S. E. Huether, V. Brashers, & N. Rote (Eds.), *Pathophysiology: The Biologic Basis for Disease in Adults and Children* (8th ed., pp. 379-425). Elsevier)

Think about what the clinical manifestations would be for a minute. If the kidneys don't work, fluid can't be filtered out properly, which will result in fluid retention. Electrolyte disorders would also result, as the kidneys are essential in retaining and excreting them. Classic symptoms include:

- hypertension
- edema
- hematuria
- oliguria
- azotemia

Acute glomerulonephritis can result in nephritic syndrome. Nephritic syndrome is common with bacterial infections (streptococcus) and autoimmune disease (lupus) and is due to the inflammatory response causing white blood cells to accumulate in the glomerulus and causing damage to the glomerular filtration barrier. This inflammatory response changes the glomerular membrane and makes the capillaries extremely permeable, causing red blood cells and some proteins to leak out. The key findings in nephritic syndrome are gross hematuria (cola-colored urine) and pyuria (pus).

Nephrotic syndrome commonly results from membranous or segmental glomerulosclerosis. Minimal change syndrome (children) is also a common cause. With nephrotic syndrome, there is a destruction of the glomerular epithelium, specifically the podocytes. With this destruction, large protein molecules, such as albumin, antithrombin (needed to stop clotting), and antibodies can escape. Because so much protein escapes, the liver tries to compensate by producing lipoprotein. However, the lipoprotein eventually escapes as well, causing lipiduria. The key findings in nephrotic syndrome are massive proteinuria, lipiduria, and albuminemia (low blood albumin). Microscopic amounts of hematuria may be found but are not a major finding.

Both nephrotic and nephritic syndromes have hypertension, edema, oliguria, and azotemia as manifestations. These syndromes can lead to AKI. If glomerulonephritis is not treated, it can go on to become chronic, causing permanent damage to the kidneys and resulting in CFR.

Glomerulonephritis → nephritic/nephrotic syndrome → chronic glomerulonephritis → renal failure

Acute Kidney Injury

AKI (or acute renal failure) occurs when there is an acute, often reversible disease process or injury to the kidney. There are three categories of AKI (Fig. 4.4):

- Prerenal—damage caused by decreased renal blood flow (e.g., heart failure, hemorrhage, dehydration, shock, vasoactive medications)
- Intrarenal—damage that occurs within the kidney (ischemic injury from prerenal injury, nephrotoxic drugs, acute glomerulonephritis, acute pyelonephritis, intrarenal obstruction, acute tubular necrosis [ATN])
    - ATN occurs when intrarenal damage occurs to nephron tubules
        - Initiation phase: asymptomatic, initial insult
        - Extension phase: Inflammation and lack of kidney perfusion
        - Maintenance phase: increased blood urea nitrogen (BUN)/creatinine, electrolyte disorders. Oliguria may occur. If so, ATN is more severe, and can lead to renal failure, coma, death.
        - Recovery phase: diuresis, decreasing BUN/creatinine, electrolyte disorders
- Postrenal—obstruction. In order to cause AKI, obstruction must occlude both kidneys, both ureters, or the uterovesical junction.

Chronic Kidney Disease

CRF can result from damage from any of the previous renal disorders discussed and can result in end stage renal failure (ESRD). The disease progresses slowly and does not show symptoms until few nephrons are left. Common causes are diabetes, hypertension, glomerulonephritis, and autoimmune diseases. To understand the clinical manifestations of CRF, it's important to know the functions of the kidneys first, and then the dysfunctions are more obvious (Fig. 4.5).

Clinical manifestations associated with CRF:

- Fluid, electrolyte, and acid-base disorders → hyperkalemia
- Fluid retention → hypertension → heart failure
- Azotemia → uremia → pruritus, skin breakdown, confusion, immune cell dysfunction
- High urea levels → delayed gastric emptying and changes to gut biome → nausea, vomiting → erosion and ulcerations of esophagus, stomach, bowel
- Lack of thrombopoietin → lack of platelets

However, factor VIII increases due to uremia → increased clotting

- Lack of erythropoietin → anemia
- Acid-base balance → kidneys cannot secrete H^+/retain or produce bicarbonate → acidosis
- Kidneys cannot activate vitamin D → low serum calcium → hyperparathyroidism → osteodystrophy (calcium taken from bone)

Study Guide for Chapter 4

Make sure that you have your class notes and textbooks on hand to answer these questions. A concept map is included to help you diagram and link disease concepts together.

Anatomy and Physiology of the Kidney

1. What labs do we use to assess kidney function? What are the normal values?

____

____

____

____

2. Which labs are most indicative of kidney issues?

____

____

ACUTE KIDNEY INJURY

TYPES of AKI	PRERENAL	INTRARENAL	POSTRENAL
MECHANISM	• Reduced blood flow to the kidneys	• Damage to kidney tubules, glomerulus, or interstitium	• Obstructed urine flow
CAUSES	• Hypovolemic states (hemorrhage, GI loss, renal loss, severe burns, sepsis) • Systolic heart failure • Hypoalbuminemia • Medications (NSAIDs, ACE-inhibitors, ARBs, Cyclosporine, & iodinated contrast	• Acute tubular necrosis • Nephrotoxins (aminoglycosides, methotrexate, lead, ethylene glycol, radiocontrast dye) • Rhabdomyelisis • Glomerular disease • Acute insterstitial nephritis	• Kidney stones • Benign prostatic hyperplasia • Prostatic cancer • Intra-abdominal tumors

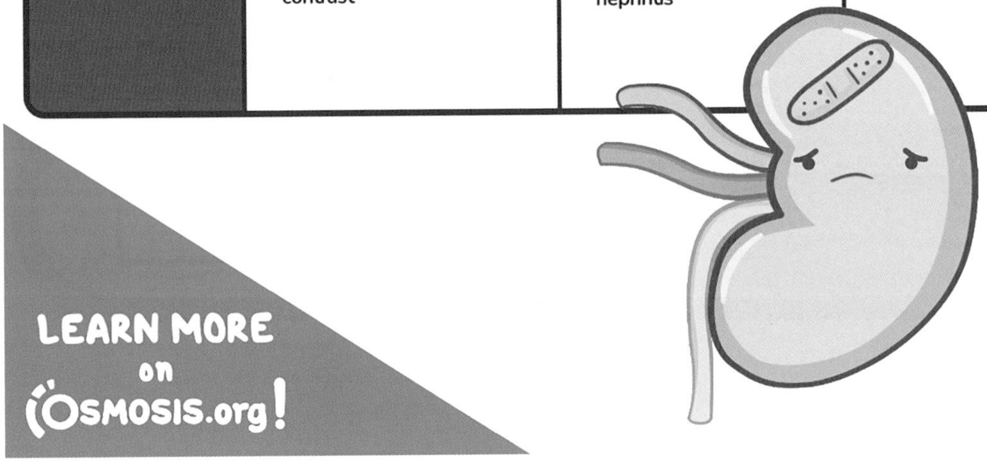

• **Fig. 4.4** Types of acute renal injury. *ACE,* Angiotensin-converting enzyme; *AKI,* acute kidney injury; *ARBs,* angiotensin 2 receptor blockers; *GI,* gastrointestinal; *NSAIDs,* nonsteroidal anti-inflammatory drugs. (From https://www.facebook.com/Osmoselt/photos/a.293866334077588/2605673802896818/?type=3.)

3. If they kidneys do not function as normal, what symptoms would the client have? What complications could result?

4. What hormones and vitamins do the kidneys secrete or affect?

Disorders of Renal Function

5. How do race-based medicine and GFR play a role in diagnosing kidney failure?

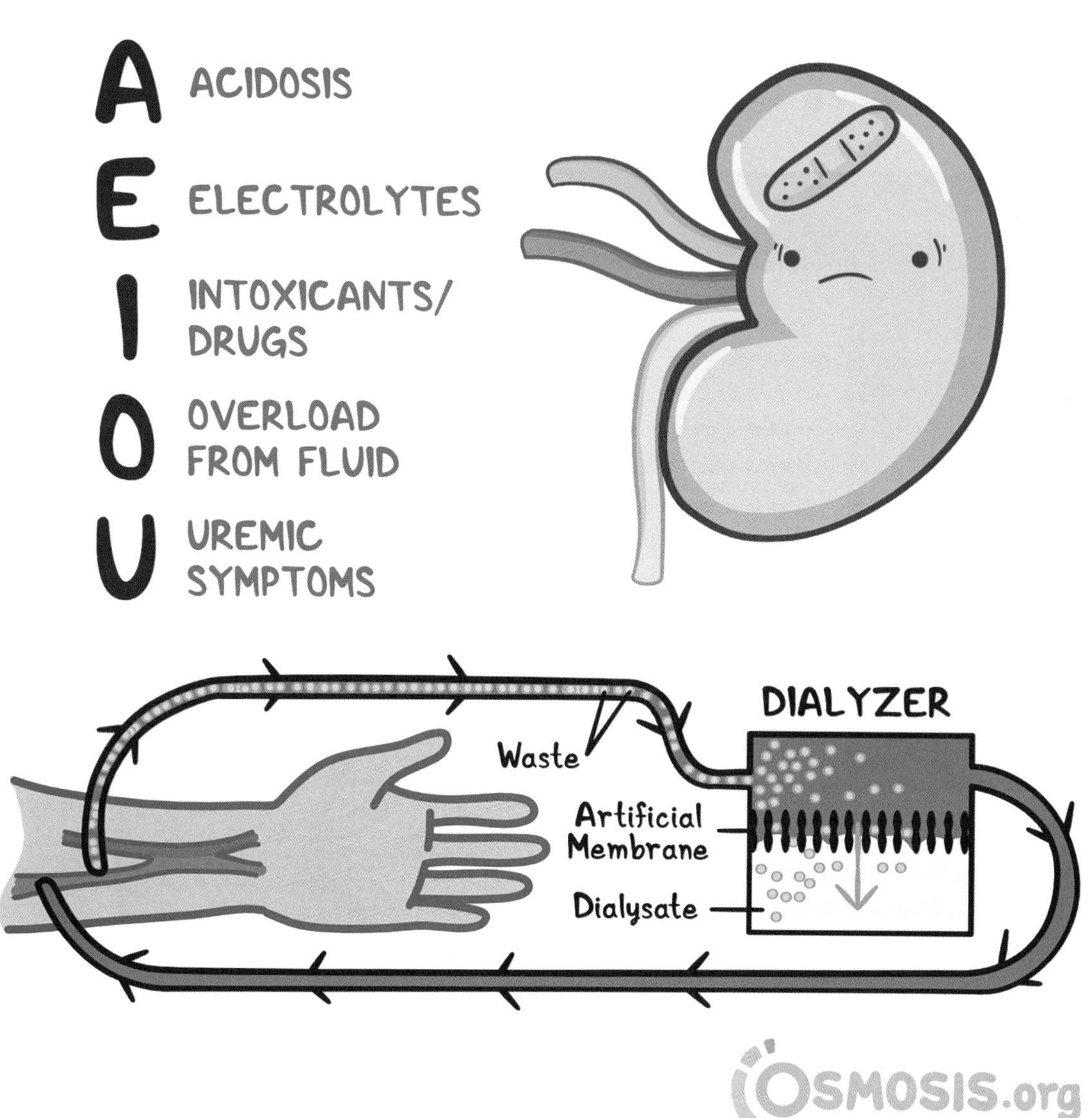

• **Fig. 4.5** Outcomes of Chronic renal failure. (From https://www.facebook.com/Osmoselt/photos/a.293866334077588/1936639006466971/?type53.)

6. What role do immune mechanisms play in glomerular disorders?

7. What causes glomerulonephritis? What are the symptoms? What is the difference between acute and chronic glomerulonephritis?

8. What causes nephrotic syndrome? Is it a disease? What are the symptoms?

9. What causes acute and chronic pyelonephritis? What are the symptoms?

Obstructions

10. What are the common causes of urinary tract obstruction? How do urinary tract obstructions impact the kidney? How do they impact the client?

11. Describe hydronephrosis and hydroureter. What are the complications?

12. How does an enlarged prostate lead to an obstruction?

13. Describe the varied causes of kidney stones and how they can result in pain and infection.

14. What is a neurogenic bladder? What issues does a client with this face?

Acute Kidney Injury and Chronic Kidney Disease

15. What are the differences between acute renal failure and chronic kidney disease?

16. Describe the three types of acute renal failure (prerenal, intrarenal, postrenal). What are their causes?

17. What is acute tubular necrosis? Describe the stages. What does this cause?

18. What other disorders (fluid/electrolyte imbalances, disorders of other symptoms) would you expect to see in clients with renal failure? Why?

19. Who is most at risk for kidney failure?

Disorders of the Bladder and Lower Urinary Tract

20. How does the body typically protect itself from urinary tract infections?

21. How does nursing care impact the risk of UTIs?

22. What are the differences between upper and lower tract UTIs?

Concept Map

Use this concept map to link each disease to its pathophysiology, diagnostics, causes, risk factors, complications, and clinical manifestations together. This way, you will be able to see the whole picture of the disease.

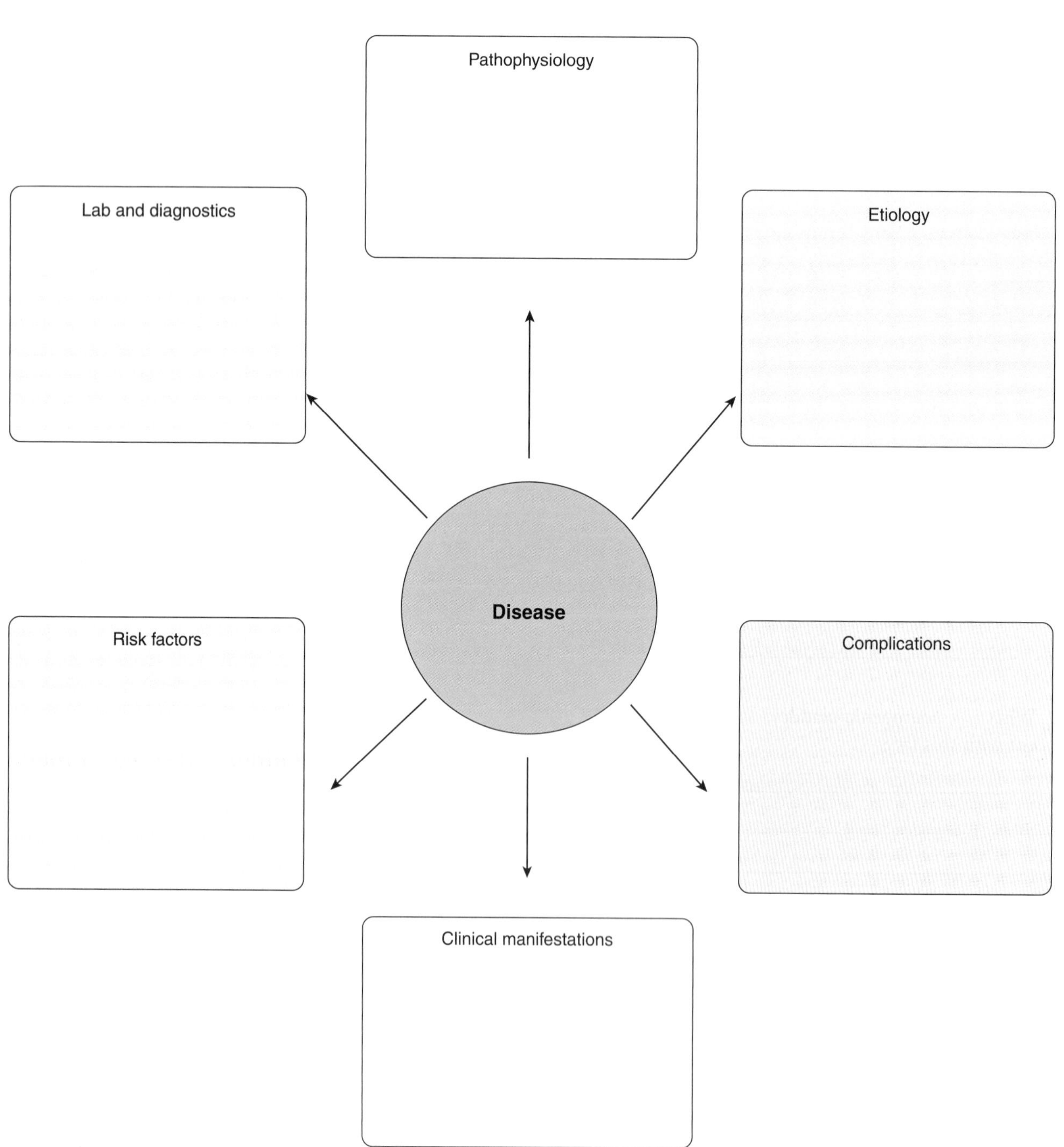

Case Studies for Chapter 4

Make sure that you have your class notes and textbooks on hand to answer these questions.

Case Study 4.1

An 85-year-old cis-female client (she/her) with a history of mild to moderate dementia comes to her provider with her daughter (she/her), with whom she lives. Her daughter reports that the client seems more confused and sleeping more than usual. The provider asks if the client's urine is cloudy or has a foul odor. The daughter says that she has noticed a strong odor coming from her mother's urine.

1. As the nurse, what would you notice about this client? How would you interpret this?

2. What condition do you think that the client has? Does she show typical symptoms? Why or why not?

3. Does the client's dementia play a role in this disorder? Why or why not?

4. What lab tests would you expect the provider to order?

Two weeks later, the client is hospitalized with fever, lethargy, nausea, and severe bilateral flank pain.

5. How has the client's condition progressed? Explain the pathophysiology.

6. What lab results would you expect to see?

7. How would this condition be treated?

The client's creatinine and blood urea nitrogen (BUN) continue to rise. The client is diagnosed with acute kidney injury.

8. Why type of acute kidney injury (AKI) would the client most likely have? Explain the pathophysiology and complications.

Case Study 4.2

An 18-year-old Black cis-male (he/him) visits a clinic located in a rural community. He reports swelling around his eyes and bilateral lower leg edema that started a week prior. He states that he has not seen a doctor for years, but decided to come to the clinic when he started seeing blood in his urine. His vital signs are: 178/94; 94 beats/minute; 18 breaths/minute.

1. As the nurse, what would you notice about the client's symptom history and vital signs?

2. What disorder might this client have? Explain what may have caused this issue and what symptoms support your diagnosis.

3. What role, if any, would social determinants of health play in this case?

Bloodwork and urine analyses are performed.

Labs

Result

Creatinine
1.8 mg/dL
Blood urea nitrogen
72 mg/dL
Serum sodium
135 mg/dL
Serum potassium
5.2 mg/dL
Low-density lipoprotein (LDL)
178 mg/dL
Serum albumin
2.0 g/dL
Hemoglobin
9 g/dL
Urine analysis
+ Protein
+ Red blood cells
White blood cell count
14 million/mm^3

4. What do you notice about the labs? How do these values support your diagnosis?

5. How would you treat someone with this disorder?

Case Study 4.3

Josie, a 62-year-old White, nonbinary individual (they/them), arrives at an urgent care center, with symptoms of vomiting, paleness, and shaking. They are immediately taken back to an exam room where Josie tells the nurse that they have not urinated in 12 hours. The nurse quickly assesses them and finds that Josie's abdomen is quite distended and painful. The nurse explains to Josie that catheterization is necessary. When going to catheterize Josie, the nurse finds out that they are assigned male at birth (AMAB) and expresses surprise, which makes Josie uncomfortable. The nurse has great difficulty inserting the catheter, but is finally successful, with immediate output of two liters of dark, red urine. The nurse sends off a urine sample and urine culture.

1. What do you notice about Josie's condition? How would you interpret these findings and make a diagnosis?

2. Did the nurse respond appropriately? How could the nurse have made Josie more comfortable?

3. How would this condition lead to acute kidney injury (AKI)? What type of AKI would this lead to?

Josie is transferred to the emergency room. Their labs are taken and an IV is inserted.

Labs

Result

Blood osmolality
285 mOsm/kg
Blood urea nitrogen (BUN)
124 mg/dL
Creatinine
1.4 mg/dL
Glomerular filtration rate (GFR)
53 mL/minute/1.73m^2
White blood cell (WBC) count
11 mg/dL
Urine analysis (UA)
+Red blood cells
−Protein
Urine specific gravity 1.03
Urine culture (UC)
Pending

Looking at Josie's labs:

4. Do the labs support a diagnosis of AKI? Why or why not?

5. What complication(s) may arise in Josie's case?

Case Study 4.4

Maria is a 57-year-old Brazilian trans-female (she/her) with a history of hypertension and type 2 diabetes mellitus (T2DM). She has been taking her medications for hypertension and T2DM, but her blood sugar has continued to increase. On her last visit, her provider wanted her to start taking insulin. The provider stated that Maria was starting to show signs of kidney damage.

1. How is diabetes related to chronic renal failure?

2. Which lab tests would indicate that Maria was in the beginning stages of renal failure?

3. The provider tells Maria that she needs to eat healthier and suggests limiting salt, meat, beans, and rice. Maria is dismayed as these are staples of her diet. She asks you, "Do I have to get rid of these foods? What will I eat?" How would you answer her?

Ten years later, Maria's renal failure has progressed. She has been admitted to the hospital with confusion, severe anemia, and vertebral fractures.

4. Explain the pathophysiology behind her symptoms.

5. During her hospitalization, the provider tells Maria and her family that her heart is failing. Her partner asks, "I don't understand why her heart is failing. She has issues with her kidneys." How would you reply?

5 Hematological Disorders

Hematological disorders, or blood disorders, encompass platelet, red blood cell (RBC), and white blood cell (WBC) disorders. In this chapter, we will talk mainly about platelet disorders, coagulation disorders, and RBC disorders. WBC disorders are mainly cancers such as leukemias and lymphomas. As cancer was covered in Chapter 2, we will not spend as much time on this topic.

Knowing the serum values of platelets, RBCs, and WBCs is key. This is a memorization task that you can do with flashcards. The values you should know are in Table 5.1.

Platelet and Coagulation Disorders

As you may already know, platelets (thrombocytes) are part of hemostasis, or the clotting process, or coagulation cascade, forming clots in areas of injury to isolate those areas or stop bleeding. Think for a moment—too many platelets will cause too many clots, or hypercoagulability. Too much clotting could block blood vessels, causing myocardial infarctions, strokes, and embolisms. This is a condition called thrombocythemia and can be caused by inflammatory diseases and cancer. It would logically follow that too few platelets would lead to excessive bleeding and hemorrhaging, a condition called thrombocytopenia. To understand why this disorder occurs, we need to go back to anatomy and physiology.

The bone, liver, and spleen are crucial to platelets and the clotting process. Bone marrow contains cells called megakaryocytes, which produce platelets. Platelets are stored in the spleen until they are needed. They can bind with fibrinogen and phospholipids to form a stable clot. Platelets contain granules that cause platelet adhesion and aggregation,

TABLE 5.1 Complete Blood Count Values

Type of Cell	Measurement	Value
Red blood cell (RBC) count	Total number of RBCs/mL	Assigned male at birth (AMAB): 4.1–6.1 million/mL Assigned female at birth (AFAB): 4.0–5.0 million/mL
Mean corpuscular volume (MCV)	Reflects volume/size of RBCs	84–96 fL
Mean corpuscular hemoglobin concentration (MCHC)	Concentration of hemoglobin in each RBC	32–36 g/dL
Percentage of reticulocytes (RET)	Immature RBCs; index rate of RBC production	0.5%–1.5%
Hematocrit (Hct)	% of blood by volume made up of RBCs	AMAB: 42%–52% AFAB: 36%–48%
Hemoglobin (Hgb)	Measures the hemoglobin content of blood	AMAB: 14–17 g/dL AFAB: 12–16 g/dL
Platelets (PLT)	Total number of PLTs/mL	150,000–400,000 cells/mL (150–400)
White blood cells (WBC)	Total number of WBCs/mL	4000–11,000 cells/mL (4–11)
Prothrombin time (PT) *warfarin	Time needed for clotting (intrinsic pathway)	10–15 seconds
Partial thromboplastin time (PTT) *heparin	Time needed for clotting (extrinsic pathway)	25–35 seconds

*Please note that the CBC of transgender males and transgender females receiving hormone therapy will reflect their chosen gender, not their gender assigned at birth.

vasoconstriction, and vessel repair. Platelets are activated by mediators in the blood plasma and blood vessel endothelium.

- Plasma contains inactive clotting proteins that are produced by the liver. Some clotting factors are vitamin K, prothrombin, and calcium.
  - Clotting factors are activated one by one during the coagulation cascade.
- von Willebrand factor (vWF) is an important mediator produced by the endothelium that helps platelets bind to the injured tissue.

The liver not only produces clotting proteins, but it also stores and activates vitamin K, which helps to synthesize clotting proteins. When there is a vitamin K deficiency (newborn) or liver damage, clotting is affected, and bleeding can occur. The liver also helps to filter out old RBCs.

There are two clotting pathways: intrinsic and extrinsic. The intrinsic pathway is activated by blood vessel damage. The clotting factors are in the vessel, but the coagulation pathway is slower and longer, reflected by the partial thromboplastin time (PTT). The extrinsic pathway is activated by tissue factor, released when there is a tissue injury. This is a bigger stimulus, and the clotting pathway is much faster, reflected by the prothrombin time (PT). Both pathways work together to bring about hemostasis. Note that both the intrinsic and extrinsic pathways meet at the common pathway (Fig. 5.1).

When considering anticoagulants, different anticoagulants work on different pathways (heparin → intrinsic, warfarin → extrinsic).

The steps of hemostasis (clotting) (Fig. 5.2):

Eventually the clot retracts, and the clot dissolves, revealing new skin.

Plasminogen → activated by tissue plasminogen activator (t-PA) → plasmin → clot dissolution

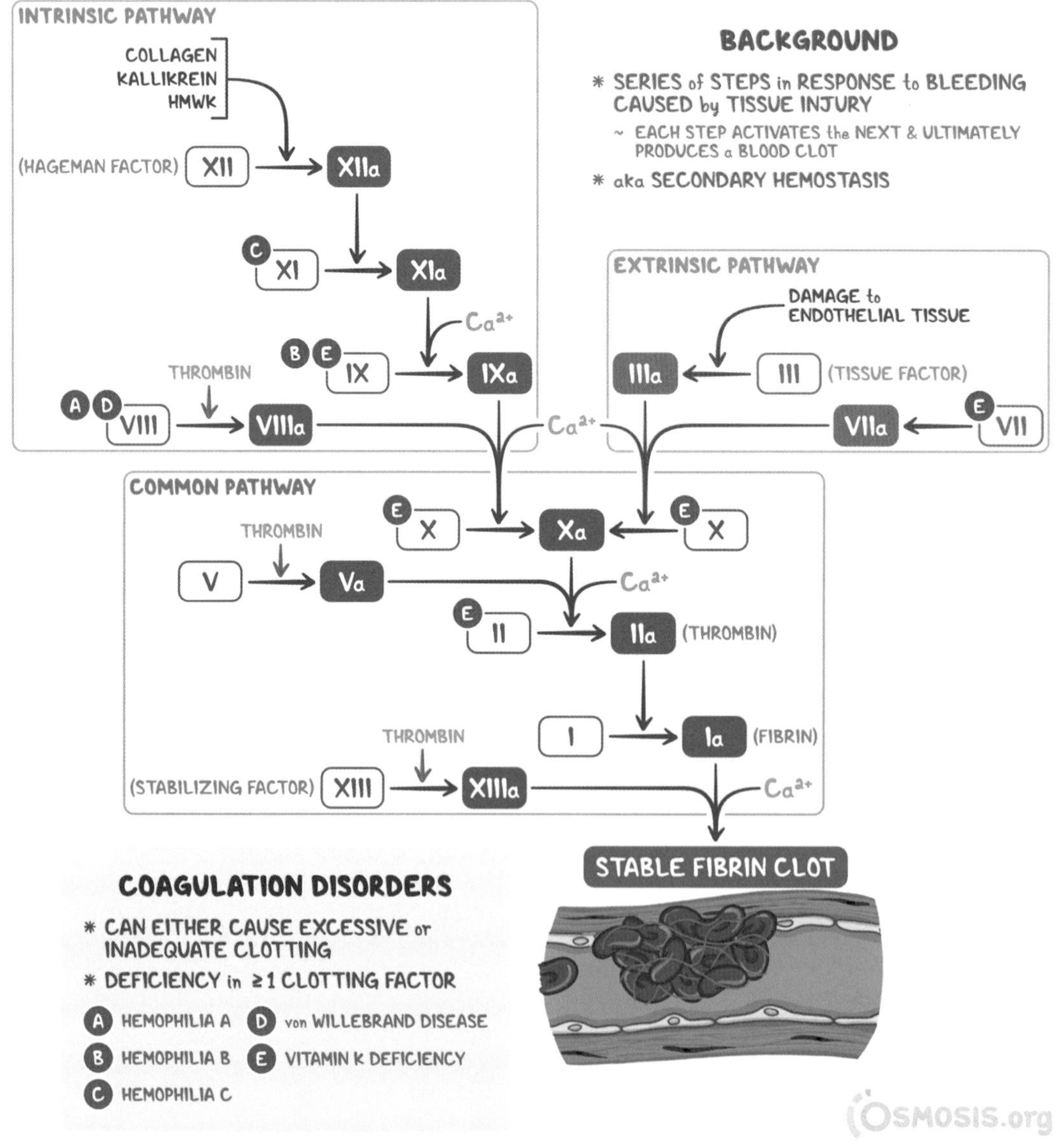

• **Fig. 5.1** Clotting pathway. (From https://www.osmosis.org/answers/coagulation-cascade.)

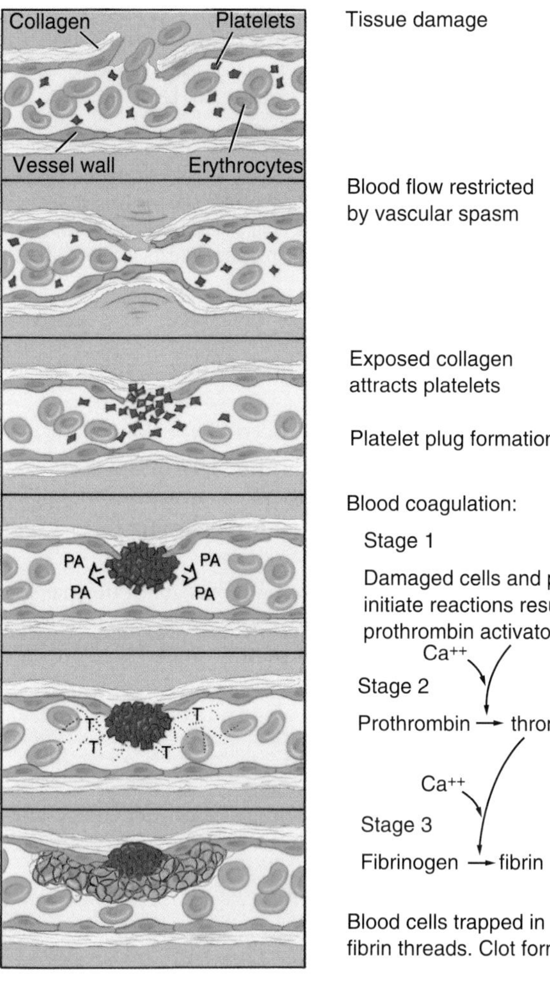

• **Fig. 5.2** Hemostasis Steps of Clotting (From Diehl, M. O., Shiland, B. L., & Klieger, D. M. (2003). *Medical assistant: Urinary, blood, lymphatic and immune systems with laboratory procedures—Module E* [2nd ed.]. Elsevier, Fig 4.6.)

Thrombocytopenia refers to low platelet count. There are many different causes for thrombocytopenia, such as chemotherapy, autoimmune disease, certain medications, or genetic disorders.

Types of thrombocytopenia:

- Immune thrombocytopenic purpura
  - Antiplatelet autoantibodies form after infection, destroying platelets
  - Causes microhemorrhages on skin, called purpura
- Drug-induced thrombocytopenia
  - Medications that cause platelet destruction, platelets to get used up, or the body to stop producing platelets
  - Example: heparin
- Thrombotic thrombocytopenic purpura
  - Deficiency of enzyme ADAMTS13, which breaks down vWF
  - Excess vWF causes clotting throughout the body
  - Platelets get used up, causing thrombocytopenia

All types of thrombocytopenia have similar clinical manifestations. Again, think logically. If you don't have platelets, you can't clot! Try and picture a person who cannot clot.

Some general manifestations:

- Bleeding
- Bruising
- Petechiae (pinpoint hemorrhage)
- Purpura (blood pooling under skin)
- Hematochezia and melena (blood in stool)
- Hematemesis (blood in vomit)
- Epistaxis (nosebleed)
- Intracranial bleeding
- Hematuria (blood in urine)
- Menorrhagia (heavy menstrual flow)

Coagulation Disorders

Difficulties with coagulation can arise from treatments, disease and inflammatory responses, or genetic mutations. For example, chemotherapy often destroys bone marrow, destroying platelets in the process. A disorder that causes severe clotting issues is disseminated intravascular coagulation (DIC). DIC is a systemic inflammatory response to disorders, such as cancer, shock, trauma burns, and liver failure. As you may remember from Chapter 1, inflammation causes clotting. When you have a disease process that causes systemic inflammation, that causes systemic clotting. Once that happens, all the platelets and clotting factors are used up and the patient starts to hemorrhage. DIC has a very high mortality rate. Recognizing and treating it early is important.

- Client may suffer from stroke symptoms and hypoxia due to clotting.
- The first signs of DIC are often bleeding from surgical, intravenous (IV), and venipuncture sites.

Labs to look for with DIC:

- Decreased platelets
- Decreased fibrinogen
  - Fibrin creates mesh for a stable clot
- Increased D-dimer
  - D-dimer is a protein fragment from a blood clot
- Increased PT and PTT
  - Clotting times

Inflammation → clotting factors are activated → uncontrolled clot formation → depletion of platelets and clotting factors →severe hemorrhaging

von Willebrand disease is a genetic, autosomal dominant disease that is a mutation on chromosome 12. This disease affects the vWF, which is a protein involved in clotting. Remember that the vWF is necessary for platelets to bind to the endothelium and start the clotting process. With this disease, there is a deficiency or absence of functional vWF. This affects clotting, but typically has symptoms such as epistaxis, bleeding from mouth and gums, gastrointestinal (GI) bleeding, and menorrhagia. Bleeding typically resolves; if not, clotting promoters (e.g., desmopressin [DDAVP]) are infused.

Hemophilia A is another genetic disorder; it is an X-linked recessive disorder that causes coagulation factor VIII deficiency. A common example of this is the high incidence of hemophilia A in royal blood lines. Because of the close genetic ties between married couples, the disorder was passed through the royal blood line, predominantly affecting assigned males at birth, with assigned females at birth typically acting as carriers. Unlike von Willebrand disease, hemophilia often causes severe bleeding, either with injury or spontaneously. Clients with this disease bruise very easily, can bleed into the joints (hemarthrosis), and are at risk for intracranial bleeding. Hemarthrosis requires immobilization, ice, and compression to stop the bleeding. If left untreated, hemophilia will cause hemorrhage, circulatory shock, and death. Infusion of factor VIII in fresh frozen plasma can be used to treat this.

Red Blood Cell Disorders

RBCs, also called erythrocytes, are cells that carry oxygen. Each RBC has hemoglobin, which is made up of four polypeptide chains. Each chain holds an iron-containing heme unit. When oxygen levels are low and more RBCs are needed, the kidneys secrete a hormone called erythropoietin (EPO). This stimulates the bone marrow to produce reticulocytes, which are immature RBCs. Reticulocytes mature to RBCs in 1 to 2 days.

When an RBC is old or damaged, it is destroyed by the spleen. The heme units are broken down by the liver, which recycles or stores the iron. The heme groups are converted to bilirubin, which the liver conjugates into a water-soluble form. Bilirubin is reused in bile or excreted in feces (dark color due to bilirubin). If there is excessive RBC destruction, bilirubin piles up (bilirubinemia) because the liver cannot conjugate all of it and make bile. This causes the bilirubin to leak out into the blood, causing jaundice (yellowing). This is filtered by the kidneys, resulting in bilirubinuria (dark urine). Because the liver is not conjugating bilirubin, bile production decreases, and the color of the feces changes to gray.

Most of the RBC disorders we think about are anemias. All anemias cause a lack of circulating RBCs, which means a lack oxygen to tissues. Think about what a lack of oxygen means as far as clinical manifestations.

Common Clinical Manifestations of Anemia

- Pallor (grayish skin and pale conjunctiva in melanated skin)
- Shortness of breath (lack of oxygen)
- Fatigue (lack of oxygen)
- Weakness (lack of oxygen to muscle)
- Headache (lack of oxygen to brain)
- Palpitations/angina (lack of oxygen to coronary arteries)
- Syncope (fainting)
- Jaundice (increased bilirubin in blood due to RBC destruction)
- Splenomegaly and hepatomegaly (increased rate of RBC destruction)
- Loss of appetite

NOTE

When we talk about cyanosis and pallor, it is important to understand that individuals who are melanated will show cyanosis and pallor differently.

- Skin may be ashen, gray, or yellow in color.
- Conjunctiva may be paler than usual.
- Checking palmar surfaces may also reveal a lighter than usual color.
- Pulse oximetry is also less accurate in people of color. Oximetry readings can be higher than actual oxygenation levels in individuals who are melanated. This may result in delayed treatment and distress for clients.

When we talk of anemias, there are five major anemias (Fig. 5.3):

- Iron-deficiency anemia (microcytic/hypochromic)
- Anemia of chronic disease (normocytic/normochromic)
- Megaloblastic anemia (macrocytic/normochromic)
- Aplastic anemia (normocytic/normochromic)
- Hemolytic anemia

Normocytic and normochromic RBCs are of normal size and normal color. Microcytic RBCs are smaller than normal and macrocytic RBCs are larger than normal. Hypochromic RBCs are paler than normal.

Iron-Deficiency Anemia

The most common type of anemia is iron-deficiency anemia. This occurs because of:

- low iron intake
- blood loss (hemorrhage)
- malabsorption

Iron stores in the liver are slowly depleted, resulting in small, pale RBCs. Iron-deficiency anemia has all the common clinical manifestations of anemia. Some hallmark signs are:

- koilonychia (spoon nails)
- glossitis (inflamed tongue)
- cheilitis (inflamed lips)
- pica (compulsive eating of nonfood)
- cold sensitivity

Labs for iron-deficiency anemia would show low hematocrit, low hemoglobin levels, low iron levels, and low mean corpuscular volume (MCV). Treatment would depend on the underlying cause (low iron, GI bleeding). Iron supplements and transfusions may help address this anemia.

Anemia of Chronic Disease

Anemia of chronic disease is the second most common type of anemia. It is caused by chronic, inflammatory diseases, such as:

- cancer
- autoimmune diseases (e.g., rheumatoid arthritis)
- kidney disease
- chronic liver disease
- coagulation disorders

Inflammation results in increased cytokines, increased phagocyte (macrophage) activation, and iron sequestration,

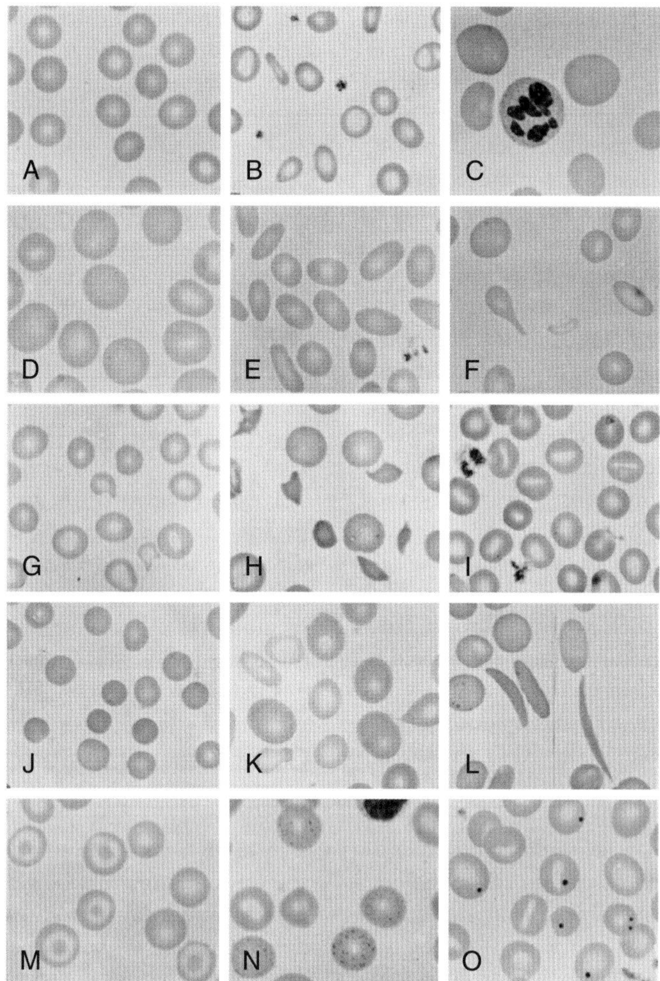

• **Fig. 5.3** A. Normal, B. hypochromic-microcytic, and C. macrocytic anemias. (From Power-Kean, K., Zettel, S., El-Hussein, M. T., Huether, S. E., & McCance, K. L. (2022). *Huether and McCance's understanding pathophysiology, Canadian Edition* (2nd ed.). Elsevier. Fig. 21.2A–C.)

which cause RBCs to be underproduced and have shorter life spans. Serum iron and transferrin levels also drop. RBC production is impaired because of decreased EPO production and decreased bone marrow responsiveness to the hormone. RBCs start out normocytic but can become microcytic. Labs would show low hemoglobin and low hematocrit levels. Clinical manifestations would include underlying disease symptoms and general symptoms of anemia. Treatment may include iron supplementation, EPO, and addressing the underlying disease.

Hemolytic Anemia

Hemolytic anemia is the third most common type of anemia. This type of anemia is caused by premature destruction of RBCs. Extrinsic hemolytic anemia is acquired, meaning that RBCs are destroyed due to outside factors, such as:

- drugs
- toxins
- mechanical injury (artificial heart valves)
- DIC
- renal disease
- immunohemolytic disease
- cancers

Extrinsic hemolytic anemia develops rapidly, and clinical manifestations include the common anemia symptoms, as well as the manifestations of the underlying condition. It can be life threatening. A severe complication would be acute tubular necrosis, as the kidneys become overloaded with bilirubin (hyperbilirubinemia), causing dark urine. Ultimately, acute tubular necrosis can cause kidney cell injury and death. Treatments include addressing the underlying condition, RBC transfusions, immunosuppressants and immunoglobulins, and splenectomy to remove an enlarged spleen.

Intrinsic Hemolytic Anemia

Sickle cell anemia and thalassemia are both considered intrinsic hemolytic anemias. They are both caused by autosomal recessive genetic disorders, which result in abnormal hemoglobin synthesis. Sickle cell disease causes abnormal hemoglobin structures. Thalassemia causes an underproduction of hemoglobin. Both diseases are thought to be adaptations to protect individuals living in endemic regions from malaria.

In the United States, sickle cell anemia is more common than thalassemia, although thalassemia is more common globally. We will focus on sickle cell anemia in this chapter. Although sickle cell anemia is an autosomal recessive disease, individuals with one of the sickle cell alleles are carriers. Sickle cell anemia is endemic in areas such as the Mediterranean, Central America, South America, the Middle East, India, and Africa, not just in people of Aftrican descent! It is an incurable disease and can be fatal, although a complete bone marrow transplant may be able to cure sickle cell disease. However, that is not a viable option for most.

Sickle cell anemia is typically diagnosed in infancy and early childhood. Genetic testing is often done at birth, although it is not a consistent practice. In fact, even though it is a prevalent genetic disorder, less resources are dedicated to it, compared to genetic diseases such as cystic fibrosis. This may be attributed to the fact that it is wrongly considered a "Black disease" and structural racism is at play.

With sickle cell disease, the affected genes produce abnormal hemoglobin (HbS). HbS causes the RBC to stiffen, elongate, and can block blood vessels, causing episodes of hypoxia and pain. These RBCs are fragile and die prematurely. Sickling does not always occur; without it, patients are asymptomatic. However, lack of oxygen, dehydration, infection, stress, fatigue, and exposure to cold can cause RBCs to sickle. The sickling causes the RBCs to stick together and block the blood vessel. This leads to hypoxia and pain in sickle cell crisis. This vaso-occlusive pain can occur anywhere in the body, most often in the back, chest, arms, legs, and abdomen, resulting in pain, swelling, fever, tachypnea, pallor, and jaundice (hemolysis of RBCs). Gradually all body systems are involved (Fig. 5.4). Complications would be:

- pulmonary infarctions
- stroke
- heart failure
- acute chest syndrome
  - most common acute issue
  - caused by fat emboli (released by bone marrow), infection, pulmonary infarct
  - chest pain, dyspnea, wheezing, accessory muscle use, fever
  - most common cause of death
- blindness
- renal failure

Diagnostic labs include peripheral blood smear, sickling test, and skeletal x-rays. Preventative care is important, as individuals with the disease are more prone to illness due to poor circulation. Prophylactic antibiotics (penicillin) between the ages of 2 and 5 years and vaccinations are recommended to prevent infections such as pneumonia. Oxygen, rest, fluid, and pain management are recommended treatments during a sickle cell crisis. Hydroxyurea is a medication that can reduce the frequency of sickle cell crises. Other medications treat the anemia associated with sickle cell disease. Treatments include bone marrow transplants and transfusions.

NOTE

Sickle cell clients often face discrimination when being treated during a crisis, particularly because many people of color have this disease. Often reports of pain are disbelieved, and they are undermedicated or not medicated at all. Remember that hypoxia is extremely painful and, as nurses, we need to listen to our patients.

Megaloblastic Anemia

This type of anemia can be caused by cobalamin (vitamin B_{12}) deficiency or folic acid deficiency. When these deficiencies occur, RBC DNA synthesis is affected, causing the cells to become very large, irregularly shaped and have fragile cell membranes. These membranes break as they squeeze through small vessels, causing RBCs to die prematurely.

Hallmark: large cells, MCV >100 fL

Cobalamin Deficiency

Cobalamin or vitamin B_{12} deficiency is caused by low intake of B_{12}, autoimmune disease, and malabsorption (GI surgery, inflammatory bowel disease). Vitamin B_{12} is found in meats and dairy products, so clients without access to these foods or vegans are at high risk of developing this deficiency. Vitamin B_{12} is absorbed in the stomach. It binds with intrinsic factor, which is secreted by the parietal cells in the stomach. Without parietal cells and intrinsic factor, B_{12} cannot be absorbed. There are autoimmune and congenital diseases where parietal cells and intrinsic factor are affected. This is called pernicious anemia.

Cobalamin deficiency has all the general symptoms of anemia, along with glossitis and cheilitis.

Hallmark symptom: neurological damage. Numbness, tingling, muscle weakness, confusion, depression, and altered mental status are all severe neurological symptoms. If B_{12} deficiency is not corrected, the neurological issues will become permanent.

Folic Acid Deficiency

Folic acid deficiency has a very similar presentation to cobalamin deficiency with large, fragile RBCs. The lack of folic acid causes faulty DNA synthesis and abnormal RBC production. Folic acid is found in cruciferous vegetables and fruits. Causes of folic acid deficiency are:

- malnutrition
- low intake
- alcohol use
- malabsorption
- pregnancy
  - need to supplement

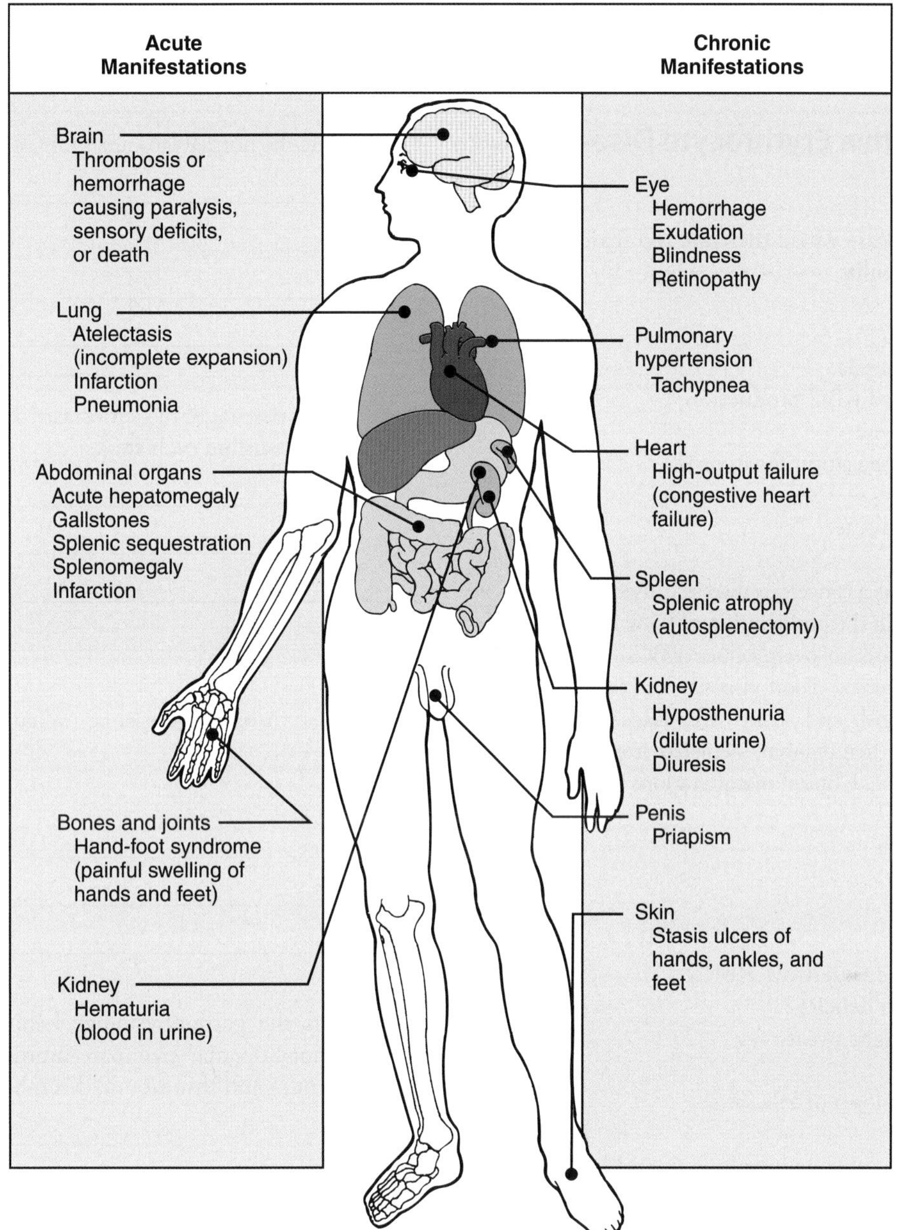

• **Fig. 5.4** Sickle cell disease effects. (From McCance K.L., & Huether S.E. (2019). Pathophysiology (8th ed.). Elsevier.)

- spina bifida may result (incomplete closure of fetal neural tube)

The clinical manifestations are the same as in cobalamin deficiency, except for one important difference—there are no neurological manifestations. Treatment would be to supplement folic acid.

Aplastic Anemia

Aplastic anemia is hypocellular bone marrow → pancytopenia. Pancytopenia is the deficiency or absence of all bone marrow cells—platelets, RBCs, and WBCs. This can happen due to inherited genetic reasons. This is because of a random mutation and seen in children and young adults.

Acquired aplastic anemia is typically due to autoimmune disease. The body's immune system acts against and destroys the bone marrow. This is common in older adults and is acute and severe. Causes include:

- autoimmune disease, such as lupus
- certain drugs and chemicals
- infections, such as HIV
- chemotherapy and radiation
- pregnancy

The first symptoms to manifest are typically due to low platelets (bleeding) and low WBCs (infections). Symptoms of anemia are typically dyspnea and fatigue. Complications can be hemorrhaging, heart failure, sepsis, and acute leukemia. It can be diagnosed by a complete blood count (CBC) and bone marrow biopsy. Treatment is to treat underlying disease and symptoms.

Myeloproliferative Erythrocyte Disorder—Polycythemia

Polycythemia is a disease where there are too many RBCs.

Relative polycythemia:

- Dehydration
- Vomiting/diarrhea

Absolute polycythemia:

- Primary—increased RBC production
  - Polycythemia vera
- Secondary—compensation for hypoxia
  - High altitudes
  - Chronic lung disease
  - Smoking

Polycythemia vera is a cancerous disease caused by a genetic mutation that results in the proliferation of bone marrow cells. The bone marrow starts to overproduce RBCs, WBCs, and platelets. There is increased blood viscosity, causing the blood flow to become sluggish and sticky. This leads to increased hematocrit, increased hemoglobin, depleted iron stores, and increased blood volume. Clinical manifestations include:

- dizziness
- shortness of breath
- hypertension
- headache
- fatigue
- splenomegaly (spleen destroys RBCs)
- hearing and vision deficits
- weight loss and night sweats
- joint pain
- severe itching (buildup of bile salts)
- venous stasis
- dusky extremities, mucous membranes, and lips

Complications include:

- thromboembolism; after platelets are used up, hemorrhage
- peptic ulcer disease
- myelodysplastic syndrome → acute myelogenous leukemia

Polycythemia vera is malignant and incurable. Treatments are supportive to treat symptoms. Phlebotomy, to reduce RBC volume, and hydroxyurea, to suppress bone marrow, are common treatments.

Study Guide for Chapter 5

Make sure that you have your class notes and textbooks on hand to answer these questions. A concept map is included to help you to diagram and link disease concepts together.

1. What roles do the liver, spleen, and kidneys play in hematological disorders?

____

____

____

____

2. What are the normal lab values for CBC and clotting times?

____

____

____

____

3. What are the stages of hemostasis? Describe the components and outline each stage.

____

____

____

____

4. What is thrombocytopenia? What complications can occur?

____

____

____

____

5. What is the pathophysiology behind heparin-induced thrombocytopenia? Compare immune thrombocytopenic purpura and thrombotic thrombocytopenic purpura.

____

____

____

____

6. What causes von Willebrand disease? What are the manifestations and complications?

____

____

____

____

7. What causes hemophilia A? What are the manifestations and complications?

____

____

8. Describe the RBCs of iron-deficiency anemia. What are the major causes and manifestations of iron-deficiency anemia?

9. Describe the RBCs of megaloblastic anemia. What are causes of cobalamin deficiency (B_{12}) and folic acid deficiency? Compare and contrast the manifestations. Who would be at risk for each?

10. What is aplastic anemia? What are the causes?

11. What happens to the RBCs in sickle cell anemia? Why? What complications can occur?

12. Describe what happens in DIC.

13. Describe primary and secondary polycythemia. What are the manifestations/complications of polycythemia vera?

14. How do you assess pallor and skin in people of color?

15. How does darkly pigmented skin affect pulse oximetry?

STUDY TIPS

You may want to try using a T-chart to differentiate between the different thrombocytopenias and different anemias.

	Cobalamin (B_{12}) deficiency anemia	Folic acid deficiency anemia
Cause?		
Pathophysiology?		
Symptoms?		

Concept Map

Use this concept map to link each disease to its pathophysiology, diagnostics, causes, risk factors, complications, and clinical manifestations together. This way, you will be able to see the whole picture of the disease.

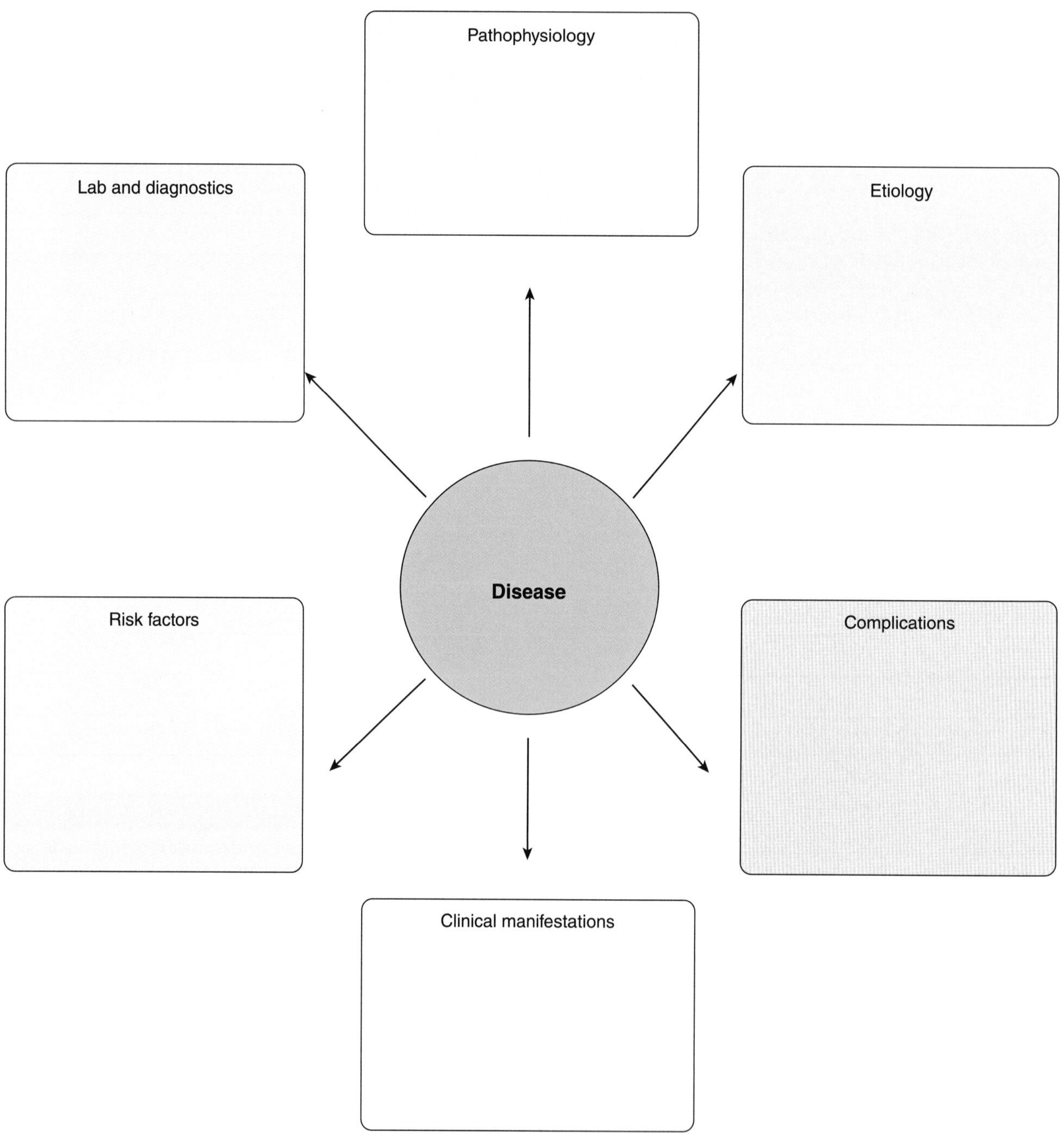

Case Studies for Chapter 5

Make sure you have your class notes and textbooks on hand to answer the questions.

Case Study 5.1

Leo, a 54-year-old Black cis-male (he/him), has come to his provider because he feels weak and dizzy. He tells the nurse that he almost "passed out" when he got up from bed to take a shower. Leo has a past medical history of atrial fibrillation, deep vein thrombosis, and takes medication to prevent clots.

On assessment:

Vital signs	Blood pressure: 88/40; respiratory rate: 24 breaths/minute; heart rate: 110 beats/minute, irregular; oxygen saturation: 94% on room air
Skin	Grayish cast to skin, cool to touch, cap refill >2 seconds
Cardiac	Atrial fibrillation, irregular heartbeat, systolic murmur
Respiratory	Dyspnea on exertion
Gastrointestinal	Regular diet. Loss of appetite. Dark stools noted
Neurological	Alert and oriented x4, fatigued, anxious
Extremities	Cool to touch, dry. 2+ edema noted to right lower extremity. No edema noted on left lower extremity

1. As the nurse, what would you notice about Leo's assessment?

____

____

____

____

2. How would you interpret the assessment? What do you think is the specific cause of Leo's weakness and dizziness?

____

____

____

____

3. What orders would you anticipate from the provider? (Labs)

____

____

____

____

The nurse receives the results of Leo's labs.

Labs	Results
Hgb	9 g/dL
Hct	26%
MCV	70 fL
WBC	11,000
PLT	175,000
RET	1.7%
PT	25 seconds

4. What is Leo's specific diagnosis? Support your answer with the lab results.

____

____

____

____

5. Leo tells the nurse, "I eat lots of protein. Why do I have this condition?" How can the nurse respond?

____

____

____

____

6. The provider orders an endoscopy and a colonoscopy. Why would these be ordered?

____

____

____

____

7. How would Leo's condition be treated?

____

____

____

____

Hct, Hematocrit; *MCV,* mean corpuscular volume; *PLT,* platelets; *PT,* prothrombin time; *RET,* percentage of reticulocytes; *WBC,* white blood cell.

Case Study 5.2

Krishna is a 75-year-old South Asian female (she/her/hers). Her daughter Soma (she/her/hers) brings her to the provider because she is concerned about Krishna's increasing confusion and forgetfulness over the past month. Soma tells the provider that Krishna has not been drinking much fluid and tends to get urinary tract infections. Krishna has a past medical history of hypertension, hyperlipidemia, and is prediabetic. She has adopted a plant-based diet because of this.

On exam, Krishna appears alert and oriented, although she is hard of hearing, has a language barrier, and has difficulty understanding all the questions posed to her. Soma acts as an interpreter for her mother and states that Krishna has no pain or distress, just fatigue and some numbness and tingling to her extremities occasionally. Blood and urine tests are ordered, as well as a chest x-ray and head CT scan.

1. Looking at Krishna's past medical history and her symptoms, what might be some reasons for her confusion?

____

____

____

____

Labs/Imaging	Result
Hgb	7.5 g/dL
Hct	24%
MCV	128 fL
WBC	12 g/dL
Serum glucose	116 mg/dL
UA	Normal, clear, yellow, no bacteria
UC	Pending
Chest x-ray	Normal
Head CT	Normal

2. Looking at the results, what do you think the diagnosis of the patient is? Support your answer with the lab results.

____

____

____

____

3. Soma is surprised by the results and says to the nurse, "I really don't understand how my mom has this disorder. She has never had this before. What could this come from?" What are three questions the nurse can ask to find out possible causes of this disorder?

____

____

____

____

4. Krishna wants to know more about her condition and how to treat it. As the nurse, how would you explain things so that Krishna is able to understand?

____

____

____

____

CT, Computed tomography; *Hct,* hematocrit; *Hgb,* hemoglobin; *MCV,* mean corpuscular volume; *UA,* urinary albumin; *UC,* urinary creatinine; *WBC,* white blood cell.

Case Study 5.3

Bella is a 1-year-old Brazilian child (she/her) transported by ambulance to the emergency room for seizures and difficulty breathing. Her parents, who have recently emigrated from Brazil, have accompanied her, and a Portuguese interpreter is on hand to translate. After Bella is stabilized and tests are run, the provider lets the parents know that she had a stroke, which was caused by sickle cell anemia. Neither of her parents have the disease.

1. As the interpreter translates, Bella's father starts to cry. He tells the interpreter that he and her mother don't have the disease and does not understand how Bella has this disease. He asks how she got sickle cell disease (SCD) and says that this disease only happened to people of African descent. How would you address his question?

____

____

____

____

2. Explain the pathophysiology behind SCD and the conditions that would cause red blood cells to change shape.

____

____

____

____

3. Is sickling permanent? Which symptoms occur with sickling episodes?

____

____

____

____

4. How is this disease treated?

5. Bella's parents tell the nurse (through the translator) that they recently moved from Brazil, they do not have family or friends locally, and that they do not have a lot of resources. How can this impact Bella's care? How can the nurse intervene?

Case Study 5.4

Vicky is a 32-year-old White cis-female (she/her) who comes to the clinic because she is having frequent nosebleeds, easy bruising, and petechiae on both lower extremities. Her vital signs are within normal limits; she has no complaints or pain, dyspnea, or any other discomfort. She states that she had a bad viral infection a few weeks earlier. The provider orders a complete blood count (CBC).

Labs	Result
Hgb	13 g/dL
Hct	36%
MCV	90 fL
WBC	11,000
PLT	70,000
RET	1.7%
PT	20 seconds

Hct, Hematocrit; *Hgb,* hemoglobin; *MCV,* mean corpuscular volume; *PLT,* platelets; *PT,* prothrombin time; *RET,* percentage of reticulocytes; *WBC,* white blood cell.

1. What do you notice about Vicky's symptoms and how they correspond to her labs?

2. The provider orders an antiplatelet antibody test, which comes back as abnormal. What diagnosis would you infer from these data? Explain the pathophysiology.

3. Would you treat this disorder? Why or why not?

4. Is this an acute or chronic issue? What complications could result?

6

Cardiac Disease Part 1

Cardiac disorders are sometimes intimidating to nursing students. The cardiac system often seems very mysterious and complicated to students, but when you break it down, the system is not as complex as it may seem at first. Before starting this chapter, there are two things that you need to do. First, you must review the anatomy and physiology of the heart. You will not be able to understand the disorders without understanding how the heart works. Second, make sure that you have a good grasp of the material in the preceding chapters. Fluid and electrolytes, renal, and hematology all have a lot to do with the cardiac system. You'll see, there's a method to the madness!

Review

- Structure of the heart (Fig. 6.1)
- Heart valves
- Cardiac cycle
- Coronary arteries
  - Remember that the coronary arteries feed the heart during diastole (ventricles are resting/filling). This is because during systole (ventricles contracting) arteries are constricted and the aortic valves are open, transporting blood to the rest of the body.
  - With myocardial infarction (MI) (heart attack), it is the coronary arteries that are occluded.
- Electrical activity of the heart (myocytes can produce and transmit electrical impulses)
  - Heart conduction system
    - Sinoatrial node (SA node): pacemaker of heart
    - Atrioventricular node (AV node)
    - Bundle of His
    - Left and right bundle branches
    - Purkinje fibers
  - Contraction of the heart—depolarization and repolarization of myocardium (cardiac muscle)
    - The inside of a myocyte (cardiac muscle cell) is negatively charged compared to the outside of the cells. Cellular pumps, such as the sodium/potassium pump, maintain this gradient.
    - Myocytes can independently:
      - produce electrical stimuli (automaticity)
      - respond to electrical stimuli (excitability)
      - transmit electrical stimuli (conductivity)
      - contract with electrical stimuli (contractility)
    - With electrical stimulus that causes depolarization, the sodium and voltage-gated calcium channels open and let positive ions into the cell, causing depolarization → action potential
    - When a certain charge is reached, the channels close and repolarization begins; active transport pumps remove sodium and calcium from inside the cell and potassium diffuses out, restoring the negative charge.
    - There is a refractory period afterwards as the cell restores its resting potential.
    - Electrocardiograms (ECGs) measure this electrical activity.
  - Preload—amount of blood in ventriclesat the end of disatole
  - Afterload—the resistance that the left ventricle must overcome to push blood into the aorta and to the rest of the body
  - Peripheral vascular resistance - measures how hard it is for blood to flow through peripheral blood vessels (the more they are vasoconstricted, the higher the resistance)

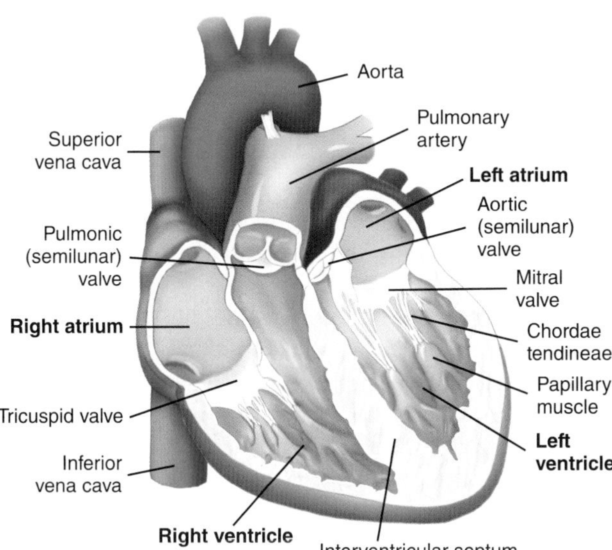

• **Fig. 6.1** Structures of the heart. (From Harding, M. M., Kwong, J., Hagler, D., & Reinisch, C. (2022). *Lewis's medical-surgical nursing: Assessment and management of clinical problems* (12th ed.). Elsevier. Fig. 35.2.)

Atherosclerosis

The biggest culprit in cardiac disease is atherosclerosis. Atherosclerosis is an inflammatory disease caused by hyperlipidemia (fats) and fibrin (scar tissue) in blood vessels throughout the body, causing these vessels to harden and narrow.

Hyperlipidemia is a major risk factor in cardiovascular disease. Genetics, lifestyle, diet, medications, and social determinants of health and equity influence this condition.

- Low-density lipoprotein (LDL)—carries cholesterol to the cells/tissues—bad
- Very-low-density lipoprotein (VLDL)—carries triglycerides and suppresses plasmin—bad
- High-density lipoprotein (HDL) carries cholesterol from the cells/tissues to the liver to be excreted in bile—good

LDL carries cholesterol and plays a huge role in damaging the endothelium (inner lining of vessels) and provoking inflammatory and immune responses (Fig. 6.2). It is also the main building block of the atherosclerotic plaques described below.

NOTE

Atherosclerosis is an inflammatory and immune response to blood vessel damage. It can take place in vessels at any place throughout the body (brain, extremities, gastrointestinal tract, lungs) not just the heart!

- Endothelial injury
- Increase in vessel permeability
- Inflammation and migration of monocytes and platelets
- Excess of LDL infiltrates the intima (inner lining of vessel)
- T-lymphocytes and macrophages infiltrate the intima (immune response)
- Macrophages release toxic oxygen radicals, which oxidize LDL
- Macrophages engulf oxidized LDL and become foam cells
- As foam cells accumulate and die, they become fatty streaks and form lipid cores
- Smooth muscle cells accumulate over the fatty necrosed lipid core and form a cap
- An atheroma or a plaque is formed

Plaques are raised, grayish-white, and they protrude into the lumen and can obstruct the blood vessel. Depending on the size of the lipid core and the thickness of the cap, the plaques can be either a stable lesion (small core and/or thick cap) or an unstable lesion (large core and/or thin cap). Unstable lesions will continue to grow and can eventually rupture, which will result in a clot formation, occluding the vessel more and more, causing ischemia, pain, and turbulent blood flow.

Peripheral Arterial Disease

Peripheral arterial disease (PAD) is caused by atherosclerosis to the extremities, typically the legs. Remember, atherosclerosis can affect arterial vessels anywhere in the body. Atherosclerotic plaques can occlude vessels in the extremities, causing pain and tissue ischemia (remember- hypoxia causes pain!). The risk factors for PAD are the same as for atherosclerosis; however, diabetes and smoking are the two biggest risk factors. PAD develops gradually, which makes sense as atherosclerotic plaques develop gradually.

Symptoms are the "6Ps"

- Pain
- Pallor
- Pulselessness
- Paresthesia (numbness and tingling)
- Paralysis
- Poikilothermy (coolness)

Clients experience intermittent claudication, or pain with activity/movement. Circulation is affected, so you will see dependent rubor. This is when gravity causes blood to rush to the extremity when arms or legs are down. Gravity helps blood circulate through the extremity. When arms/legs are raised, the client experiences hypoxia and pain. Affected extremities are usually thin, shiny, hairless, with muscle atrophy. Arterial ulcers, small, often gangrenous, can develop on the ankle and toes. Treatment includes exercise until claudication (pain), anticoagulants, and surgery to remove the plaques or bypass the occluded vessels.

Aneurysm

Aneurysms are caused by a weakening of vessel or heart chamber walls.

This weakening can be caused by:

- atherosclerosis
- hypertension
- smoking
- infections
- trauma
- connective tissue disorders

Aneurysms can happen anywhere in the body. The most common aneurysm is an aortic aneurysm, specifically an abdominal aortic aneurysm (AAA) (Fig. 6.3).

Aortic aneurysms:

- Usually asymptomatic
- Location and size determine symptoms
- Surgery to repair once aneurysm is greater than 5 cm

AAA:

- Most common
- Over 50 years of age
- Pulsating abdominal mass is the first sign
- An abdominal bruit can be auscultated and thrill can be palpated (felt)
- Dull lower back and scapular pain

Aortic dissection (false aneurysm):

Aortic dissections are not aneurysms but are a degeneration and "ripping" of the medial layer of the vessel. This causes hemorrhaging into the blood vessel, and depending on where the aneurysm is and interventions, circulatory shock can occur.

Risk factors:

- Hypertension
- Assigned male at birth
- Age 40 to 60 years

Symptoms:

- Ripping sensation in abdomen and back
- Cool, pulseless extremities

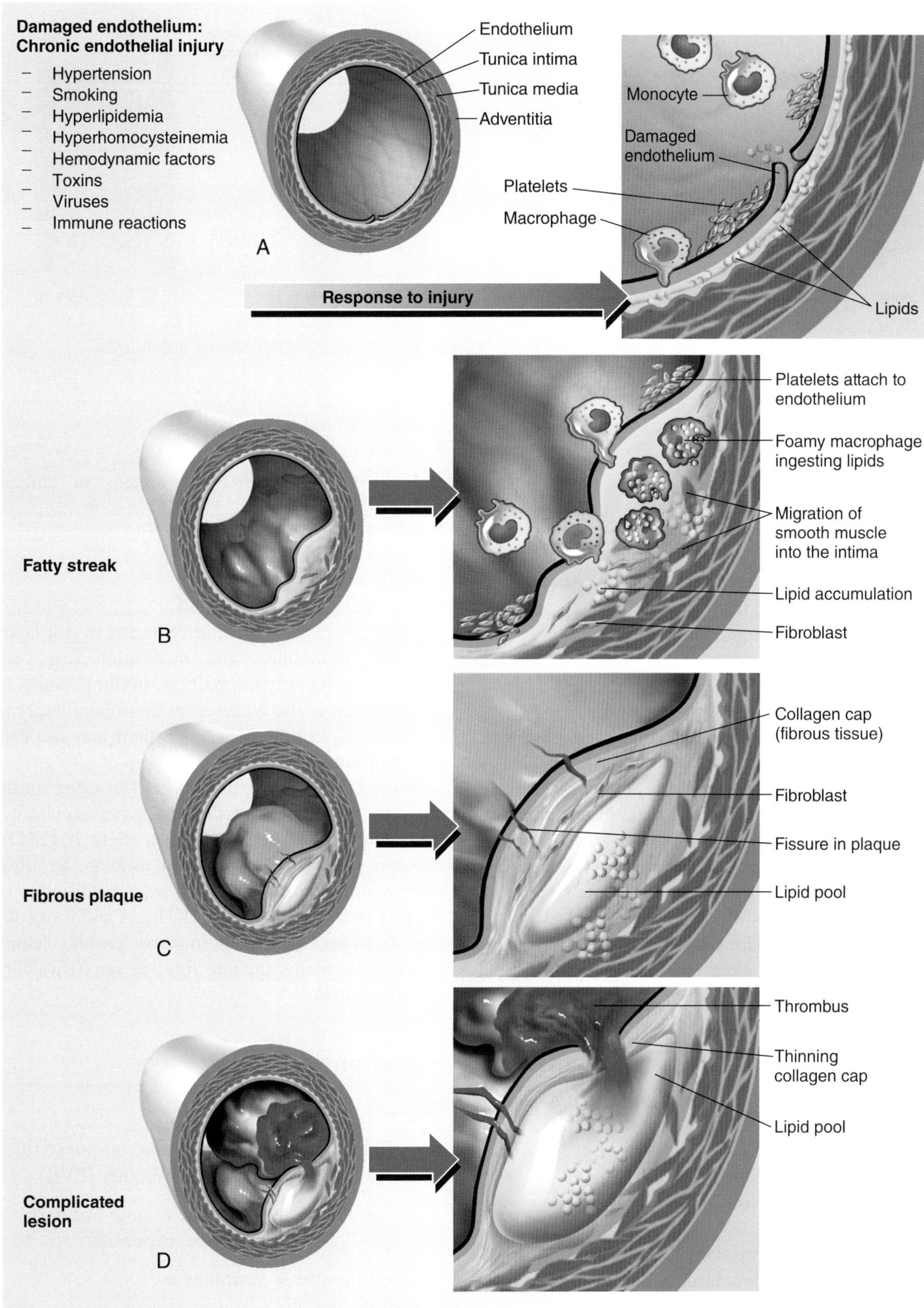

• **Fig. 6.2** (A, B, C, D) Development of atherosclerosis. (From Huether, S., & McCance, K. (2019). Understanding Pathophysiology (7th ed.). p. 600 [Figure 26.7]. Elsevier.)

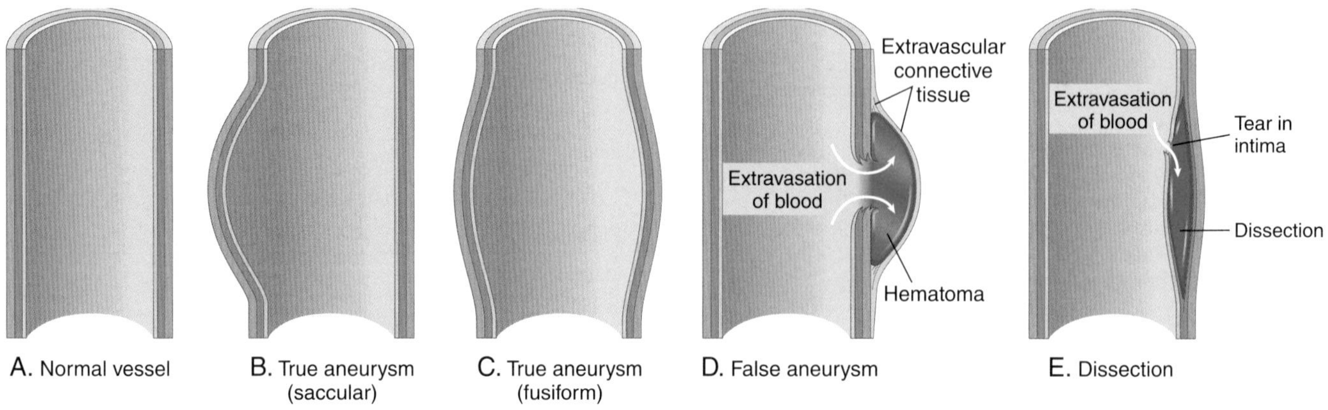

• **Fig. 6.3** Types of aneurysms. (From Kumar, V., Abbas, A.K., & Aster, J.C. (2021). Robbins and Cotran pathologic basis of disease (10th ed.), Elsevier.)

- Blood pressure differences between right and left side
- Hypotension
- Neurologic deficits, paralysis
- Decreased urine flow

Aneurysms can be detected by ultrasound, magnetic resonance imaging (MRI), computed tomography (CT) scan, and angiography. Often, an aneurysm is an incidental finding. Treatment could range from lifestyle changes (small, asymptomatic) to surgery (large, symptomatic).

Chronic Venous Insufficiency

Chronic venous insufficiency occurs when there is an obstruction to moving blood from the veins back to the heart. Veins are larger and more elastic, so blood can pool easily in the veins. Blood typically moves back by skeletal muscle pumps (movement). The valves in the veins prevent the blood from flowing back. If the valves are damaged and/or the client is immobile, blood will tend to pool in dependent areas, such as the legs. These are the clients with large edematous legs, with dark, brawny looking skin. With venous insufficiency, there is a lack of circulation, blood pooling, and red blood cell (RBC) death. This also increases the probability of clots forming, or deep vein thrombosis (DVT).

Signs and symptoms:

- Edema (can be weeping)
- Hyperpigmentation (dark, brawny color from dead RBCs and iron [hemosiderin])
- Necrotic tissue
- Dry, red, flaky skin (stasis dermatitis)
- Large, wet ulcers on medial and distal lower legs, typically painless

Treatments involve compression, Unna boots, and skin grafts. Ulcers can be very slow healing due to the lack of circulation.

Deep Vein Thrombosis

As said before, chronic venous insufficiency can lead to formation of thrombi, or a DVT. The triad of Virchow is a tool to assess risk for developing thrombi.

Triad of Virchow

- Injury to blood vessel
  - Atherosclerotic plaques
  - Trauma, toxins
- Abnormalities of blood flow
  - Turbulence
  - Stasis
- Hypercoagulability of blood

With DVTs, clots form in veins due to risk factors such as stasis, immobility, and medication (e.g., estrogen). Clients may report pain, redness, swelling, and warmth in the affected leg. This is caused by the inflammatory response of the vessel wall. However, the client may not experience any symptoms at all.

With DVTs, prevention is key, meaning ambulation, adequate hydration, and alternating pressure boots for clients who are bedridden. When a client has a DVT, the opposite is true. It is important to keep the affected extremity immobile. You do not want to dislodge the clot, because it can travel back to the heart and lungs and cause complications such as pulmonary emboli (clot in the lungs). Treatments include inferior vena cava filters and anticoagulants.

Hypertension

Formulas to know:

Blood pressure (BP) = cardiac output (CO) × peripheral vascular resistance (PVR)

Cardiac output = stroke volume (mL/beat) × heart rate (beats/minute)

Blood pressure is controlled by:

- intrinsic receptors
  - osmoreceptors
  - baroreceptors
  - chemoreceptors
- nervous system
  - parasympathetic
    - acetylcholine

- decreased heart rate, vasodilation, bronchoconstriction
- sympathetic
  - catecholamines (epi and norepinephrine)
  - increased heart rate, vasoconstriction, bronchodilation
- hormonal (short term)
  - renin-angiotensin-aldosterone system (RAAS)
    - causes vasoconstriction, sodium reabsorption, water reabsorption, thirst, triggers sympathetic response
  - vasopressin (antidiuretic hormone)
    - vasoconstriction
    - causes kidneys to conserve water only (not sodium)
- kidneys (long term)
  - RAAS
    - retention of water and sodium, vasoconstriction, increases BP
  - natriuretic peptides—atrial natriuretic peptide and B-type natriuretic peptide
    - diuresis of sodium and water, decreases BP

Diagnosing of Hypertension

The American Heart Association guidelines for the diagnosis of hypertension are shown are Table 6.1.

Hypertension is not diagnosed with just one visit. Typically, high readings after two or three visits would result in a diagnosis of hypertension. Blood pressure should be taken when:

- the client has rested for 5 to 10 minutes
- the client has not smoked or had a caffeinated beverage or food item within 30 minutes
- the client is sitting, and arms are at heart level and relaxed

White coat syndrome, or increased blood pressure while at the provider's office, is a common issue. To address this, providers often have clients take their blood pressure at home and record the readings.

Primary hypertension is the most common (90%–95% of cases). This means that an external condition or disease has not caused the hypertension. Nonmodifiable risk factors are:

- genetics
- age
- social determinants of health
  - toxic stress
  - gender-affirming therapy—testosterone
- insulin resistance

Modifiable risk factors are:

- high salt intake
- obesity
- alcohol use
- smoking

Secondary hypertension (5%–10% of cases) is caused by a different primary condition or disease.

- Renal disease—increases RAAS, fluid retention
- Endocrine disease—increased aldosterone (Na/fluid retention) or increased glucocorticoids
- Pheochromocytoma—tumor-secreting catecholamines
- Coarctation of the aorta—increased afterload
- Drugs—decongestants, contraceptives, cocaine, testosterone

TABLE 6.1 Diagnosis of Hypertension[a]

Category	Systolic	Diastolic
Normal	<120	<80
Elevated	120–129	<80
Stage 1 hypertension	130–139	80–89
Stage 2 hypertension	≥140	≥90
Hypertensive crisis	>180	>120

[a]You must know these values and check the American Heart Association website regularly for updates. https://www.ahajournals.org/doi/10.1161/HYPERTENSIONAHA.120.15026.

NOTE

Hypertension is not dependent on race and different medications and treatments should not be given to clients because of race! In fact, heart disease in clients of color is diagnosed at a much later stage than for White clients and treatments are also often not as aggressive as those given to White clients. Please be aware of this in your practice and speak up!

Hypertension can be asymptomatic. However, the danger of hypertension is the damage it causes to vital target organs.

- Heart—left ventricular hypertrophy (due to increased afterload) → heart failure, arrhythmias, cardiac arrest
- Blood vessels— chronically elevated pressure → causes increased arterial stretch → aneurysms, atherosclerosis, coronary artery disease (CAD)
- Kidney—scarring and damage to small vessels → nephrosclerosis → diabetic nephropathy
- Brain—scarring and damage to vessels leads to:
  - stroke—hemorrhagic and ischemic
  - hypertensive encephalopathy
  - vascular dementia
  - hypertensive retinopathy → blindness

A severe complication that can develop from secondary hypertension, or more commonly, non-adherence to blood pressure-reducing medication, is hypertensive crisis. This is when a client's systolic blood pressure is 180 mm Hg or over and/or the diastolic blood pressure is 120 mm Hg or over. When a client has blood pressure in this range without symptoms, it is called hypertensive urgency. Hypertensive emergency is when the client not only has blood pressures in this range, but also displays target organ damage, such as hypertensive encephalopathy (severe headache, confusion, visual disturbances, seizures), heart failure, or renal failure (increasing creatinine and decreasing glomerular filtration levels).

As clients age, they are more prone to hypertension. More than 75% of clients 70 years of age and older have hypertension.

This can be due to several issues. The myocardium and blood vessel walls stiffen and increase resistance; the left ventricle can hypertrophy due to the increased resistance; and baroreceptors, osmoreceptors, and chemoreceptors are not as sensitive. Catecholamine receptors lose sensitivity as well. All of this can lead to orthostatic hypotension.

Coronary Artery Disease

With CAD, atherosclerosis is the biggest risk factor. The other modifiable and nonmodifiable risk factors are the same as those discussed for atherosclerosis and hypertension.

> **NOTE**
>
> For transgender individuals undergoing estrogen therapy, there is an increased risk of unhealthy weight and hyperlipidemia, both of which lead to atherosclerosis and coronary artery disease (CAD).
>
> Social determinants of health play a huge role in the CAD disease progression. Within marginalized populations, psychological stressors can lead to unhealthy habits, such as smoking. Socioeconomic status is directly correlated with diet, access to green spaces, and ability to exercise. All these factors can lead to type 2 diabetes mellitus, hypertension, hyperlipidemia, and obesity, which ultimately result in CAD.

Atherosclerotic lesions are found in the coronary arteries, the blood vessels that feed the heart. The right coronary artery, the left anterior descending artery (LAD), and the left circumflex artery are the arteries typically affected in CAD. The LAD is known as the "widowmaker," because it perfuses the left ventricle and septum. An occlusion here can have a bad outcome.

As you know, atherosclerosis causes lesions that can occlude the coronary artery. If the lesion is small, with a thick cap and a small core, it is called a stable lesion. With this kind of lesion, clients are only symptomatic during exertion. The lesion is small and stable; at rest, cardiac function is fine. However, once the client starts to exert themselves, they will start to feel chest pain, or angina, as they are not getting enough blood through the coronary artery to perfuse the heart. A stable lesion causes chronic ischemic heart disease. The stable angina goes away with rest or nitroglycerin.

Angina is the chest pain that occurs when the heart is not being perfused. The pain can be substernal or epigastric and often radiates to the jaw or shoulders. Shortness of breath, skin color change, anxiety, diaphoresis, and nausea often accompany angina. You must keep in mind that clients who are assigned female at birth, older age, or immunocompromised may have different symptoms such as indigestion; fatigue or no symptoms at all; called silent ischemia.

If the lesion is large, with a thin cap and a large core, it will rupture and create a large clot that can partially or completely occlude the vessel. This is called an unstable lesion. With an unstable lesion, the client may feel angina at rest because the occlusion is so large. This type of angina is called unstable angina. This can then progress to a non–ST-elevation myocardial infarction (NSTEMI) or an ST-elevation myocardial infarction (STEMI). It is important to note that a STEMI can occur without any warning and not be preceded by stable or unstable angina.

It's best to think about CAD as a progressive disease. Chronic ischemic heart disease evolves to become acute coronary syndrome (unstable angina, NSTEMI, STEMI).

Chronic ischemic heart disease → unstable angina → myocardial infarction

How will you know if the client has acute coronary syndrome? You would look at the client's ECG and their serum biomarkers. The client would experience unstable angina and ECG changes, such as T-wave inversion, ST-segment depression, ST-segment elevation, and pathological (deep) Q waves.

But you need to distinguish between unstable angina and an MI. That's where serum biomarkers come in. Serum biomarkers are proteins that are released during the death of the myocardial tissue. These proteins then diffuse into the blood, and we can measure them to see if an MI has occurred. Creatinine kinase-MB and troponin (I and T) are the serum biomarkers that are specific to the cardiac muscle. Of these two, elevated troponin levels are the gold standards to indicate that an MI has occurred.

An MI can result from either a partially occluded coronary vessel (NSTEMI) or a fully occluded coronary vessel (STEMI). With an MI, a client can experience crushing chest pain, anxiety and a feeling of doom, weakness, shortness of breath, and nausea and vomiting. Clients with diabetes may not experience pain due to neuropathy. Older clients and assigned females at birth may experience weakness and fatigue as their main symptoms. When a client is experiencing an MI, the critical priority is reperfusion. An MI causes loss of contractile functions and may lead to severe arrhythmias, which affect circulation. The longer the heart is not perfused, the greater is the damage to the myocardium. Once treated, the myocardium does heal; however, the damaged and scarred area will not be able to contract and relax normally, which can cause complications such as arrhythmias and heart failure.

Study Guide for Chapter 6

Make sure that you have your class notes and textbooks on hand to answer these questions.

1. What is the relationship between blood volume and blood pressure in the circulatory system?

____

____

____

____

2. Define the term *hemodynamics* and describe the effects of blood pressure (afterload, preload, stroke volume, cardiac output).

____

____

____

____

3. Explain how cardiac output and peripheral vascular resistance interact in determining systolic and diastolic blood pressure.

4. Describe the role of the autonomic nervous system (ANS) in the control of circulatory function. How does the ANS help regulate our blood pressure?

5. Describe the neural, humoral, and renal mechanisms for short-term and long-term regulation of blood pressure.

6. What is the definition of hypertension? Differentiate between primary and secondary forms of hypertension. What target organs are affected in hypertension? How?

7. What is the difference between hypertensive urgency and emergency?

8. Define the term orthostatic hypotension. Explain how fluid deficit, medications, aging, disorders of the ANS, and bed rest contribute to the development of orthostatic hypotension.

9. Characterize the pathology of venous insufficiency. How does venous insufficiency relate to the development of stasis dermatitis and venous ulcers?

10. What risk factors are associated with venous thrombosis and what are its manifestations? What is the importance of Virchow triad?

11. Describe blood flow in the coronary circulation and relate it to the metabolic needs of the heart.

12. List the types of lipoproteins and state their function in terms of lipid transport and development of atherosclerosis.

13. What are the risk factors for atherosclerosis?

14. How does atherosclerosis develop? Describe the process.

15. What are the differences in pathology between fixed atherosclerotic lesions, unstable plaque, and thrombosis with obstruction?

16. How would you distinguish among the following acute coronary syndromes: unstable angina/NSTEMI and STEMI in terms of pathology, symptomatology, ECG changes, and serum cardiac markers?

17. State the signs and symptoms of acute arterial occlusion. How does PAD develop? What are the risk factors? What are the clinical manifestations?

18. Why do aortic aneurysms occur? Discuss the clinical manifestations.

STUDY TIP

Make T-charts for groups of diseases.
Example:

	Chronic venous insufficiency	Peripheral arterial disease
Cause?		
Pathophysiology?		
Symptoms?		

Concept Map

Use this concept map to link each disease to its pathophysiology, diagnostics, causes, risk factors, complications, and clinical manifestations together. This way, you will be able to see the whole picture of the disease.

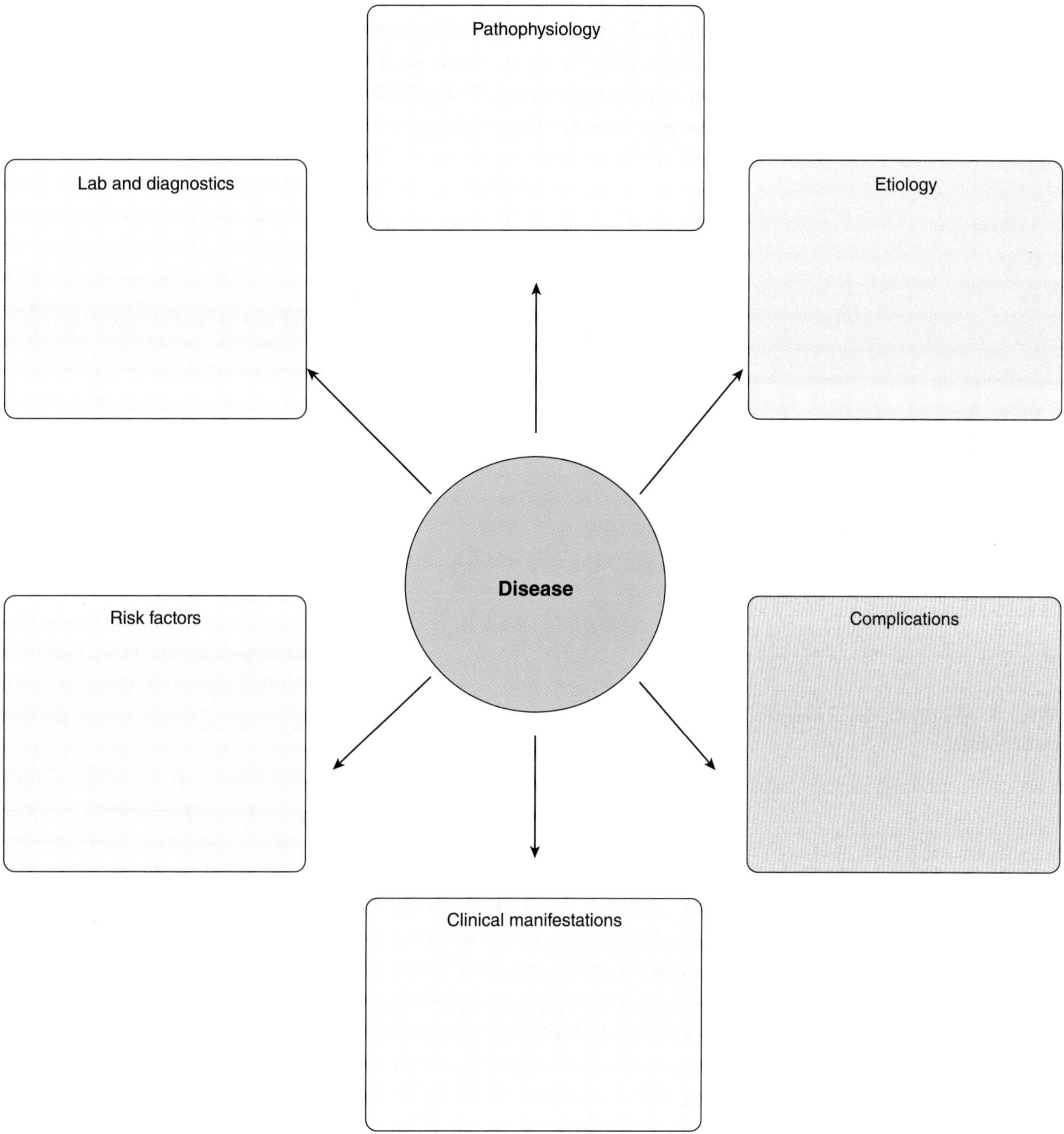

Case Studies for Chapter 6

Make sure you have your class notes and textbooks on hand to answer the questions. A concept map is included to help you to diagram and link disease concepts together.

Case Study 6.1

Myra is a 75-year-old Latinx trans-female (she/her). She is overweight and has a history of hypertension and hyperlipidemia. She has been prescribed medications for her hypertension and hyperlipidemia, but states that she often forgets to take them. She has come to the urgent care clinic because of a persistent, worsening headache and blurry vision.

On assessment:

Blood pressure	200/140 mm Hg
Respiratory rate	26 breaths/minute
Pulse	110 beats/minute
Oxygen saturation	95%
Height	5′2″
Weight	175 pounds

1. Looking at Myra's history and assessment, what are you concerned about?

2. What do you think Myra's diagnosis is? What could have caused this?

3. What complications could result from this?

4. What would you want to discuss with Myra? What may some of her barriers be?

Myra returns 6 weeks later for follow-up. She has started to take her medications more regularly, but states that she feels occasional chest pressure with exertion, which resolves with rest.

5. What do you think Myra's condition has evolved into? What would you relate this to Question 2? Explain the pathophysiology?

6. What tests would you run to confirm the diagnosis?

Four months later, you see Myra brought by ambulance to the emergency room with crushing chest pain, nausea, and diaphoresis.

7. What would you diagnose her with now? How is this different from Question 5?

8. What lab tests would confirm this?

9. What is the priority?

10. What complications would you see?

Case Study 6.2

A 62-year-old Asian cis-male (he/him) has been brought to the emergency room with severe lower back pain radiating to the abdomen. He tells the provider and the nurse that he felt a sudden "ripping pain" in his lower back and rated the pain 10/10.

On assessment, the nurse finds the client's blood pressure to be 80/42 mm Hg on the left and 146/70 mm Hg on the right. The client's lower extremities are cool to touch, and pedal pulses are absent.

1. What do you think is happening to the patient? Explain your diagnosis.

2. Why are the blood pressures in both arms different? Why are the extremities cool to touch?

The client is scheduled for an emergent computed tomography (CT) scan. Prior to this, the nurse notices that he is becoming more confused and lethargic.

3. Why do you think these symptoms are occurring?

4. How would you treat this condition?

Case Study 6.3

A 49-year-old client (they/them) has just gotten off a plane, after a 10-hour flight. When the client gets home, they feel some pain in their right calf. They go to the urgent care clinic to have the pain checked. An ultrasound is done, and the client is found to have a deep vein thrombosis (DVT) in the right calf.

1. What may have caused the DVT to occur? Explain the pathophysiology.

2. Could the DVT have been prevented? How?

3. How would you explain the condition and treatment to the client?

The client is sent home on anticoagulant therapy. A few days later, they are brought to the emergency room with severe shortness of breath, anxiety, and tachycardia.

4. What do you think the client's diagnosis is now? Explain.

Case Study 6.4

A nursing student (he/him) comes into the room to assess a client. He finds the client sitting on the edge of the bed, with feet dangling over the edge. When the student tries to get the client back into bed, the client gets agitated and angry and states that it is too uncomfortable to get back in bed. The student notices that the client's legs are thin, shiny, and dark red.

1. What would you diagnose the patient with? Explain the pathophysiology.

2. What are some risk factors causing this condition?

3. What complications could you expect with this client?

Case Study 6.5

A 70-year-old Latinx cis-female (she/her) comes to the urgent care clinic with complaints of lower back and abdominal pain. You are her nurse. As you assess her pain, you notice that she has a quivering abdominal mass.

1. How would you assess the mass? What findings would you expect?

2. What would you diagnose this client with? Is this an emergent condition? Why?

7 Cardiac Disease Part 2

In this chapter, we will be talking about pericarditis, endocardial and valvular disorders, cardiomyopathy, and heart failure. Remember that cardiac diseases are on a continuum. If these diseases progress, heart failure will result.

Pericarditis

Pericarditis is an inflammation of the pericardium caused by cancer, infection, kidney disease, radiation, trauma, COVID-19, and myocardial infarction (MI).

- Serous (pericardial effusion) or fibrinous (sticky, scar tissue) exudate can fill the pericardial space.
- This can constrict the heart and restrict the movement, affecting cardiac output, leading to obstructive shock.
- Dressler syndrome
  - Autoimmune inflammation of pericarditis a few weeks after MI
  - Immunosuppressants
- Symptoms
  - Stabbing chest pain, worse with deep breath, coughing, and lying down
  - Low-grade fever
  - Restrictive pericarditis → friction rub
  - Feel better sitting up and leaning forward
  - Can lead to pericardial effusion
- Pericardial effusion consequences
  - Pulsus paradoxus
  - Jugular distension
  - Decreased cardiac output and heart failure
  - Cardiac tamponade (if rapid exudate buildup)
- Cardiac tamponade—rapid accumulation of exudate
  - Beck triad—caused by exudate
    - Hypotension → decreased cardiac output
    - Muffled heart sounds → due to fluid
    - Jugular venous distension → backup of blood
  - Medical emergency—surgical decompression

Endocardial Disorders

Infective Endocarditis

Infective endocarditis occurs when a pathogen is introduced directly into the bloodstream. Some of the causes of this disorder are Staphylococcus infections, peripherally inserted central catheter (PICC) lines, central lines, intravenous (IV) drug use, and periodontal disease. Patients who are immunodeficient (e.g., HIV/AIDS, diabetes mellitus, and alcohol use disorder) may also suffer from this disorder. Endocarditis can also become chronic, causing destruction and dysfunction of heart valves.

- Bacteria travel to the heart and form loose, bulky vegetative lesions on the valves.
- These lesions are made up of bacteria, fibrin, platelets, antibodies, and other cell debris.
- These lesions can break off, sending bacteria through the bloodstream.
- These lesions can form emboli and occlude blood vessels.
- Acute endocarditis—fever, chills, night sweats, arthralgia, fatigue
- Chronic endocarditis—dyspnea, cough, edema, emboli, petechiae, murmurs, arrhythmias.
- Interventions—blood culture, antibiotics, echocardiogram, valve replacement

Rheumatic Heart Disease

Rheumatic heart disease is caused by an untreated strep infection. The strep infection then develops into rheumatic fever, which is a systemic, inflammatory, immune-mediated disease. Children (5–15 years old) are typically affected.

Symptoms are systemic: fever, polyarthritis, erythema marginatum, and chorea.

The body's immune system eventually attacks the endocardium, as it mistakes the heart's antigens for the pathogen (molecular mimicry). This is now rheumatic heart disease (Fig. 7.1).

- The initial endocardial lesion is called an Aschoff body.
- This can cause the valves to dysfunction, and vegetative lesions to form.
- The autoimmune response affects all layers of the heart, causing pancarditis.
- Murmurs, arrhythmias (any change in the heart can result in arrhythmias), and pericardial friction rub can occur.

Like infective endocarditis, rheumatic heart disease can become chronic and cause permanent deformity of valves.

- Interventions
  - Strep culture, antibiotics, erythrocyte sedimentation rate, electrocardiogram (ECG)

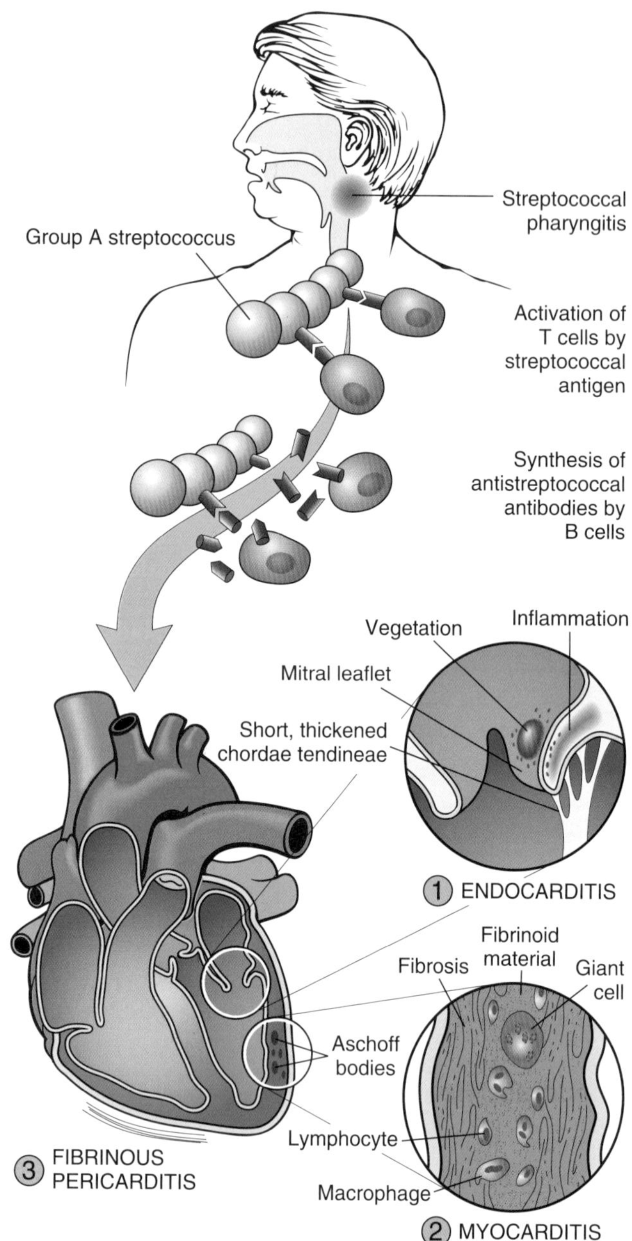

• **Fig. 7.1** Acute rheumatic heart disease. (From Damjanov, I. (2012). Pathology for the health professions (4th ed.). Saunders.)

- Steroids and nonsteroidal anti-inflammatory drugs (NSAIDs) for inflammation
- Valve replacement

Valvular Disorders

When valves are stenotic or regurgitant, the heart must work harder to compensate (Fig. 7.2). Concentric hypertrophy increases myocytes and other support cells, thickening the ventricle and causing a more forceful contraction. This is commonly seen in the left ventricle, as it works harder against resistance to push blood into the aorta. This can also be seen in the right ventricle when there is pulmonary hypertension, and the right ventricle must push harder to get blood into the pulmonary artery. Eccentric hypertrophy is an elongation, or "stretching out" of the myocardium, typically affecting the ventricles. This occurs when there is volume overload. The ventricular wall becomes stressed and is thinner and weaker, unable to contract well.

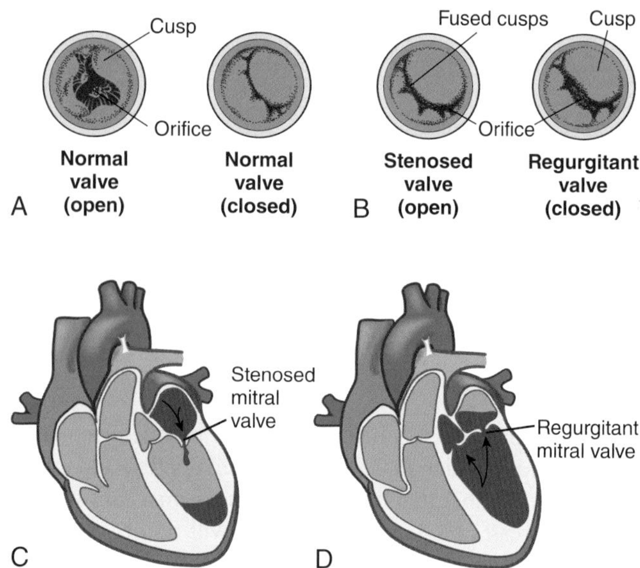

• **Fig. 7.2** Valvular stenosis and regurgitation. (McCance K.L., & Huether S.E. (2018). Pathophysiology: the biologic basis for disease in adults and children. Elsevier Health Sciences.)

Compensation, although effective at first, ends up increasing myocardial oxygen demand and myocardial ischemia. Eventually, this weakens the heart muscle, decreases contractility, and decreases cardiac output. The change in the structure of the heart leads to change in the electrical activity and increased risk of arrhythmias.

Diagnosis is made by medical history, physical exam, and echocardiogram. Treatment for severe valve disorders is valve replacement.

Mitral Valve Stenosis

- Causes: rheumatic heart disease, congenital disorders
- Cardiac abnormalities: narrowed mitral valve, left atrial dilation, atrial arrhythmia (atrial fibrillation), thrombi, diastolic murmur (atria contract), decrease in cardiac output
- Clinical manifestations: fatigue, weakness, angina, palpitations, pulmonary congestion, dyspnea, orthopnea
- Diagnosis: echocardiogram, cardiac catheterization, ECG
- Treatment: blood thinners, echocardiogram

Mitral Valve Prolapse

- Causes: Marfan syndrome, genetics, Grave disease, Ehler-Danlos syndrome
- Cardiac abnormalities: mucinous degeneration of valve, enlarged, leaky mitral valve, systolic murmur (ventricular contraction)
- Clinical manifestations: typically, asymptomatic. Signs and symptoms of autonomic dysfunction. Sympathetic

nervous system (SNS) stimulation (tachycardia, dyspnea, anxiety, fatigue, dizziness)
- May progress to mitral valve regurgitation (MVR)
- Diagnosis: echocardiogram, cardiac catheterization, ECG
- Treatment: no stimulants (caffeine, nicotine), beta-blockers, valve replacement

Mitral Valve Regurgitation

- Causes: mitral valve prolapse, infective endocarditis, rheumatic heart disease, MI
- Cardiac abnormalities: leaky mitral valve (does not shut), increased preload, eccentric hypertrophy, left atrial dilation, atrial fibrillation, thrombi, systolic murmur (ventricular contraction)
- Clinical manifestations: pulmonary congestion, heart failure
- Diagnosis: echocardiogram, cardiac catheterization, ECG
- Treatment: blood thinners, valve replacement

Aortic Valve Stenosis

- Causes: Congenital disease, calcifications (aging), atherosclerosis, rheumatic heart disease
- Cardiac abnormalities: narrowed aortic valve, systolic murmur (ventricular contraction), concentric hypertrophy, increased afterload, arrhythmias
- Clinical manifestations: angina, dyspnea, syncope, pulmonary congestion, left-sided heart failure symptoms
- Diagnosis: echocardiogram, cardiac catheterization, ECG
- Treatment: medications, valve replacement

Aortic Valve Regurgitation

- Congenital: genetics, Marfan syndrome
- Causes: congenital: genetics, Marfan syndrome
- Acquired (acute): trauma, aneurysm, aortic dissection
- Acquired (chronic) infective endocarditis, rheumatic fever, hypertension
- Cardiac abnormalities (acute): sharp increase in left end diastolic volume
- Clinical manifestations (acute): pulmonary edema, sudden death
- Cardiac abnormalities (chronic): leaky aortic valve, diastolic murmur (ventricular relaxation), left ventricle eccentric hypertrophy, left atrial dilation, increased stroke volume, decreased cardiac output, arrhythmias
- Clinical manifestations (chronic): heart failure (dyspnea, orthopnea), Corrigan and Quincke's pulses, widened pulse pressure, sympathetic response (tachycardia, anxiety, palpitations)
- Diagnosis: echocardiogram, cardiac catheterization, ECG
- Treatment: valve replacement

Cardiomyopathies

Arrhythmogenic Right Ventricular Dysplasia

- Causes: genetics (autosomal dominant), assigned male at birth (AMAB) affected more often
- Cardiac abnormalities: right ventricle muscle tissue is replaced with adipose or fibrinous tissue. Right ventricle is dilated.
- Clinical manifestations: ventricular arrhythmias, palpitations, dizziness, heart failure, sudden death (especially in young athletes who are AMAB)
- Diagnosis: familial history, echocardiogram, ECG, cardiac magnetic resonance imaging (MRI), cardiac computed tomography (CT)
- Treatment: medication for heart failure and arrhythmias, defibrillator, ventricular assist device, heart transplant

Hypertrophic Cardiomyopathy

- Causes: genetic (autosomal dominant), most common cause of young athlete sudden death
- Cardiac abnormalities: mutations in genes that code for muscle fibers, making cardiac muscle weaker. Severe hypertrophy of left ventricle, thickening of ventricular septum, leading to aortic outflow obstruction with contraction (Fig. 7.3)
- Clinical manifestations: dyspnea, chest pain, syncope, atrial and ventricular arrhythmias, heart failure, sudden death
- Diagnosis: family history, echocardiogram, ECG
- Treatment: medications, defibrillator/cardioverter, surgery

Myocarditis

- Causes: inflammation and immune response to infection, medication, and autoimmune disease. Note: Myocarditis is a well-known symptom of COVID-19.
- Cardiac abnormalities: immunologic response to cardiac injury (molecular mimicry) leading to inflammation of myocardium
- Clinical manifestations: fever, chills, nausea, vomiting, muscle, and joint pain would be prodromal symptoms; heart failure and MI symptoms may occur
- Diagnosis: echocardiogram, ECG, cardiac biomarkers, chest x-ray
- Treatment: typically supportive, self-limiting disease; oxygen, rest, antibiotics—in severe cases, heart transplant may be necessary

Dilated Cardiomyopathy

- Causes: genetic, infections, medications, toxins, alcohol, chemotherapy
- Cardiac abnormalities: progressive dilation of heart chambers' contractile dysfunction; the heart becomes severely enlarged and flabby, with wall thinning and dilation of all four chambers (Fig. 7.3)
- Clinical manifestations: heart failure, low ejection fractions, thrombi, emboli; MVR and cardiac arrhythmias are common, sudden death may occur
- Diagnosis: echocardiogram, ECG, medical history
- Treatment: medications to reduce work of the heart, biventricular pacemaker, cardioverter/defibrillator, heart transplant

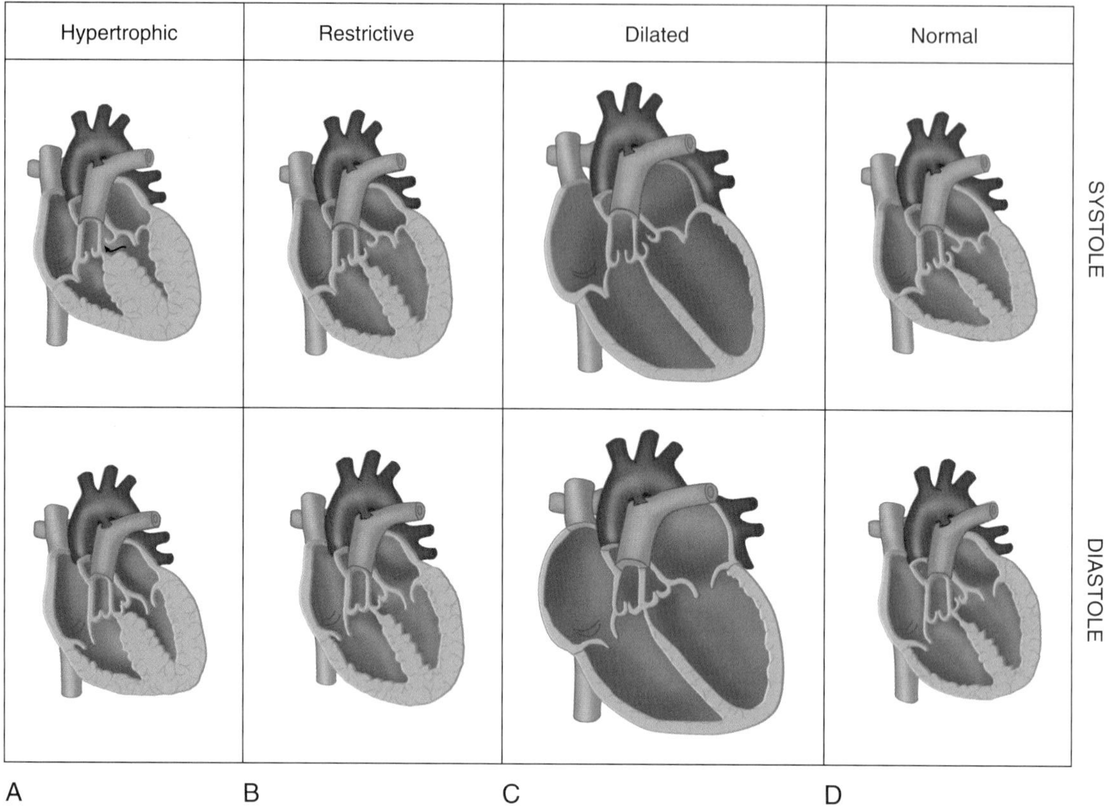

• **Fig. 7.3** Cardiomyopathies. (From Urden, L. D., Stacy, K. M., & Lough, M. E. (2023). *Priorities in critical care nursing* (9th ed.). Elsevier. Fig. 11.18.)

Takotsubo Cardiomyopathy (Broken Heart Syndrome)

- Causes: stress, profound psychological and emotional stress; typically found in older assigned females at birth
- Cardiac abnormalities: catecholamines cause the left ventricle to be "stunned," unable to contract; the left ventricle can be seen to "balloon" out during contractions
- Clinical manifestations: symptoms of MI; chest pain, diaphoresis, anxiety, etc.; ECG may show ST elevation
- Diagnosis: cardiac catheterization shows no disease, serum biomarkers are not as elevated as in an MI
- Treatment: resolves with supportive care

Heart Failure

Heart failure is a condition caused by the cardiac diseases we discussed in both this chapter (Chapter 7) and Chapter 6. Heart failure results in decreased cardiac output, due to a decrease in inotropy (contractile force), preload, and afterload. The left ventricle contracts and pushes a fraction of the blood it contains into the aorta. This is called the ejection fraction (EF) and EF of 50% to 75% is normal.

When there is heart failure, compensation mechanisms are in place (Fig. 7.4). The Frank-Starling mechanism states that when the stroke volume increases, the increased stretch of the heart causes an increased force of contraction. This leads to increased preload by initiating the renin-angiotensin-aldosterone system (RAAS), which causes increased secretion of angiotensin 2 and aldosterone, causing fluid retention. The SNS is activated, increasing vasoconstriction, heart rate, and contractility. Angiotensin 2 also causes vasoconstriction. These forms of compensation are initially helpful. However, over time, this chronic compensation damages the heart. It can cause ventricular hypertrophy, arrhythmias, increase preload and afterload, and may lead to sudden death.

> **NOTE**
>
> Compared to assigned males at birth, persons of color and assigned females at birth are less likely to receive heart transplants or ventricular assist devices. They were also less likely to receive appropriate heart failure, pacemaker, or defibrillator therapy.

Systolic Heart Failure

This is caused by impaired cardiac contractility due to myocardial dysfunction. This reduces ejection fraction below 40%. The heart muscle would be observed to be thick and weak.

Diastolic Heart Failure

This is caused by the inability to fill the ventricles during diastole. The ejection fraction is preserved because the left ventricle increases the force of contraction to maintain the

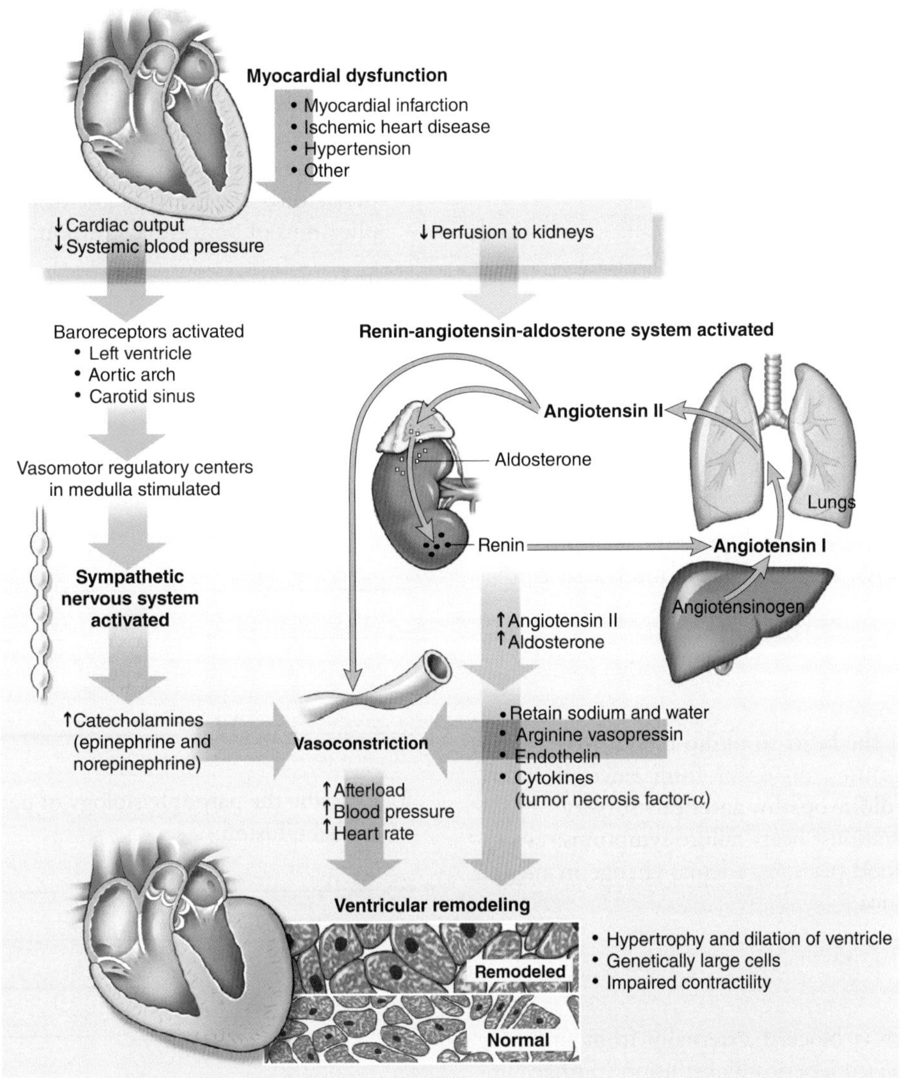

• **Fig. 7.4** Heart failure compensation mechanisms. (From Huether, S., & McCance, K. (2019). Figure 26.31 p. 621 Understanding Pathophysiology (7th ed.). Figure 26.31, p. 621. Elsevier.)

cardiac output. The heart muscle would be observed to be thick and stiff.

Left-Sided Failure (Left Side → Lung)

In left-sided heart failure, the left ventricle does not accept enough blood and/or is unable to pump enough blood. Blood backflows into the lungs. The capillaries fill with blood and the capillary filtration pressure is high. The blood shifts from the blood vessels to the lung tissue and alveoli, causing pulmonary edema.

- Clinical manifestations: pulmonary congestion, pulmonary edema, cyanosis, hypoxia, dyspnea, orthopnea, cough with frothy sputum, paroxysmal nocturnal dyspnea
- Diagnosis: history, physical exam, echocardiogram, brain natriuretic peptide (BNP) levels
- Treatments: medications (positive inotropes, medications to reduce preload, afterload, and sympathetic response), implanted cardioverter/defibrillator, heart transplant

Right-Sided Failure (Right Side → Body)

In right-sided heart failure, the right ventricle is not able to pump adequate volume of blood into the pulmonary circulation, via the pulmonary artery, due to right ventricle infarct, left heart failure, pulmonary hypertension, or lung disease. This results in a backflow of blood through the venous system and into the body. As the lungs are not oxygenating enough blood to send to the left heart, eventually, cardiac output will decrease and there will be left-sided heart failure as a result.

- Clinical manifestations: fatigue, ascites, hepatomegaly, splenomegaly, anorexia, constipation, dependent edema, jugular venous distension
- Diagnosis: history, physical exam, ECG, echocardiogram, BNP levels
- Treatments: medications (positive inotropes, diuretics, medications to reduce preload, afterload, and sympathetic response), implanted cardioverter/defibrillator, heart transplant

Cor Pulmonale

Cor pulmonale is right-sided heart failure caused by pulmonary disease resulting in pulmonary hypertension. Because the pressure is high in the lung vessels, the right ventricle workload increases and the right ventricle hypertrophies and fails. Manifestations, diagnosis, and treatments are the same as in right-sided heart failure.

Shock

Circulatory

- Cause: decrease in blood volume by more than 15%; this can be due to dehydration, hemorrhage, or third spacing
- Clinical manifestations: restlessness, agitation, confusion, tachycardia, low blood pressure, clammy skin, weak thready pulse, decreased urine, decreased cardiac output, coma

Cardiogenic

- Cause: failure of the heart to pump blood; MIs are the most common cause; can occur from valve disorders, arrhythmias, cardiomyopathy, and heart surgery
- Clinical manifestations: heart failure symptoms; cyanosis, decreased blood pressure, edema, change in mental status, and dyspnea

Obstructive

- Cause: the heart is blocked externally from pumping blood; this can be from pericardial effusion (cardiac tamponade), tension pneumothorax, tumors, or pulmonary embolism
- Clinical manifestations: compression of the heart, resulting in jugular venous distension, muffled heart sounds, and low blood pressure

Distributive

- Cause: systemic vasodilation; this causes blood to move from vessels to the tissue. Anaphylaxis, sepsis, and neurogenic shock can cause this.
- Clinical manifestations: symptoms depend on the specific cause; common symptoms may be tachypnea, tachycardia, hypotension, altered mental status.

NOTE

All types of shock can result in acute respiratory distress syndrome, kidney injury, bowel ischemia, disseminated intravascular coagulation ischemia, and hypoxia. Multiple organ dysfunction syndrome also may result.

Study Guide for Chapter 7

Make sure that you have your class notes and textbooks on hand to answer these questions. A concept map is included to help you to diagram and link disease concepts together.

1. Describe pericarditis. What is the difference between pericarditis and pericardial effusion? What are the complications of pericardial effusion?

___

___

___

___

2. What are the components of Beck triad? When would you look at this?

___

___

___

___

3. Describe the pathophysiology of pericarditis and of pericardial effusion.

___

___

___

___

4. What is cardiac tamponade? Describe the clinical manifestations of the disorder, including pulsus paradoxus.

___

___

___

___

5. Discuss endocarditis, its symptoms, and complications.

___

___

___

___

6. Explain the etiology of rheumatic heart disease and its acute and chronic complications.

___

___

7. Differentiate between the five valvular disorders. (This is a good time to use T charts!).

8. Explain compensation mechanisms for valvular disorders.

9. Differentiate between the following: arrhythmogenic right ventricular dysplasia; myocarditis; hypertrophic, dilated, and takotsubo cardiomyopathies.

10. Discuss ventricular remodeling.

11. Explain the mechanisms behind heart failure (SNS, RAAS).

12. Understand the difference between systolic and diastolic heart failure.

13. Distinguish between left and right heart failure.

14. Describe pulmonary edema.

15. Differentiate between the causes of hypovolemic, distributive, cardiogenic, and obstructive shock.

16. Describe the clinical manifestations of the different types of shock.

STUDY TIPS

T-charts.
Example:

	MVS	MVP	MVR	AVS	AVR
Cause					
Murmur					
Cardiac symptoms					

AVR, Aortic valve regurgitation; *AVS,* aortic valve stenosis; *MVP,* mitral valve prolapse; *MVR,* mitral valve regurgitation; *MVS,* mitral valve stenosis.

Concept Map

Use this concept map to link each disease to its pathophysiology, diagnostics, causes, risk factors, complications, and clinical manifestations together. This way, you will be able to see the whole picture of the disease.

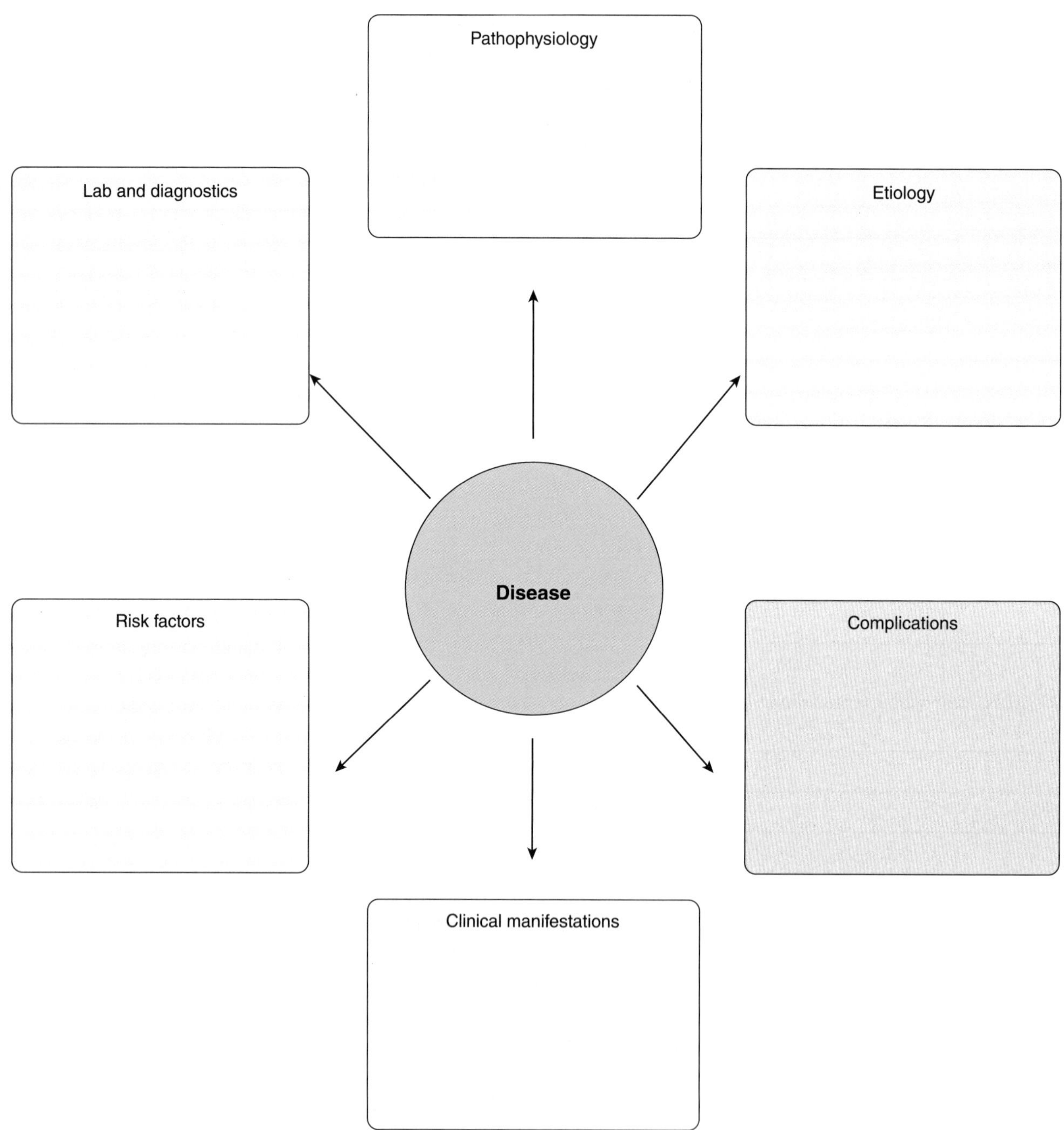

Case Studies for Chapter 7

Case Study 7.1

Jess is a 19-year-old transgender individual (he/him). He came to the emergency room with complaints of chest pain and dyspnea. Jess does not have a known history of heart disease, but has not seen a provider for a few years, as he had a falling out with his family and has been staying with friends and in and out of shelters. When the provider asks about his health history, Jess says that he has had bad sore throats sometimes but that he was otherwise healthy. When the provider auscultates Jess' heart, the provider hears a diastolic murmur.

1. What condition/disease do you think Jess has?

2. How did Jess get this condition/disease? Explain the pathophysiology.

3. What complications would you be worried about? Why?

4. How do the social determinants of health and equity affect Jess' case?

Case Study 7.2

Nevil is a 38-year-old Navajo cis-male (he/him). He is at his provider's office for a physical exam. Nevil has Marfan syndrome, and he states that he has been experiencing palpitations and dizziness intermittently. The provider auscultates his heart and lungs and hears a systolic murmur.

1. Why might Nevil be experiencing palpitations and have a murmur? Explain the pathophysiology.

2. What would be some things Nevil can do to avoid these symptoms?

Ten years later, Nevil, now 48 years old, comes back to his provider for a cardiology exam. He states that he is increasingly short of breath, especially at night. He is fatigued and states that his heart feels like it is "fluttering."

3. Has Nevil's condition progressed? What would his diagnosis be? Explain the pathophysiology behind Nevil's symptoms.

The provider explains to Nevil that if the condition continues to progress, he may need surgery, or his heart may fail. Nevil is upset and says, "I don't understand why I need surgery. How can this cause my entire heart to fail?"

4. Explain why Nevil's condition could progress to heart failure.

Case Study 7.3

Mia is a 16-year-old Black cis-female (she/her) athlete who just made the varsity lacrosse team. Prior to starting the season, the school required a complete physical exam, including a cardiac exam and electrocardiogram (ECG), for all school athletes.

1. Why would the school require a cardiac exam and ECG?

Mia is diagnosed with hypertrophic cardiomyopathy. She asks, "Can I still play lacrosse?"

2. What would you say to Mia?

Case Study 7.4

A 65-year-old client, who was hospitalized with COVID-19, was treated with steroids and antivirals, and discharged. A few days later, the client was brought to the emergency room with a cough, low-grade fever, sharp chest pain, and worsening shortness of breath. On exam, the provider heard diminished breath sounds in both lungs and could not hear the heart sounds clearly when auscultating. The client was sent to get a chest x-ray with oxygen. While getting the x-ray, the client coded. An emergency department nurse, who responded to the code, noticed jugular vein distension.

1. What do you think caused the code? Explain the pathophysiology.

The code team leader suspects that the client went into shock.

2. What type of shock did the client experience? Explain.

8 Pulmonary Disease Part 1

Pulmonary Background

First, let's go through some of the anatomy and physiology of the lung. When we talk about lung compliance , we are talking about the ease of lung inflation on inspiration, and elastic recoil is how well the lungs spring back into place on expiration.

- Compliance = change in volume/change in pressure

The bronchioles have goblet cells (produce mucous), cilia, and mucous glands to protect them from pathogens and debris. A mucociliary blanket covers the bronchioles and traps pathogen.

The alveoli are where gas exchange takes place (Fig. 8.1). The alveoli have their own macrophages, type I, and type II alveolar cells. Type II alveolar cells produce both type I and II cells and secrete surfactants A, B, C, and D. Surfactants B and C are important because they lower the surface tension inside the alveoli. This means that the alveoli only partially collapse during expiration, allowing the alveoli to fill more easily on inspiration. Surfactants A and D act as chemokines. Surfactants B and C are distributed through the pores of Kohn, so that air and surfactant can move freely to equalize. However, infection can also spread easily through the pores of Kohn.

Tidal volume, air that moves in and out of the lungs, is typically about 500 mL. Of that, the lungs use 350 mL. The 150 mL remaining in the nose, pharynx, and airways do not participate in gas exchange (dead space). Residual volume is the air left in the lungs after expiration (1200 mL). Lung capacity is the amount of air that can be held in the lungs (6000 mL). Incentive spirometry measures the inspiratory capacity and is used to help clients who are immobilized to deep breathe.

> **NOTE**
>
> Lung capacity is often falsely underestimated in people of color due to race-based medicine. Incentive spirometers use a race correction, or ethnic adjustment, to supposedly correct for lower lung capacities in Asian and Black individuals. However, this difference has been debunked by scientists. Despite this, many facilities and organizations are continuing to use race correction algorithms for lung capacity.

Pulmonary Gas Exchange

Ventilation is the movement of air in and out of the lungs. Perfusion is the movement of oxygenated blood throughout the body. Diffusion is when gas exchange takes place. The difference in pressure of CO_2 and O_2 on either side of the membrane forms a concentration gradient, resulting in a transfer of CO_2 and O_2 between the alveoli and capillaries.

Respiratory issues are often caused by ventilation and perfusion mismatch (Fig. 8.2). This means that the person may be able to ventilate (breathe in and out), but perfusion (blood circulating through the lungs) may be blocked. This is called ventilation with perfusion, of a high V (ventilation)/Q (perfusion) ratio. This typically happens with pulmonary emboli and vasoconstriction in the lungs. Perfusion without ventilation or low ventilation to perfusion (low V/Q ratio) occurs with airway obstructions, such as atelectasis and mucus plugs.

Hypoxemia

Hypoxemia is a reduction of PaO_2 in the blood. This can be caused by hypoventilation, impaired diffusion (pulmonary edema and pneumonia), and mismatching of ventilation and perfusion (chronic obstructive pulmonary disease [COPD]). It is monitored by chemoreceptors in the peripheral vessels (aortic arch, carotid arteries). The chemoreceptors activate when the PaO_2 is lower than 60 mm Hg (hypoxic drive). This leads to tissue hypoxia.

Hypoxemia symptoms:

- Mild—change in vital signs (heart rate [HR], respiratory rate [RR], pulse oximetry)
- Pronounced—altered mental status
- Severe—cyanosis, stupor, coma
- Chronic

Diagnosis:

- Observation
- Pulse oximetry
- Arterial blood gas (ABG)
- Lactate levels

Treatment: identify cause and treat

Hypercapnia

Hypercapnia is an increase of $PaCO_2$ in the blood. It is monitored by chemoreceptors located in or near the medulla. These receptors are activated by high CO_2 levels, which then cause increased respirations. Hypercapnia can be caused by many different diseases affecting breathing and

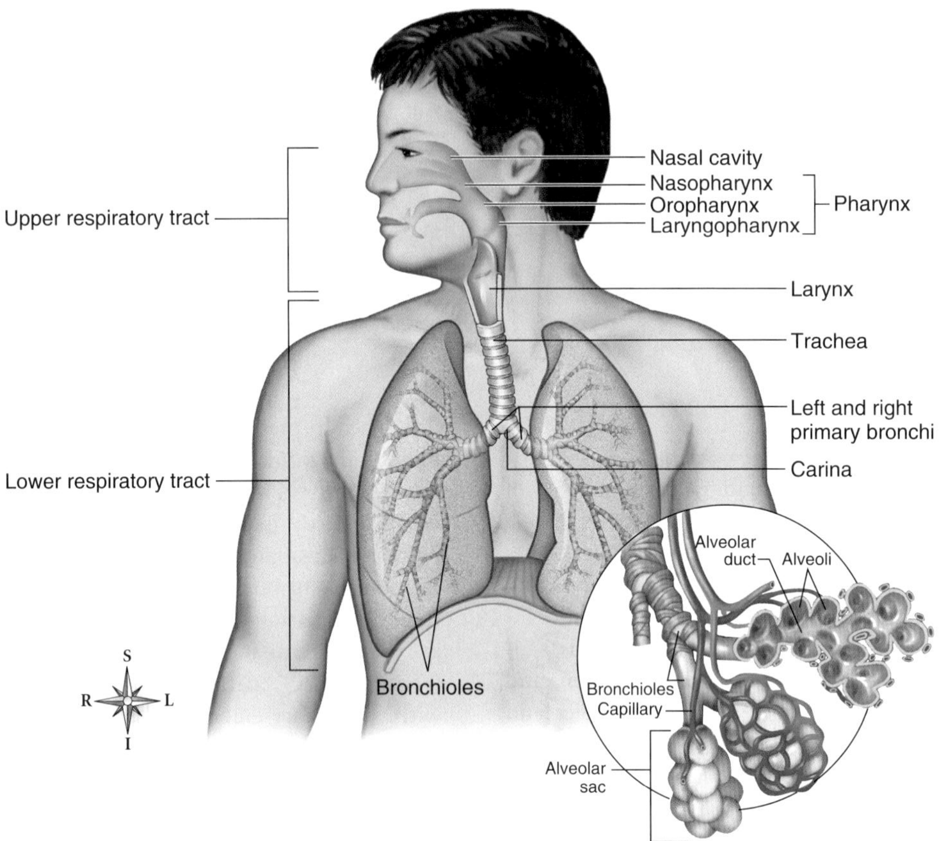

• **Fig. 8.1** Structure of the pulmonary system. (From Patton, K.T., & Thibodeau, G.A. (2016). Structure & function of the body (15th ed.) Mosby.)

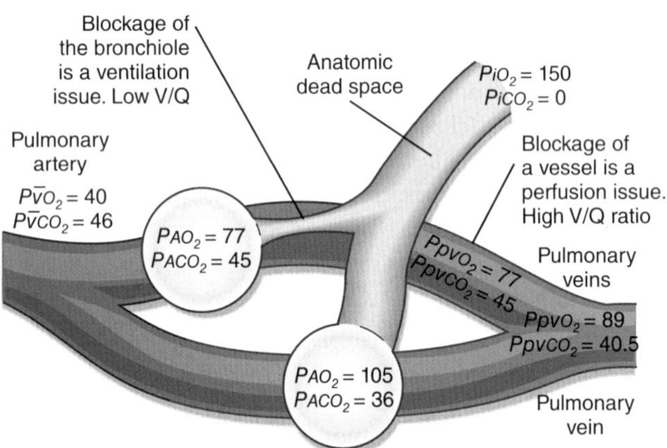

• **Fig. 8.2** Ventilation-perfusion mismatch. (From Harding, M. M., Kwong, J., Hagler, D., Reinisch, C. (2022). *Lewis's medical-surgical nursing: Assessment and management of clinical problems* (12th ed.). Elsevier. Fig. 32.4.)

causing hypoventilation: cancer, neurodegenerative disease, COPD, injury, age.

Symptoms

- Tachycardia
- Agitation
- Restlessness
- Cerebral vasodilation (headache)
- Altered level of consciousness

Diagnosis: ABG

Treatment: treat underlying cause

Hypoxia

Hypoxia is the resulting oxygen deficiency in the tissues from hypercapnia and hypoxemia. Regional hypoxia in the lungs can occur with vasoconstriction in a specific region of the lung. It can also occur with a localized airway obstruction, such as a mucus plug or atelectasis. Generalized hypoxia occurs when there is vasoconstriction throughout all vessels of the lungs.

Causes:

- High altitudes (thinner air, lower PaO_2)
- Lung disease
- Circulatory shock
- Acidosis

Pleural Effusion

The lungs are encased in by the parietal and visceral pleura. There is typically a little bit of fluid between the two layers, so that they can move smoothly. However, with disease, fluid overload, trauma, obstruction, and inflammation, an abnormal amount of pleural fluid can collect, called pleural effusion.

Types:

- Exudate—yellowish, clear, proteins, leukocytes
- Transudate—clear, fluid overload
- Empyema—infection in pleural space, purulent, yellow green

- Chyle—lymph fluid from blockage, milky white
- Sanguineous—hemothorax, blood

Manifestations
- Dyspnea
- Crackles
- Dull sounds on percussion
- Fever
- Increased white blood cells
- Pleuritic pain

Diagnosis: x-rays, computed tomography (CT) scan, bronchoscopy
Treatment: removal of fluid by chest tube, surgery

Pneumothorax

A pneumothorax is a puncture in the lung, which lets air escape into the pleural space. This causes the lung to collapse (Fig. 8.3).

Spontaneous Pneumothorax

Air-filled blisters, or blebs, can occur in tall, thin, healthy individuals. These blebs are typically located at the top of the lungs. Individuals with Marfan syndrome and smokers are also at risk.

When these blebs rupture, it causes air to escape into the pleural space, making the pressure positive, which makes it harder for the lung to expand (compliance). This can cause partial or total lung collapse.

Secondary Pneumothorax

This can occur with chronic obstructive lung diseases, such as emphysema. Air is trapped in the alveoli due to the loss of elastic recoil, which means that air cannot be expired. Air pressure continues to build with each inhalation. Eventually, the alveoli can "pop" and cause lung collapse.

Traumatic Pneumothorax

Traumatic pneumothoraxes can be penetrating or nonpenetrating. A penetrating pneumothorax can be caused by a stabbing or gunshot wound. A nonpenetrating pneumothorax can be caused by blunt trauma to the chest.

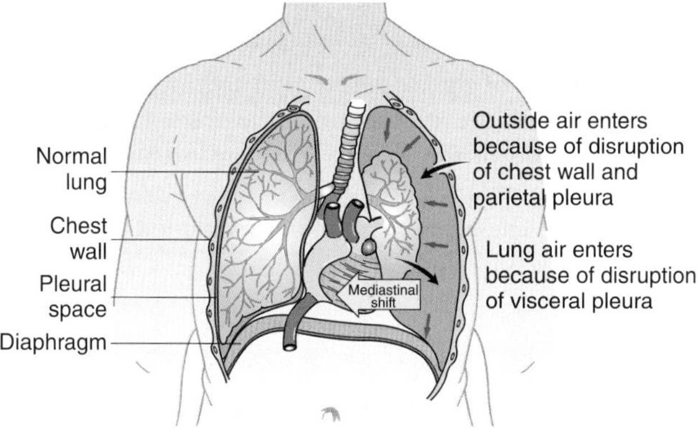

• **Fig. 8.3** Pneumothorax. (Rogers, J. (2022). *McCance & Huether's pathophysiology: The biologic basis for disease in adults and children* (9th ed.). Mosby. Fig. 35.3.)

Clinical manifestations:
- Sudden pain on one side of the chest
- Tachypnea
- Dyspnea
- Absent breath sounds
- Hyperresonance
- Hypoxemia
- Subcutaneous emphysema
- Drop in O_2 saturation

Diagnosis: chest x-ray, chest CT, physical exam
Treatment: monitoring if only a partial collapse, oxygen, chest tube, needle decompression
Complications: tension pneumothorax

Tension pneumothorax can occur with any type of pneumothorax, though most commonly with traumatic pneumothoraxes. There is a rapid rise in pressure in the intrapleural cavity, which acts as a one-way valve, letting air in, but not out. As the lung collapses, the pressure in the intrapleural cavity builds up and compresses the unaffected lung and heart. Eventually, the unaffected lung collapses and the heart is unable to beat effectively. This causes a deadly decrease in cardiac output and obstructive shock. This is a medical emergency and requires needle decompression to get rid of the air or fluid in the pleural space.

Atelectasis

Atelectasis refers to the collapse of alveoli. This can be caused by:
- an obstructed airway and absorption of air from the affected alveoli
- compression of the lung (e.g., tumor)
- deficiency or lack of surfactant

Clinical manifestations
- Shortness of breath
- Tachypnea
- Tachycardia
- Lower readings on the pulse oximeter

Diagnosis: chest x-ray or CT scan
Treatment: monitoring, deep breathing, and oxygen
Prevention: deep breathing, incentive spirometry, drinking fluids, and early ambulation are encouraged

Aspiration Pneumonitis

Aspiration pneumonitis or aspiration pneumonia is not a disease, but a condition caused by difficulty swallowing, difficulty breathing, and decreased consciousness. It is the inflammation and infection that occurs within the lung when the client inhales regurgitated gastric contents.

Causes: lung disease, stroke, seizures, dementia, gastroesophageal reflux disease (GERD), neuromuscular disease, narcotics, anesthesia
Clinical manifestations:
- Choking
- Wheezing

- High fevers
- Tachycardia
- Dyspnea

Diagnosis: chest x-ray, lung consolidation can be seen
Treatment: intravenous (IV) antibiotics are used to treat

Restrictive Lung Disease

Restrictive lung diseases are diseases and conditions which affect compliance or expansion of the lungs. This affects ventilation and gas exchange.

Conditions leading to restrictive lung disease: sarcoidosis, pneumonia, pulmonary fibrosis, amyotrophic lateral sclerosis, obesity, and scoliosis.

Climate Change and Pulmonary Disease

NOTE

Climate change directly affects and causes pulmonary disease and increased death rates. Wildfires, extreme weather, and air pollution can directly affect pulmonary health and exacerbate pulmonary diseases like asthma, COPD, and allergies. Increased air pollutants can cause inflammation and, eventually, lung cancer. Looking at the social determinants of health, it is the marginalized communities that suffer most from climate change and have the least access to medical care, safe housing, education, and healthy food.

Obstructive Pulmonary Diseases

Asthma

Asthma can be extrinsic (epigenetic, antibody/antigen reaction) or intrinsic (nonimmune stimulation of mast cells). Nonimmune asthma can be caused by respiratory infections, exercise, cold air, hyperventilation, or inhaled irritants. Genetics, climate change, and social determinants of health increase the risk of asthma. Note: race is not a risk factor.

Diagnosis: pulmonary function tests, chest x-rays, ABGs, and triggers to asthma may be identified. Early phase asthma consists of mast cell activation, chemical mediator (histamine) release, bronchoconstriction, and increased mucus production by goblet cells (Fig. 8.4).
Symptoms

- Expiratory wheezing
- Chest tightness
- Dyspnea
- Tachycardia
- Tachypnea
- Nonproductive cough

Late phase asthma consists of the influx of inflammatory cells, cytokines, prostaglandins and leukotrienes, edema, increased capillary permeability, decreased mucus clearance, and airway hyperresponsiveness and closure.
Symptoms

- Distant breath sounds
- Inspiratory and expiratory wheezing
- Word fatigue

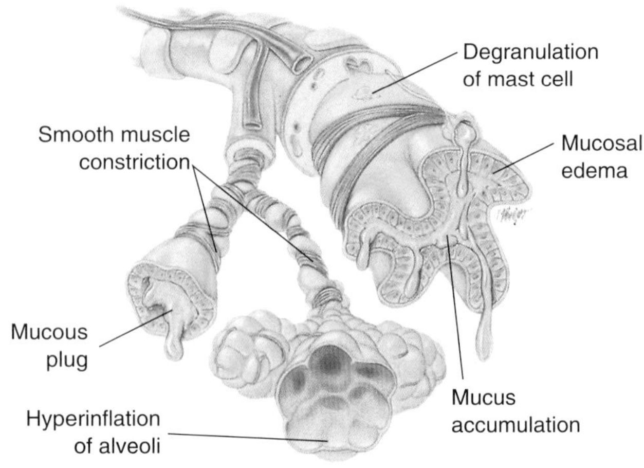

• **Fig. 8.4** Asthma. (Modified from Des Jardins, T., & Burton, G.G. (1995). Clinical manifestations and assessment of respiratory disease, (3rd ed.). Mosby)

- Accessory muscle use
- Can lead to changes in structure of the airway and respiratory failure

Treatment: bronchodilators, nebulizers, and steroids. Severe cases may need mechanical ventilation.

Chronic Obstructive Pulmonary Disease

COPD is most often caused by smoking but can also be caused by air pollution. Social determinants of health and climate change add to the risk factors. COPD consists of emphysema and chronic bronchitis. Clients may have either of these conditions or both, resulting in a mismatching of ventilation and perfusion and destruction of lung tissue (Fig. 8.5).

Emphysema

Emphysema is the destruction of the alveoli and elastic tissue of the lungs. It is typically caused by smoking. Smoking causes an inflammatory response, which releases an enzyme called elastase. Elastase breaks down elastin in the lungs, which decreases elastic recoil. In healthy individuals, an enzyme called alpha-1 antitrypsin is secreted, which inhibits the action of the elastase. However, smoking leads to decreased levels of alpha-1 antitrypsin and increased actions of elastase. With the destruction of the elastic fibers in lung tissue and walls of the alveoli, the lungs become hyperinflated and expiration is prolonged.

Diagnosis: chest x-rays, pulmonary function tests, reflex testing for levels of alpha-1 antitrypsin
Symptoms

- Dyspnea
- "Pink" appearance (pink puffer)
- Tachypnea
- Barrel chest (from hyperinflation)
- Thin appearance (all effort goes into breathing)
- Prolonged expiration (pursed lip breathing)

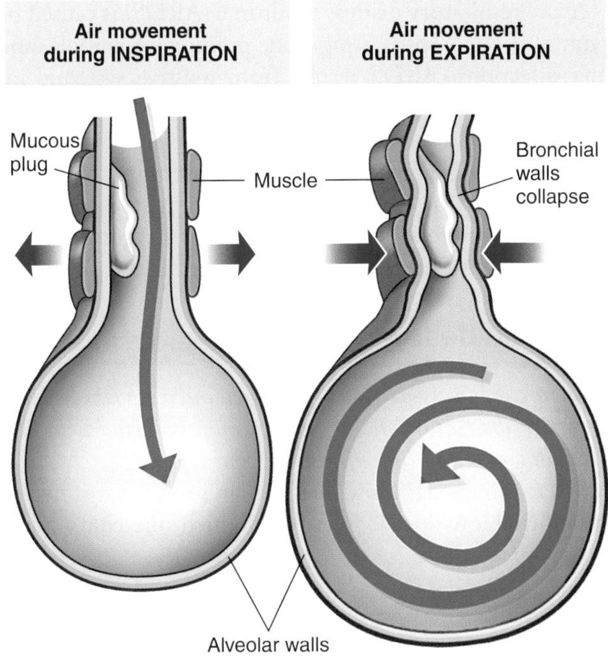

• **Fig. 8.5** Air trapping in chronic obstructive pulmonary disease. (McCance, K. L. (2019). Cancer Epidemiology. In K. L. McCance, S. E. Huether, V. Brashers, & N. Rote (Eds.), Pathophysiology: The Biologic Basis for Disease in Adults and Children (8th ed.). Elsevier. pp. 379-425.)

- Decreased breath sounds
- Tripod positioning

Treatment: bronchodilators, nebulizers, steroids, oxygen, smoking cessation, diet, exercise

Chronic Bronchitis

Chronic bronchitis results in airway obstruction due to narrowing (bronchospasm) of the airway and hypersecretion of mucus. Chronic irritation of the bronchi causes an inflammatory response and an increase in goblet cells and a hypertrophy of mucus glands (Fig. 8.6). Inflammation of the airways results in scarring, fibrosis, and narrowing of the airways. The overproduction of mucus and decreased airway clearance block the smaller airways, causing hypoxemia, and create a hospitable environment for respiratory infection (pneumonia).

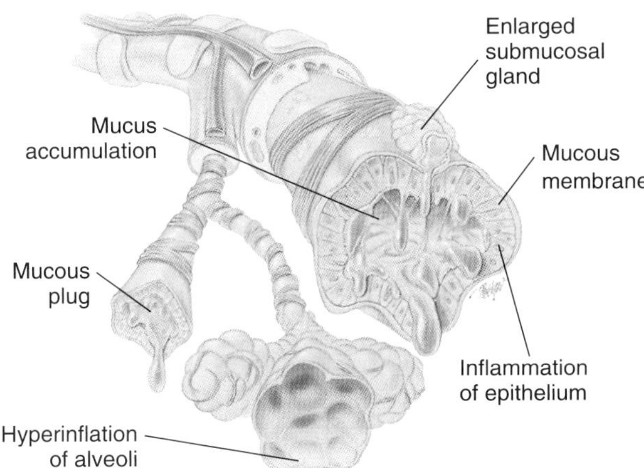

• **Fig. 8.6** Chronic bronchitis. (Modified from Des Jardins, T., & Burton, G.G. (1995). Clinical manifestations and assessment of respiratory disease (3rd ed.)., Mosby.)

With a clinical diagnosis, having a chronic productive cough for 3 consecutive months over a period of 2 years would demonstrate chronic bronchitis. Chronic bronchitis would also cause diffuse pulmonary vasoconstriction. This would lead to ventilation-perfusion mismatch, and ultimately, cor pulmonale (right-sided heart failure due to lung disease). In cor pulmonale, the diffuse vasoconstriction of the lungs causes the right ventricle to work harder and ultimately fail.

Diagnosis: pulmonary function tests, chest x-rays, and chest CT scans

Symptoms

- Weight gain and hypoxemia→ cyanosis (blue bloaters)
- Secondary polycythemia (overproduction of red blood cells [RBCs] due to lack of oxygen)
- Productive (mucus-filled) cough
- Wheezing and rhonchi would be heard in the lungs

Treatment: bronchodilators, nebulizers, steroids, oxygen, smoking cessation, diet, and exercise

Cystic Fibrosis

Cystic fibrosis (CF) is an inherited, obstructive, autosomal recessive disease (chromosome 7) that affects chloride channels. The cystic fibrosis transmembrane conductance regulator (CFTR) gene mutation codes for a defective CFTR chloride channel. This defective channel does not allow chloride ions to be secreted outside the cell resulting in increased reabsorption of sodium and water, causing the mucus to become thicker on the epithelial surfaces (lungs) and stickier and viscous on secretions from the exocrine glands (pancreas). The CFTR channel works the opposite way in the skin. Chloride ions are unable to be reabsorbed, and increased chloride ions and sodium ions are secreted. Remember that water follows sodium, so water is lost as well. That is why individuals with CF may have saltier skin (sweat test).

Clients with CF are often identified at birth with blood and genetic testing. Infants can have meconium ileus, jaundice, frequent pulmonary infections, and fail to thrive. Individuals can also show symptoms much later in life, leading to a later diagnosis. However, the respiratory system is not the only organ affected. Pancreatic enzyme secretion is affected, leading to an inability to digest food properly, and having foul and fatty stools. Reproductive organ secretions are affected, leading to infertility. Liver failure, anemia, and skin diseases are also common. CF is an incurable disease with a shortened lifespan, so the emphasis is on symptom management.

Symptoms

- Fatigue
- Clubbing of fingers and toes
- Barrel chest, chronic cough
- Chronic bronchitis
- Bronchiectasis (dilated and twisting bronchioles)
- Atypical pneumonias
- Malabsorption and steatorrhea

Treatment regimens consist of home oxygen if needed, antibiotics for pulmonary infections, mucolytics, anti-inflammatories, chest physiotherapy/postural drainage, and bronchodilators. Pancreatic enzyme supplements are given so that food can be digested. A new medication that modulates and opens the chloride ion channels (Trikafta) has been approved by the FDA and is increasing lifespans of those with CF.

Pulmonary Embolism

Pulmonary emboli are obstructions that occur in the pulmonary arteries. There are different types of emboli.

- Air embolism
  - Air can escape into the blood vessels from the lungs or be injected through a central line or port.
  - Nitrogen can also accumulate in the vessels (decompression sickness).
- Amniotic fluid embolism
  - Amniotic fluid or fetal cells can escape from fetal circulation, causing an inflammatory response in the person giving birth. As you know, inflammation causes clotting!
- Fat embolism
  - Fat globules are released into the bloodstream, occluding the pulmonary vessel. This fat typically comes from long bone and pelvic fractures.
- Thrombus
  - A thrombus or vegetative lesion can break off and travel to the pulmonary arteries, causing an obstruction. Similarly, a deep vein thrombus may break off and travel to the pulmonary arteries.

A pulmonary embolus can be small, moderate, or massive. Symptoms correspond to size and degree of obstruction. A small embolus may be asymptomatic. A moderate embolus may have the hallmark signs of low-grade fever, tachycardia, low oxygen saturation, and blood-tinged sputum. A massive thrombus may result in severe dyspnea, chest pain, and sudden death.

Diagnosis: history and physical, elevated D-dimer, confirmed by a chest CT scan

Treatment: anticoagulants, thrombolytic therapy, inferior vena cava (IVC) filter

Prevention: early ambulation after surgery, alternating pressure boots, adequate fluids. IVC filters and anticoagulants can be used to existing clots

Respiratory Failure

Respiratory failure can be hypoxemic, hypercapnic, or a combination of the two. Hypoxemic respiratory failure is respiratory failure due to lack of oxygen (pO_2 <60 mm Hg). This can occur due to mismatch of ventilation and perfusion or impaired diffusion (COPD, pulmonary edema, pneumonia, and atelectasis). Restlessness, anxiety, tachycardia, and tachypnea are early symptoms. Late symptoms are bradycardia, agitation, and severe dyspnea. Hypercapnic respiratory failure is due to inadequate alveolar ventilation from the increase of carbon dioxide in the blood (pCO_2 >45 mm Hg). Narcotics, lung disease, neuromuscular disease, and decreased levels of consciousness are common causes of hypercapnia. With hypercapnia, drowsiness, disorientation, headache, dyspnea, hyperkalemia, hypotension, and low blood pressure can occur.

Acute respiratory distress syndrome (ARDS) is caused by trauma, shock, sepsis, aspiration, pulmonary emboli, and lung infections. ARDS results from massive systemic inflammation, causing lungs to become extremely edematous, and show a "white-out" on chest x-ray. This happens when both lungs are filled with exudate. Symptoms of this are severe dyspnea, tachypnea, tachycardia, and hypoxia. Treatment for respiratory failure and ARDS is oxygenation and ventilation, with treatment of underlying disease processes.

Study Guide for Chapter 8

Make sure that you have your class notes and textbooks on hand to answer these questions. A concept map is included to help you to diagram and link disease concepts together.

1. What is hypoxia? How does it manifest? What is hypercapnia? How does it manifest? Which one controls the respiratory drive?

____

____

____

____

2. Define lung compliance, elastic recoil, and surface tension.

____

____

____

____

3. What happens when lungs are not compliant? What can cause this? What happens when there is no elastic recoil? What causes this?

____

____

____

____

4. Why is surface tension so important? What lung structure(s) does it affect?

____

____

____

____

5. Define ventilation, perfusion, and diffusion.

____

____

6. How does blood get oxygenated in the lungs? Draw or write out the process.

7. What happens in perfusion without ventilation? What about ventilation without perfusion? When would these occur?

8. What are some of the pulmonary changes with age?

9. What is a pleural effusion? Where does it occur? What are the different types of effusions?

10. What is a pneumothorax? Compare spontaneous pneumothorax, traumatic pneumothorax, and tension pneumothorax. Outline the causes and complications.

11. What is atelectasis? What causes it and what are the complications?

12. How does aspiration pneumonia occur? What are the manifestations?

13. What is the difference between intrinsic and extrinsic asthma? Is asthma obstructive or restrictive?

14. What is the pathophysiology of asthma?

15. Outline the pathophysiology and differences between chronic bronchitis and emphysema.

16. What is CF? Explain the pathophysiology and how CF affects the respiratory system. What other systems does it affect?

17. What conditions can cause a pulmonary embolus? How does it manifest?

18. What is cor pulmonale? How does pulmonary hypertension cause it?

19. What are the causes of respiratory failure? How does it manifest?

STUDY TIPS

Now that you know many of the systems, try to connect them together. What are the connections between pulmonary and hematology? Pulmonary and renal? Pulmonary and cardiac?
Set up a T-chart!
Example:

	Emphysema	Chronic bronchitis
Cause?		
Pathophysiology?		
Symptoms?		

Concept Map

Use this concept map to link each disease to its pathophysiology, diagnostics, causes, risk factors, complications, and clinical manifestations together. This way, you will be able to see the whole picture of the disease.

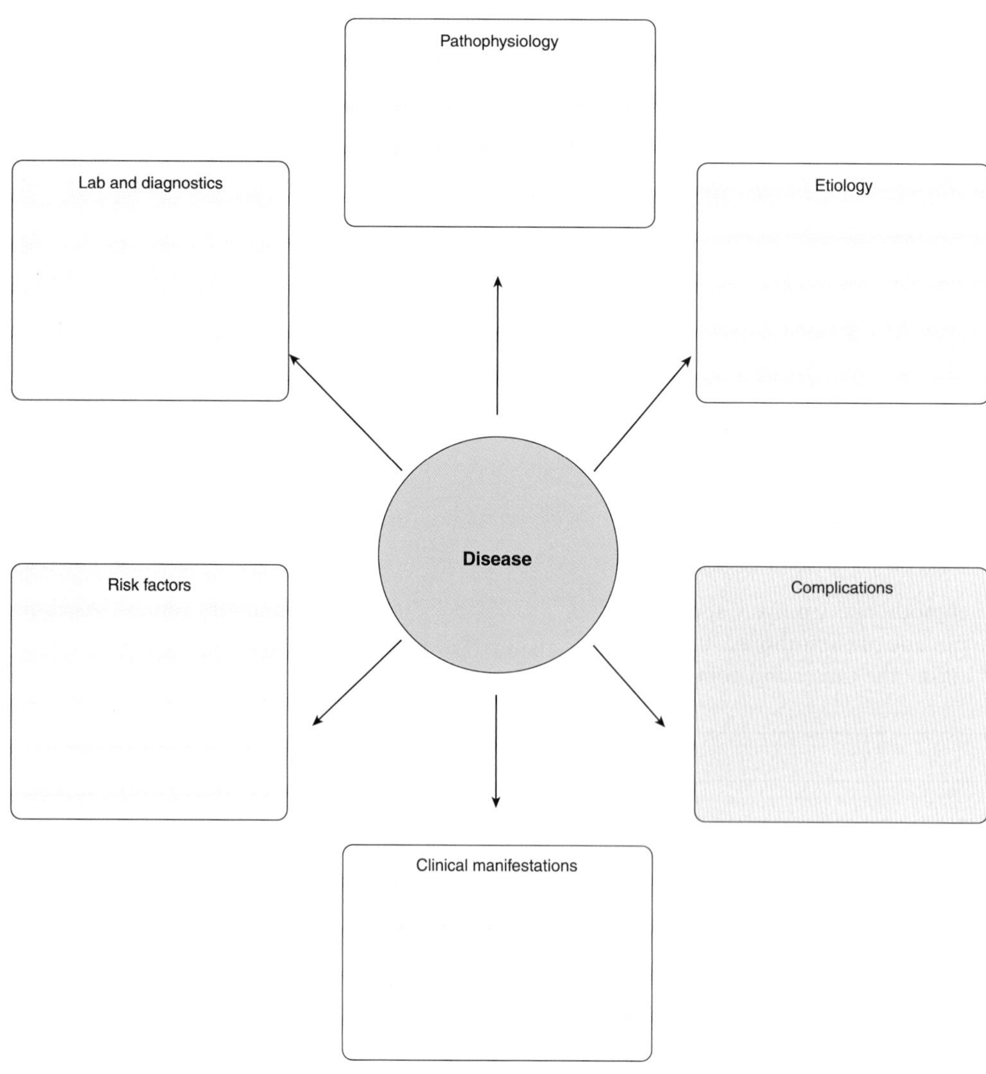

Case Studies for Chapter 8

Case Study 8.1

Kai (they/them) has a history of asthma and is having an asthma exacerbation. They are wheezing and coughing. They take their rescue inhaler, but it does not seem to be working and they are still having some difficulty breathing. Their wife wants them to go to the emergency room, but Kai refuses and says that they will go if it gets worse.

1. Should Kai wait to seek treatment? Why or why not?

2. How might climate change and social determinants of health cause increased prevalence of asthma?

Kai decides to go the emergency room that evening, as their breathing has gotten even worse.

3. Explain the pathophysiology behind early and late-stage asthma.

4. What are the symptoms of severe asthma?

Case Study 8.2

Rhea (she/her) grew up in South India. Her mother and grandmother used to cook over a charcoal fire until the kitchen was modernized with a gas stove when Rhea was a teenager. Rhea's father and uncles all smoked around her. Rhea moved to the United States when she was 18 to attend college. She finished school, got married, and had children. Rhea is now 50 years old and has come to her provider because of shortness of breath and a chronic cough.

Vital Signs	Assessment	Labs
BP: 152/78 RR: 26 breaths/minute HR: 95 beats/minute O_2 sat: 92% on room air Height 5′6″ Weight 140 pounds	Client uses she/her pronouns. Appears slightly dyspneic. Cough is productive. Lung sounds are diminished in bilateral bases, with occasional crackles on auscultation. Right extremity appears slightly edematous. Denies smoking or alcohol use	pO_2: 78 mm Hg pCO_2: 45 mm Hg Alpha-1 antitrypsin level: below normal

BP, Blood pressure; *HR,* heart rate; *O_2 sat,* oxygen saturation; *RR,* respiratory rate.

1. Looking at the data, do you think that Rhea has chronic bronchitis or emphysema? Provide evidence.

2. The provider, after assessing Rhea asks, "Are you sure you've never smoked?" Rhea denies smoking. For what other reasons could she have developed lung disease?

3. Outline the major differences between emphysema and chronic bronchitis.

Case Study 8.3

Jon (he/him) is an active 6-year-old boy. For the past few months, Jon has had frequent respiratory infections and a thick, productive cough. He has also had frequent, foul-smelling diarrhea. After doing a series of tests, Jon is diagnosed with cystic fibrosis.

1. Jon's parents are very upset. They ask, "We thought he was tested at birth for this. Why is this showing up now?" What would you say to them?

____

____

____

____

2. As a clinician, how would you explain the progression of the disease? What treatments will Jon potentially need?

____

____

____

____

3. What is the prognosis of an individual with cystic fibrosis?

____

____

____

____

Case Study 8.4

Abena (she/her) is a 15-year-old Black cis-female who comes to the urgent care clinic with shortness of breath. You are her nurse. When you take her vital signs, you notice that she is tachycardic (heart rate [HR]: 130), tachypneic (respiratory rate [RR]: 30), and her oxygen saturation is 93% on room air. She also states that she has been running a low-grade fever. She denies being anxious, is doing well in school, and enjoys sports. She has no allergies, no significant past medical history, and has not traveled. She states that she has gotten COVID three times in the past year, but it has been mild. As she is talking to you, her oxygen saturation dips to 90% on room air.

1. What do you think Abena has? What would cause this to happen?

____

____

____

____

2. What are the hallmark symptoms of this disease? How can you diagnose this?

____

____

____

____

3. What would this condition do to the V/Q ratio?

____

____

____

____

9 Pulmonary Disease Part 2

Respiratory Tract Infections

Rhinitis

Rhinovirus causes the common cold in older children and adults. Respiratory syncytial virus (RSV) and parainfluenza virus are common causes of colds in children under 3 years of age. The virus invades the upper airway and causes an inflammatory response. This leads to increased capillary permeability and mucus secretion. The cough and sore throat are caused by pharyngeal drainage. The virus also may affect the eustachian tube and ears (more so in young children) and cause otitis media and bacterial sinusitis.

Symptoms

- Rhinitis
- Cough
- Sneezing
- Congestion
- Sore throat
- Fever (in younger children)

Diagnosis: history and physical

Treatment: frequent handwashing; children pass it quickly (fingers to face). It is a virus, so there are no medications to treat it; it is self-limiting. Encourage supportive care, rest, and antipyretics.

Rhinosinusitis

Viruses (rhinovirus) causing the common cold lead to rhinosinusitis, allergic rhinitis, smoking, wet and/or cold environment. Rhinosinusitis is a viral infection of the upper respiratory tract, causing swelling and edema of the sinuses. Because of the swelling, the sinuses (ostia) are blocked, creating pockets of mucus. This is highly susceptible to bacterial growth (moist warm places!) and develop into a secondary bacterial infection.

Symptoms

- Same signs and symptoms of cold (but last longer)
- Facial pain
- Headache
- Maxillary pain
- High fever (bacterial)

Diagnosis: acute rhinosinusitis is diagnosed with signs and symptoms; chronic rhinosinusitis (episode lasting >12 weeks). It can be diagnosed by nasal endoscopy or computed tomography (CT) scan.

Treatment: if it is a viral infection, then it is self-limiting with supportive care; if it develops into a secondary bacterial infection, antibiotics will be needed.

Influenza

Influenza A, B, C, and D viruses contain single-stranded RNA made up of two glycoproteins (hemagglutinin and neuraminidase). Mutations in these glycoproteins can make the virus more transmissible and virulent, causing epidemics and pandemics. The viruses directly attack the respiratory epithelium. Viral infection starts in the upper respiratory system (destroying mucous-secreting and ciliated cells) and progresses to the lungs (causing destruction of bronchial and alveolar cells), inflaming the lungs due to the innate and immune response. Adults are infectious a day before signs and symptoms appear. Children are infectious at least a week before signs and symptoms appear. Individuals are contagious up to 10 days after onset of symptoms.

Clinical manifestations:

Early

- Headache
- Cough
- Malaise
- Runny nose
- Fever
- Nausea
- Diarrhea

Viral pneumonia can develop within a day of onset of influenza. The onset of bacterial pneumonia typically occurs 5- to 7 days after the onset of influenza.

Late

- Fever and chills
- Tachypnea
- Tachycardia
- Hypotension
- Sinusitis, bronchitis, and otitis media are common complications
- Can lead to sepsis, shock, and death

Bacterial pneumonia can occur because of the destruction of alveolar and bronchial cells. Immune defenses are down, creating a hospitable environment for infection. With bacterial pneumonia, typically the individual starts to feel better after the initial onset of influenza. Then 5 to 7 days later, they feel much worse, with the return of fever and chills, pleuritic chest pain, and a productive, purulent cough.

Diagnosis: history and physical, flu swab (nasopharyngeal); influenza is typically seen in the winter months (December to March)

Treatment: getting a yearly flu vaccine is the best way to prevent the flu. Antiviral medication may help if flu is caught early; antibiotics are not used with viral illness unless bacterial pneumonia occurs as a complication.

Tuberculosis

Tuberculosis is spread by living in proximity to people who are infected. Autoimmune diseases, such as HIV, increase the risk of getting the disease. *Mycobacterium tuberculosis* is spread by inhaling (airborne) droplets into the lower respiratory tract (lungs). Alveolar macrophages engulf the bacteria but cannot kill it initially. Macrophages initiate an adaptive immune response. This response is chronic and forms a granuloma, walling off the bacteria. The bacteria become dormant and typically die. The granuloma eventually scars and is visible on x-ray.

Tuberculosis can also attack other organs (miliary tuberculosis). In healthy individuals, tuberculosis is asymptomatic, and they develop latent tuberculosis infections, with Ghon foci (granulomas). If an individual is reinfected or the latent bacteria is activated, they can develop secondary tuberculosis with clinical disease. This typically happens when the individual is immunocompromised. Otherwise, the bacteria will be isolated and contained again. In immunocompromised individuals, tuberculosis becomes progressive and primary, with clinical disease (Fig. 9.1).

Symptoms
- Low-grade fever
- Fatigue
- Weight loss
- Cough (purulent or bloody)
- Dyspnea
- Night sweats
- Pleuritic chest pain

Diagnosis: history and physical; a sputum culture is the gold standard (acid-fast stain); chest x-ray (detects granulomas), tuberculin skin test (cannot distinguish active/latent), interferon gamma release assay (blood test)

Treatment: antibiotics, long-term, multi-drug regimen for resistant strains

Pneumonia

Pneumonia is classified by cause and setting. Typical pneumonia is caused by bacteria, such as pneumococcus. Atypical pneumonias are caused by viral and fungal (mycoplasma) infections.

Community-acquired pneumonias are caused by bacteria (*Streptococcus pneumoniae*). The onset of community-acquired pneumonia must be prior to admission to a health care facility or within 48 hours after admission. Older and immunocompromised patients are at high risk for community-acquired pneumonia, which is why pneumococcal vaccination is strongly recommended. Hospital-acquired/nosocomial pneumonia is typically caused by Gram-negative bacteria or

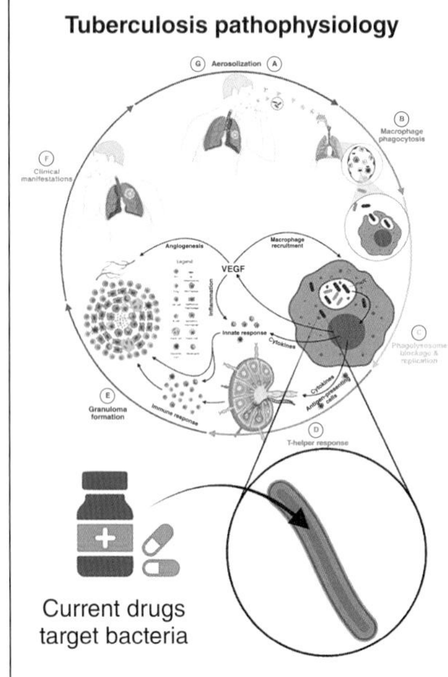

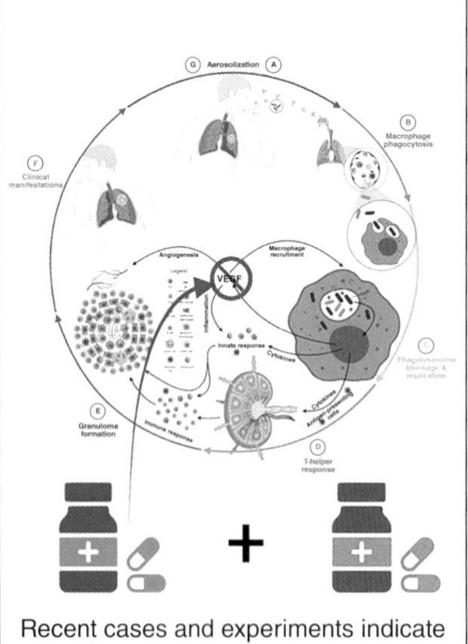

- A review of tuberculosis pathophysiology reveals only a few pharmaceutical targets.
- Current drugs focus on targeting the bacteria and its replication.
- One target revealed by analyzing tuberculosis pathophysiology is VEGF released by macrophages.
- One Anti-VEGF-A drug has shown promise in treating disseminated tuberculosis.
- Anti-VEGF and Anti-VEGFR drugs, with current FDA approval for cancer therapy, should be evaluated clinically for tuberculosis treatment.

• **Fig. 9.1** Tuberculosis pathophysiology. *FDA,* US Food and Drug Administration; *VEGF,* vascular endothelial growth factor; *VEGFR,* vascular endothelial growth factor receptor. (From Maison, D. P. (2022). Tuberculosis pathophysiology and anti-VEGF intervention. *Journal of Clinical Tuberculosis and Other Mycobacterial Diseases*, 27, 100300. https://doi.org/10.1016/j.jctube.2022.100300. https://www.sciencedirect.com/science/article/pii/S2405579422000055.)

staphylococcus. Nosocomial pneumonia is classified as such when onset is more than 48 hours after admission. Patients who are bedbound and/or intubated are at high risk for nosocomial pneumonia.

Typical Pneumonia

With typical pneumonia, bacteria enter the lower respiratory tract and damage the epithelium, cilia, and layer of mucus. This decreases the cough reflex. This accumulation of mucus and lack of cough reflex impairs the immune defenses, making it easier for bacteria to colonize the lungs. This leads to bacterial infections in the alveoli, and alveolar inflammation with exudate. Bacterial pneumonia can be seen on x-ray, as the exudate shows up as lobar consolidation.

Clinical manifestations: there is acute onset, cough, high fevers and chills, malaise, and pleuritic pain; there are fine crackles in the affected lung(s), and decreased lung sounds; the cough is productive, progressing to purulent and blood-tinged sputum

> **NOTE**
>
> Older individuals may not have typical symptoms, such as fever. Instead, they can have altered mental status, fatigue, and anorexia.

Diagnosis: history and physical, sputum culture, labs, blood culture, x-ray

Treatment: antibiotics

Atypical Pneumonia

With atypical pneumonia, viruses and fungi can infiltrate and damage the lower respiratory epithelium. This causes inflammation of the alveolar septum and lung tissue, not the alveoli. Therefore, there is no fluid buildup in the lungs or consolidation, so it may not be seen on x-ray. Clinical manifestations are typically mild, though they can progress to secondary bacterial pneumonia.

Symptoms

- Fever
- Headache
- Muscle aches
- Dry hacking cough

Diagnosis: signs and symptoms, x-ray, blood cultures, lab work

Treatment: antifungals and antibiotics for fungal or bacterial infections; if viral infection, supportive treatment

Covid-19

Coronavirus, or COVID-19 (SARS-Cov-2-2019), is transmitted by air (airborne precautions). The virus is extremely volatile and has been mutating rapidly into different strains, some of them even more transmissible and virulent than the original virus. COVID-19 is a virus with single-stranded RNA. The virus' spike protein binds to ACE2 receptors in the nose, intestines, heart, and kidneys first and then starts to replicate in the lungs (which is the reason for the lag time between symptom onset and pneumonia). Also, there are not as many ACE2 receptors in the lungs as in other organs, so the lungs take longer to infiltrate. ACE2 has multiple functions; it helps to lower blood pressure by breaking down angiotensin II, but it also helps to upregulate bradykinin production. (Remember bradykinin in Chapter 1?) once bradykinin is upregulated, a bradykinin storm occurs, and inflammatory processes accelerate quickly. Bradykinin causes pain, increases capillary permeability, and facilitates widespread clotting. Bradykinin also breaks down the blood-brain barrier. The COVID-19 virus also causes the lungs to produce hyaluronic acid, which is thick and sticky, like a gel. Therefore, it is so hard to intubate and ventilate COVID patients. Note: People who are Black and Hispanic have disproportionately high mortality rates from COVID-19!

The pathophysiology of COVID-19 correlates closely with the symptoms. Although COVID-19 may start off mild, with cough, fever, sneezing, and gastrointestinal (GI) distress, it can progress to multiorgan injury. Systemic inflammation leads to increased capillary permeability and edema of the brain, lungs, and heart. The hyaluronic acid filling the lungs can lead to a "white-out," fluid filling the lungs, which can then lead to respiratory failure. Inflammation also causes liver damage and pancreatic damage, which can lead to liver failure and diabetes. Inflammation also causes vascular damage to the kidneys (kidney failure), blood vessels, and heart. Myocarditis can occur because of viral infiltration and inflammation. There is systemic clotting as well, causing strokes, myocardial infarctions, bowel ischemia, and pulmonary emboli.

Complications: long COVID; evidence shows that the body's reaction to COVID-19 continues to wreak havoc in the body; weakness, loss of mental acuity, palpitations, insomnia, joint and muscle pain, dizziness, change in smell and taste, and chest pain are some of the many manifestations of long COVID (Fig. 9.2).

Diagnosis: signs and symptoms, x-ray, lab work, nasopharyngeal swab with polymerase chain reaction (PCR) test to confirm.

Treatment: nirmatrelvir/ritonavir and molnupiravir (oral antivirals), remdesivir (intravenous [IV] antiviral), steroids, supportive therapy; intubation and ventilation if respiratory failure is imminent; monoclonal antibodies are also authorized for use

Lung Cancer

Lung cancer is the leading cause of cancer-related death globally. Risk factors are smoking, pollution, genetics, asbestos, social determinants of health.

Non-Small Cell Lung Cancer

Squamous cell carcinoma

- Correlated strongly with smoking
- Assigned male at birth > assigned female at birth

Adenocarcinoma

- Correlated with smoking
- Commonly occurs in assigned females at birth and nonsmokers

LONG-TERM EFFECTS of COVID-19 INFECTION
* FATIGUE
* SHORTNESS of BREATH
* COUGH
* LOSS of TASTE & SMELL
* CONFUSION & DIFFICULTY CONCENTRATING
* HEADACHES & BODY ACHES
* NAUSEA or DIARRHEA
* DAMAGE to HEART, LUNGS, & KIDNEYS
* THROMBOEMBOLIC EVENTS
OSMOSIS.org
#RAISETHELINE
#FLATTENTHECURVE

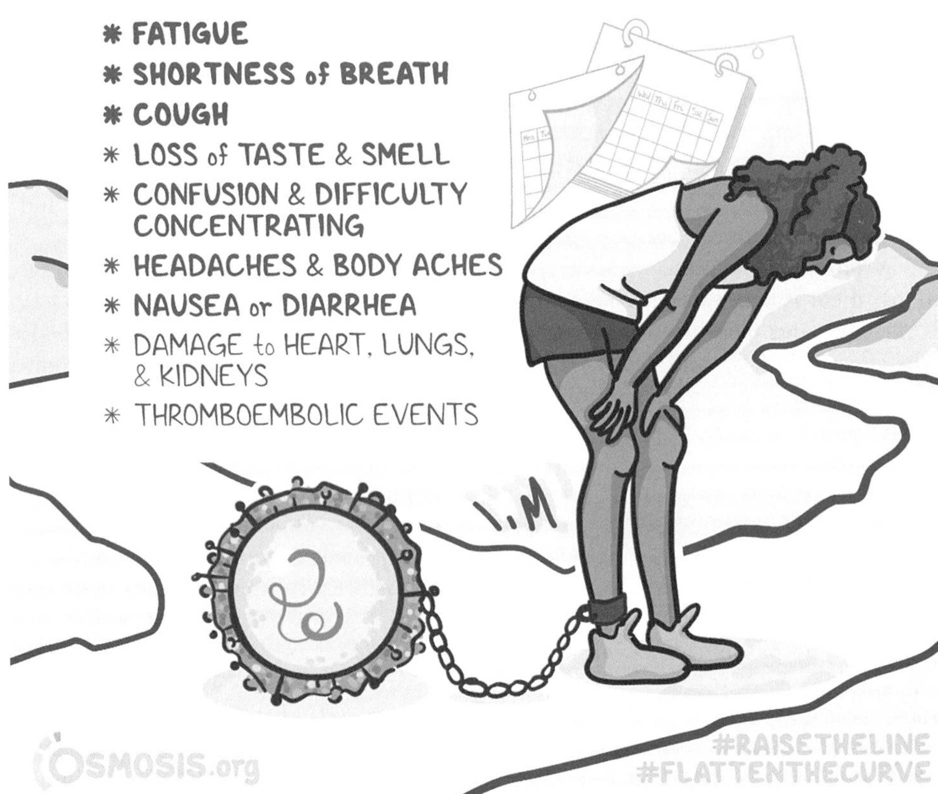

• **Fig. 9.2** Long-term effects of COVID-19. (From https://www.facebook.com/OsmoseIt/photos/a.293866334077588/2127504564047080/?type=3.)

- Poorer prognosis than squamous cell carcinoma

Large cell carcinoma

- Poor prognosis and early metastasis

Small-Cell Lung Cancer

- Small-cell lung cancers are highly malignant, often metastasizing quickly, and inoperable
- Cancer cells arise from neuroendocrine cells of the bronchi
- Strongest association with smoking
- Associated with many paraneoplastic syndromes (syndrome of inappropriate antidiuretic hormone [SIADH], parathyroid hormone [PTH], adrenocorticotropic hormone [ACTH])

Symptoms

- Nonspecific—weight loss, anorexia
- Respiratory—chronic cough, dyspnea, wheezing, hemoptysis

Complications: metastases to bone, brain, liver, and lymph; respiratory failure

Diagnosis: history and physical, x-ray, CT scan, magnetic resonance imaging (MRI), positron emission tomography (PET) scans, tumor markers

Treatment: surgery, chemotherapy, radiation, immunotherapy

Pediatric Respiratory Issues

Upper Airway Infection

Croup

Viral infection (parainfluenza virus) is seen in children from 3 months to 5 years of age. The virus invades the upper respiratory tract, initially causes upper respiratory tract infection. It then goes on to cause inflammation of the laryngotracheal tree, causing the narrowing of the subglottic area.

Symptoms

- Cold symptoms initially
- Inspiratory stridor
- Barking cough
- Dyspnea
- Retractions

Treatment: cold or warm, moist air, oxygen, steroids for inflammation, nebulized racemic epinephrine

Complications: respiratory distress, respiratory failure

Epiglottitis

Epiglottitis is caused by *Haemophilus influenzae* type B bacterial infection, typically occurring in children from 3 to 7 years of age, but may also occur in adults who have not

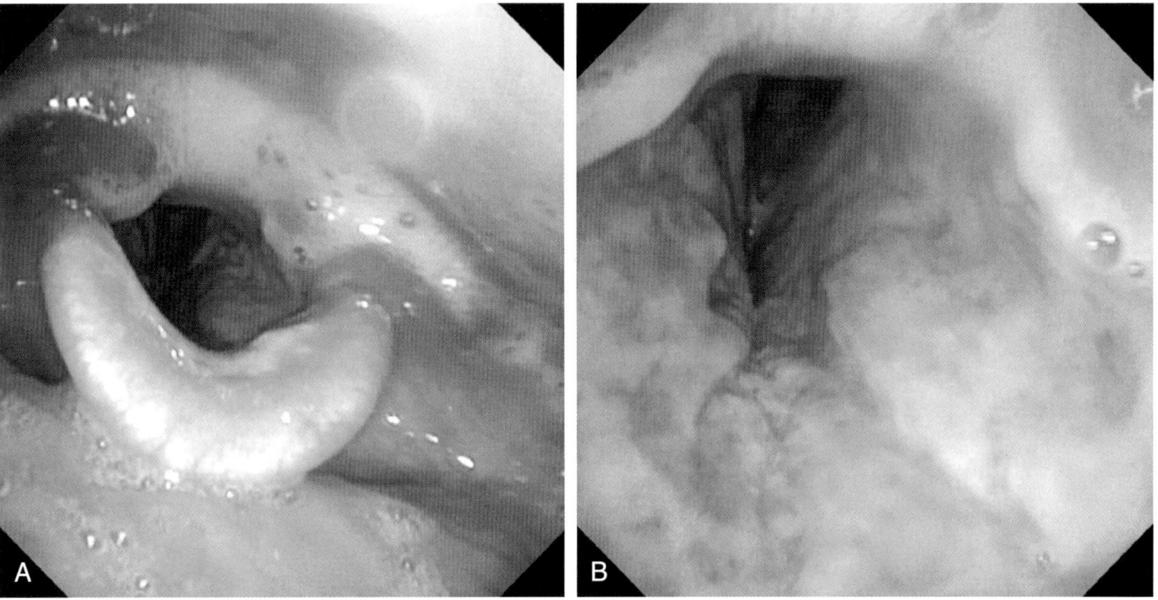

• **Fig. 9.3** Epiglottitis. (From Iwamoto, S., Sato, M. P., Hoshi, Y., Otsuki, N., Doi, K. (2023). COVID-19 presenting as acute epiglottitis: case report and literature review. *Auris Nasus Larynx*, 50(1), 165-168. https://doi.org/10.1016/j.anl.2021.12.007. https://www.sciencedirect.com/science/article/pii/S0385814621002832.)

been vaccinated or have not received vaccine boosters. It is a bacterial infection of the upper airway, causing inflammation and edema of the epiglottis and pharyngeal structures, and is an acute, rapidly progressing illness (Fig. 9.3).

Symptoms

- Severe respiratory distress
- Flaring of nares
- Inspiratory retractions
- Restlessness
- Tachycardia
- Lethargy
- Sitting up with chin forward and mouth open
- Drool
- Difficulty swallowing
- Muffled voice
- Anxiety
- Inspiratory stridor

Diagnosis: clinical signs and symptoms

Treatment: nothing by or in mouth! Immediate hospitalization is required; decrease anxiety, position for comfort; cool mist, oxygen, intravenous (IV) fluids, IV antibiotics; make intubation tray available

Complications: asphyxia, respiratory distress, respiratory failure

Lower Airway Infection

Acute Bronchiolitis

Bronchiolitis starts as a viral infection of the lower airways (RSV). The virus invades the upper respiratory system, eventually reaching the lower lobes of the lungs and causing inflammation, increased mucus production, narrowing of bronchi, and necrosis of the respiratory epithelium. The blocked and inflamed alveoli lead to alveolar air trapping. This air will eventually be completely absorbed into the lungs, causing the alveoli to collapse (atelectasis) (Fig. 9.4).

Symptoms

- Wheezing
- Dyspnea
- Irritability
- Cough
- Tachypnea
- Retractions

Diagnosis: history and physical, pulse oximetry, chest x-ray, RSV nasal swab

Treatment: oxygen, IV fluids, supportive oxygen therapy

Complications: respiratory distress and/or failure

Study Guide for Chapter 9

Make sure that you have your class notes and textbooks on hand to answer these questions. A concept map is included to help you to diagram and link disease concepts together.

1. What causes the common cold? Is there a difference between what causes colds in children and adults?

____

____

____

____

2. What are the symptoms of the common cold? How is it transmitted and prevented?

____

____

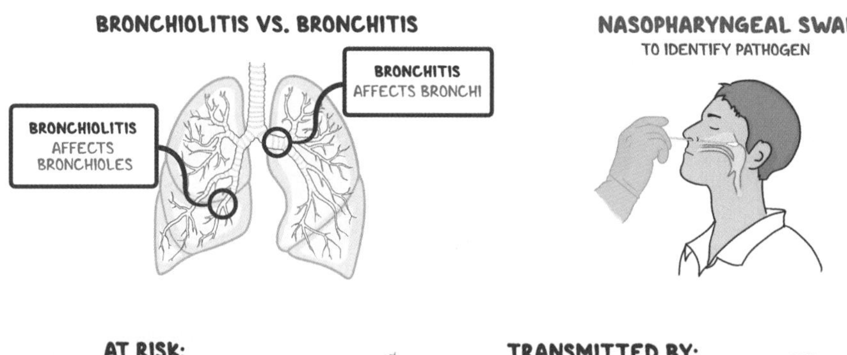

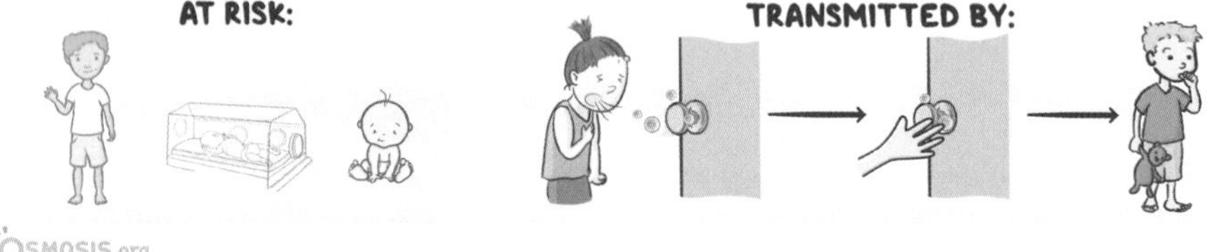

• **Fig. 9.4** Bronchiolitis. (From https://www.osmosis.org/answers/bronchiolitis.)

3. What is rhinosinusitis? What causes it and what are its manifestations?

4. How is rhinosinusitis different from the common cold?

5. What causes influenza? How does the virus attack cells?

6. What are the symptoms and complications of influenza? How is it transmitted, diagnosed, and prevented?

7. Differentiate between primary and secondary tuberculosis.

8. What causes tuberculosis? What are the symptoms? How would you diagnose it? What is a Ghon focus? What are the complications of tuberculosis?

9. What are the causes of pneumonia? What are the symptoms and complications of pneumonia?

10. Differentiate between hospital-acquired pneumonia and community-acquired pneumonia. When would you classify pneumonia as hospital-acquired or community-acquired?

11. What are the differences between non-small cell lung cancer and small-cell lung cancer? What are the types of non-small cell lung carcinoma?

12. What are the symptoms of lung cancer? What is paraneoplastic syndrome?

13. What are croup and epiglottitis? List the causes, symptoms, and complications of both. How are they different? Who is infected by these diseases?

14. When would you see bronchiolitis? What causes it? What are the symptoms and complications?

STUDY TIPS

Don't forget to draw things out and use templates or T-charts! Whatever works best for you!
Example:

	Epiglottitis	Croup
Cause?		
Pathophysiology?		
Symptoms?		

Concept Map

Use this concept map to link each disease to its pathophysiology, diagnostics, causes, risk factors, complications, and clinical manifestations together. This way, you will be able to see the whole picture of the disease.

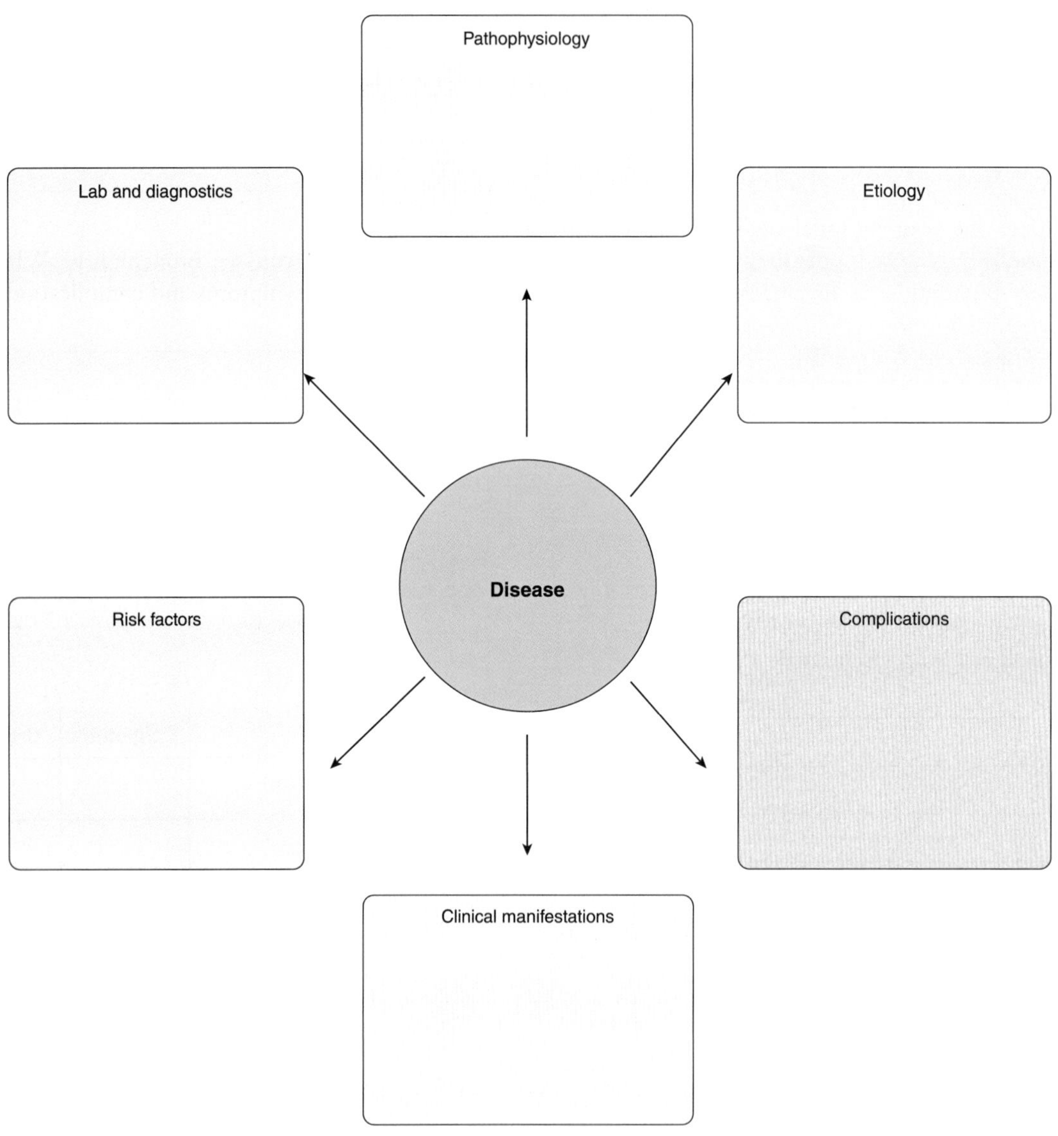

Case Studies for Chapter 9

Case Study 9.1

Indrani is a 57-year-old Malaysian cis-female (she/her). She is experiencing a cough, runny nose, low-grade fever, and diarrhea. She takes a home COVID test and she tests positive.

1. Explain the pathophysiology of the disease. Is this a definitive diagnosis? Why or why not?

____

2. What precautions should she take?

____

Indrani starts to feel better after a few days. However, after a week, she starts to experience severe dyspnea and can't seem to catch her breath.

3. What is causing these symptoms? Should she go to the emergency room right away? Explain.

Indrani ends up being hospitalized, intubated, and receives intravenous (IV) antivirals and steroids. She recovers slowly and can be discharged home after 3 weeks in the hospital. Her family notices that she is often in a "fog" and confused. A month after discharge, Indrani experiences a left-sided stroke.

4. Could her post discharge symptoms be linked to COVID? Explain.

Case Study 9.2

Callie (she/her) and her wife Susan (she/her) have brought their 3-year-old child, Sam (he/him), to the emergency room for difficulty breathing. Callie states that Sam has had a cold for the last few days but started having a cough and shortness of breath at bedtime. You are the nurse triaging the child.

Vitals	Focused Assessment
Heart rate: 110 beats/minute Respiratory rate: 40 breaths/minute Oxygen saturation: 95% on room air	Client uses he/him pronouns Client appears anxious, barking cough, stridor, tachypnea, retractions noted

1. Looking at the vitals and assessment, what diagnosis would you expect for Sam? Why?

2. What is causing the stridor, retractions, and cough? Explain the pathophysiology.

The provider orders nebulized racemic epinephrine and steroids.

3. Why would these medications be ordered?

Case Study 9.3

Dave (he/him) is a 45-year-old White cis-male who suddenly started experiencing fever and chills within the last 24 hours. He states that he has not seen his provider for years, as he is normally very healthy. He states that he does not believe in vaccinations because he feels that his immune system is "strong enough to take care of things."

Vitals	Assessment	Labs
Heart rate: 100 beats/minute Temperature: 103°F Respiratory rate: 26 breaths/minute O_2 sat: 97% on room air	Client uses he/him pronouns Client is shivering, nauseated, complaining of muscle aches and headache	Influenza A: negative Influenza B: positive COVID: negative

1. Looking at the assessment, what is Dave's diagnosis? Are his symptoms typical?

2. What would you expect the treatment to be?

Dave starts to feel better after 4 or 5 days, but then develops nasal congestion, sinus pain, brownish productive cough, and a fever. He comes back to his provider, who orders x-rays.

X-ray Report
Right lower lobe consolidation/infiltrate Maxillofacial sinuses appear inflamed and blocked

3. Why has Dave's illness progressed?

4. Is this a bacterial or viral disease? How do you know?

5. On auscultation, what lung sounds would you expect to hear?

Case Study 9.4

Gina is a 55-year-old cis-female (she/her) who works as a nurse on a med/surg floor of a hospital. She has a history of autoimmune disease (lupus) and type 2 diabetes mellitus. When she gets her annual tuberculin test, it is positive.

1. Does this mean that Gina has tuberculosis? Why or why not?

2. Describe the course of tuberculosis in a healthy individual.

Gina gets a chest x-ray and sputum culture and is diagnosed with primary progressive tuberculosis.

3. What is the difference between primary and secondary tuberculosis infection?

4. What risk factors caused Gina to develop primary tuberculosis?

Gina is put on a 6-month antibiotic regimen. However, she has difficulty with the side effects of the medication and stops taking the antibiotics early.

5. What complication(s) might Gina experience as a result?

10
Endocrine Disorders

Endocrine Glands

Let's do a quick review—hormones are chemical messengers that stimulate cells and tissues. Autocrine hormones are secreted by a cell to act on itself. Paracrine hormones are secreted by cells to nearby target cells. Endocrine glands secrete protein and steroid hormones into the bloodstream, which carries the hormones to target organs. Hormones are short-acting and there are elimination enzymes which break down hormones. When there are genetic issues or disease processes that affect hormone production or elimination, severe complications may result. In this chapter, we will be talking about endocrine disorders and their complications.

Most of our hormones are controlled by the hypothalamus and pituitary axis. The hypothalamus produces hormones such as corticotropin-releasing hormone (CRH) and thyrotropin-releasing hormone (TRH). These hormones then act on the anterior pituitary gland, which releases stimulating hormones, such as thyrotropin-stimulating hormone (TSH) and adrenocorticotropic hormone (ACTH). The hypothalamus also produces antidiuretic hormone and oxytocin, which is stored and released from the posterior pituitary gland.

When there is a hormonal disorder, we need to look at whether it is a primary, secondary, or tertiary disorder. A primary disorder is an issue with the target gland. A secondary disorder would be an issue with the anterior or posterior pituitary gland. A tertiary disorder would be an issue with the hypothalamus. These issues could be trauma-related, a tumor, or congenital/genetic disorders. In this chapter, we will be concentrating on thyroid disorders, adrenal disorders, type 1 diabetes mellitus (T1DM), and type 2 diabetes mellitus (T2DM).

Diagnostic Tests for Hormonal Disorders

Blood tests: hormone levels, antibody levels, blood glucose
Urine tests: hormone levels, metabolites
Stimulation tests
Suppression tests
Radioactive iodine uptake
Genetic testing
Imaging (i.e., magnetic resonance imaging [MRI], computed tomography [CT] scan, ultrasound)

Thyroid Gland

The follicular cells of the thyroid produce and secrete triiodothyronine (T3) and thyroxine (T4). There are higher levels of T4 which is the inactive form of the hormone. T4 is converted to T3, which is the active form. The thyroid hormones are fat-soluble, which means they need to be carried through the blood by proteins, such as albumin. The hormones increase basal metabolic rate (BMR) and cause breakdown of muscle, absorption of glucose, and catabolism of fats and cholesterol. The hormones are necessary for growth and development, sexual maturity, and central nervous system development. Thyroid peroxidase oxidizes iodide ions to produce T3 and T4.

Thyroid hormone production is controlled by a negative feedback loop, which is stimulated by stressors, such as lack of sleep and cold temperatures acting on the hypothalamus. This causes the release of TRHs from the hypothalamus, which acts on the anterior pituitary gland. The anterior pituitary gland then releases thyroid-stimulating hormones which directly stimulates the thyroid gland to release T3 and T4. However, when there is too much T3 and T4, the excess hormones act to shut down production, causing feedback inhibition to the anterior pituitary and hypothalamus.

Thyroid Disorders

Thyroid disorders are on a continuum. Normal thyroid function is called euthyroid. Decreased thyroid function is called hypothyroidism. Severe hypothyroidism can devolve to become myxedema coma. Similarly, when the thyroid is overactive, it is called hyperthyroidism. Severe hyperthyroidism is called thyrotoxicosis or thyroid storm.

One of the more common symptoms of thyroid disorder is goiter, or an enlarged thyroid gland. This can happen with hypothyroidism, hyperthyroidism, and normal function. With primary hypothyroidism, goiter can be caused by an overproduction of TSH to stimulate the thyroid gland to produce T3 and T4. The excess TSH causes hyperplasia and hypertrophy of the thyroid cells, causing the thyroid to enlarge. With hyperthyroidism, the thyroid is overproducing hormones. This effort can lead to the gland enlarging as well. With a normal thyroid gland, certain foods and medications can block iodine uptake and hormone synthesis. This leads to an "artificial" hypothyroidism, leading to goiter. Cruciferous vegetables such as Brussels sprouts and broccoli are examples. High or low iodine levels can also cause a normally functioning thyroid gland to enlarge. Toxic nodular goiters can occur, with follicular cells in the nodules overproducing thyroid hormone. Also, multinodular goiters can become quite large and occlude the airway.

Hypothyroidism

Congenital hypothyroidism is seen at birth when the newborn has an absent or defective thyroid gland. This is a condition that is tested for within 24 to 48 hours of birth. This type of hypothyroidism must be treated within the first 6 weeks of life with hormone supplementation to achieve neurotypical brain development. Clinical signs seen in infants are prolonged jaundice, large tongue, respiratory issues, sluggishness, and developmental delay. Acquired hypothyroidism, caused by thyroidectomies, iodine deficiency, head and neck radiation treatment, and autoimmune disorders, can affect thyroid hormone production and destroy the thyroid gland (Table 10.1). Assigned females at birth (AFAB) have higher rates of hypothyroidism as the thyroid gland can atrophy after age 50 years.

NOTE

In resource-challenged nations, iodine deficiency is the most common cause of hypothyroidism.

The most commonly acquired form of hypothyroidism in developing nations is Hashimoto thyroiditis. As the "itis" suggests, this is an inflammatory autoimmune disease and seen more often in AFAB than in assigned males at birth (AMAB). Antithyroid antibodies attack the thyroid gland, causing inflammation, scarring, and fibrosis, leading to an enlarged thyroid, or goiter. Initially, this causes the thyroid gland to release its stores of T3 and T4, which causes hyperthyroid symptoms and can cause thyroid storm. As the thyroid gland becomes less and less functional, production of T3 and T4 falls off and hypothyroidism ensues. Lab findings for Hashimoto thyroiditis include high TSH levels, low T4 and T3 levels, increased antithyroid peroxidase (Anti-TPO) antibodies. Decreased glucose levels may also result, as thyroid hormones cause glucose to be released in the blood.

NOTE

Once you have one autoimmune disease, you are prone to having multiple autoimmune diseases and syndromes.

TABLE 10.1 Hypothyroidism Hormone Levels

Disorders	Causes	Hormone Levels
Primary	Thyroidectomy Defective T3, T4 secretions	↓T3 and T4 ↑TSH ↑TRH ↓Radioactive iodine uptake ↑Anti-TPO antibodies (if Hashimoto)
Secondary	Anterior pituitary disease/tumor	↓T3 and T4 ↓TSH ↑TRH ↓Radioactive iodine uptake
Tertiary	Hypothalamic dysfunction	↓T3 and T4 ↓TSH ↓TRH ↓Radioactive iodine uptake

T3, Triiodothyronine; *T4,* thyroxine; *TPO,* antithyroid peroxidase; *TRH,* thyrotropin-releasing hormone; *TSH,* thyrotropin-stimulating hormone.

If hypothyroidism causes a decrease in the BMR, logically, what would you expect to see? Decreased cardiac output, bradycardia, fatigue, lethargy, dyspnea, weakness, constipation, and weight gain are some of the signs of a decreased metabolic rate. Individuals with this disorder may have hypothermia, depression, confusion, and have dry skin and muscle weakness. Severe hypothyroidism is called myxedema coma. With myxedema coma, mucous edema starts to accumulate in the face, pleural and pericardial cavities, and connective tissues. This causes periorbital edema and contributes to a mask-like effect to the face. As the client becomes more hypoglycemic and hypothermic, coma, cardiac arrest, respiratory failure, and death can result (Fig. 10.1).

Symptoms (Hint: everything goes down!):
- Fatigue and lethargy
- Bradycardia
- Weakness
- Constipation
- Weight gain
- Dyspnea
- Decreased deep tendon reflexes
- Depression
- Confusion
- Dry skin
- Brittle nails and hair
- Cold intolerance

Symptoms for myxedema coma:
- Hypoglycemia
- Hypothermia
- Mucus edema
- Coma
- Cardiac and respiratory arrest

Diagnostics: history and physical, serum TSH and T4 levels, ultrasound, CT scan

Treatment for hypothyroidism: hormone supplement (levothyroxine)

Treatment for myxedema coma: rewarming the client slowly, administering synthetic thyroid hormone, and respiratory support (intubation, continuous positive airway pressure [CPAP], bilevel positive airway pressure [BiPAP]) if needed

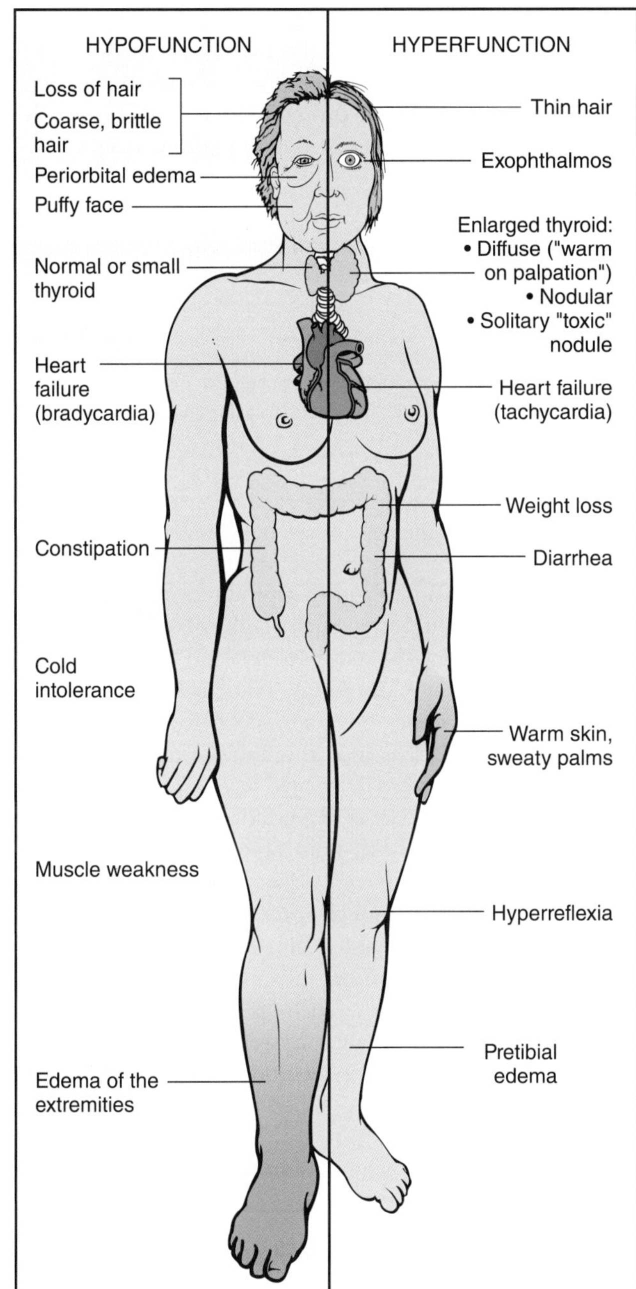

• **Fig. 10.1** Manifestations of hypo- and hyperthyroidism. (From McCance, K. L. (2019). Cancer Epidemiology. In K. L. McCance, S. E. Huether, V. Brashers, & N. Rote (Eds.), Pathophysiology: The Biologic Basis for Disease in Adults and Children (8th ed). Elsevier.)

Hyperthyroidism

Hyperthyroidism can be due to a congenital (birth) defect, but more often it is an acquired disorder. It can be caused by excessive amounts of iodine (produces more T3 and T4), thyroid adenoma, and thyroiditis (initially before gland is destroyed) (Table 10.2). However, the most common form of hyperthyroidism is an autoimmune disease called Graves' disease (Fig. 10.2).

TABLE 10.2 Hyperthyroidism Hormone Levels

Disorder	Causes	Hormone Levels
Primary	Graves disease, adenoma, thyroiditis, iodine excess	↑T4 and T3 ↓TSH ↑High radioactive iodine uptake ↑TPO ↑Thyrotropin receptor antibodies
Secondary	Issue with anterior pituitary	↑T4 and T3 ↑TSH ↑High radioactive iodine uptake
Tertiary	Issue with hypothalamus	↑T4 and T3 ↑TSH ↑TRH ↑High radioactive iodine uptake

T3, Triiodothyronine; *T4,* thyroxine; *TPO,* antithyroid peroxidase; *TRH,* thyrotropin-releasing hormone; *TSH,* thyrotropin-stimulating hormone.

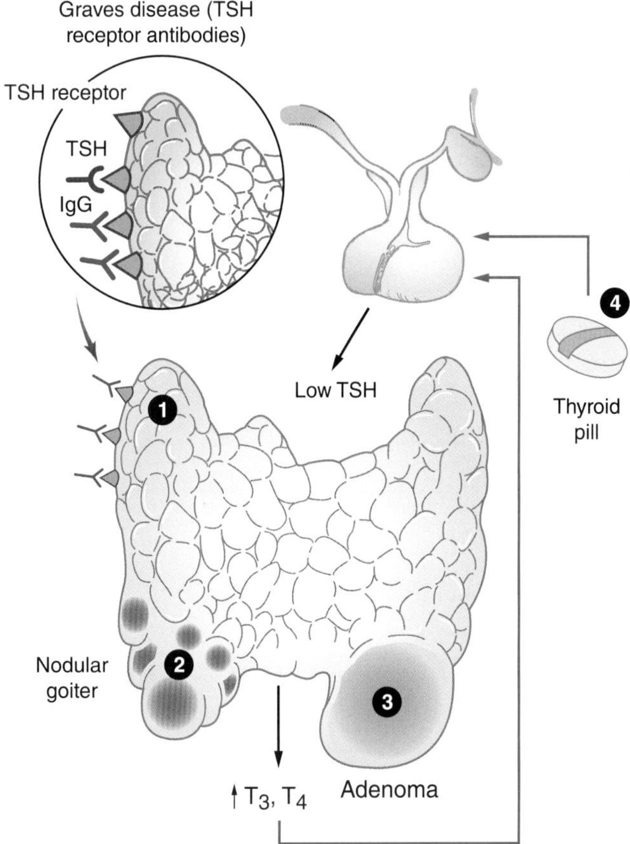

• **Fig. 10.2** Causes of hyperthyroidism. *IgG,* Immunoglobulin G; *T3,* triiodothyronine; *T4,* thyroxine; *TSH,* thyrotropin-stimulating hormone. (Adapted from Damjanov I. (2012). Pathology for the health professions, (4th ed.). Elsevier, Saunders.)

Graves disease is an autoimmune disease; the cause is unknown. This disease has exacerbations and remissions, triggered by stressful life events, trauma, surgery, and illness. In Graves disease, thyroid-stimulating antibodies bind to the thyrotropin (TSH) receptor on the thyroid gland. This blocks TSH from binding but causes the thyroid gland to produce excess amounts to T3 and T4. The negative feedback look does not work, as the autoantibodies directly stimulate the thyroid. Graves disease has a strong genetic, familial tendency. Because the thyroid is a very vascular organ, a thrill may be felt when palpating the thyroid and a bruit heard when auscultating the thyroid.

Hallmark symptoms of Graves disease are ophthalmopathy (bulging eyes), goiter (enlarged thyroid), and hyperthyroidism. Ophthalmopathy occurs because of the inflammation caused by exacerbations. The swelling and edema push the eyes out, causing them to bulge. There is a risk of dry eye, irritation, corneal ulcers, and infections because the eyes cannot close all the way. Remember that increased thyroid hormones mean an increased metabolic rate. Logically, what would happen? An increased heart rate, hypertension, increased cardiac output, dyspnea, agitation, and increased deep tendon reflexes. Gastric motility increases, so nausea, vomiting, and diarrhea are common, along with weight loss. Individuals with Graves disease often feel hot and have heat intolerance and have difficulty sleeping. Antithyroid medications can be given during exacerbations. With severe hyperthyroidism, thyroid storm can occur. Clients usually have extreme anxiety, dyspnea, chest pain, palpitations, and delirium. Hyperthermia is common, with body temperatures over 105°F (see Fig. 10.1).

Symptoms:

- Tachycardia
- Hypertension
- Dyspnea on exertion
- Agitation
- Restlessness
- Insomnia
- Increased deep tendon reflexes
- Diarrhea
- Weight loss
- Ophthalmopathy (Graves disease)
- Goiter
- Heat intolerance
- Diaphoresis
- Fine hair

Symptoms of thyroid storm:

- Very high fever
- Tachycardia
- Anxiety
- Chest pain
- Delirium

Diagnostics: history and physical, serum TSH and T4 levels, ultrasound, CT scan

Treatment for hyperthyroidism: antithyroid medications, beta-blockers, thyroidectomy

Treatment for thyroid storm: this is a medical emergency and needs to be treated right away; clients need to be cooled down; steroids can help with inflammation and can stop the conversion of T4 to T3; medications such as beta-blockers (which decrease sympathetic nervous system symptoms) and propylthiouracil (PTU) can be given; a thyroidectomy can also be performed to remove the thyroid gland

> **NOTE**
>
> If you haven't already noticed, hypo- and hyperthyroidism have opposite symptoms. That is, when you know one, you can figure out the other! With hypothyroidism, symptoms result in depressed function. With hyperthyroidism, symptoms result in increased and overactive functions. This makes it much easier to figure out clinical manifestations, rather than just memorizing them.

Adrenal Cortex

The adrenal cortex is a gland that produces and secretes 30 different steroid hormones, such as glucocorticoids (cortisol), mineralocorticoids (aldosterone), and androgens (dehydroepiandrosterone [DHEA]). Like thyroid hormones, the levels of hormones are managed through a negative feedback loop and are carried through the blood by serum proteins such as albumin. Increased levels of corticosteroids act as negative feedback to the anterior pituitary (ACTH) and hypothalamus (CRH), shutting off production.

Glucocorticoids help regulate metabolism and increase serum blood glucose through gluconeogenesis (converting noncarbohydrates to glucose). Glucocorticoids also act as an anti-inflammatory, decreasing inflammation and stress response. Mineralocorticoids, such as aldosterone, regulate sodium and potassium balance, as well as fluid balance. Too much aldosterone causes fluid retention. Androgens influence secondary sex characteristics. When there is a corticosteroid deficiency, Addison disease can result. If there is corticosteroid excess, Cushing syndrome or Cushing disease can result.

Adrenal Cortex Disorders

Addison Disease

When there is a primary, secondary, or tertiary disorder causing a deficiency in steroid hormone production, Addison disease can result (Table 10.3). The major cause of Addison disease is autoimmune disease, which destroys the adrenal cortex. Individuals with the disease do not show symptoms until over 90% of the glands are destroyed. With Addison disease all three classes of corticosteroids are deficient—glucocorticoids, mineralocorticoids, and androgens. This leads to a slow metabolic rate, hypoglycemia, and fluid loss. Think about it logically—without corticosteroids and mineralocorticoids, what would result? Low blood sugar, less immune suppression, and less fluids! So it makes sense that the hallmark signs of this disease are dehydration, weakness, fatigue, anorexia, and weight loss. With a primary disorder, the anterior secretes excess ACTH to stimulate the

TABLE 10.3 Addison Disease Hormone Levels

Disorders	Causes	Hormone Levels
Primary	Autoimmune disease Infection Trauma Medications Cancer Surgery	↓Steroid hormones ↑ACTH ↑CRH
Secondary	Anterior pituitary disease/tumor	↓Steroid hormones ↓ACTH ↑CRH
Tertiary	Hypothalamic dysfunction	↓Steroid hormones ↓ACTH ↓CRH

ACTH, Adrenocorticotrophic hormone; *CRH,* corticotropin-releasing hormone.

adrenal cortex. ACTH is very similar in composition to melanocyte-stimulating hormone, causing excessive melanin production and skin hyperpigmentation. Clients with hyperpigmentation may have patchy dark sites, or they can look like they have tanned skin.

Addison disease can develop into Addisonian crisis triggered by a sudden decrease in corticosteroids, stress, overexertion, cold temperatures, or acute infection. Other signs are pallor, hypotension (low blood volume), tachycardia, abdominal pain, fever and chills, hyponatremia, hyperkalemia, confusion, irritability, and somnolence. This is a medical emergency (Fig. 10.3).

Symptoms for Addison disease:

- Progressive weakness
- Weight loss
- Dehydration
- Fatigue
- Hyperpigmentation

Symptoms for Addisonian crisis:

- Hypotension
- Extreme dehydration
- Fever and chills
- Abdominal pain
- Nausea and vomiting
- Hyponatremia/hyperkalemia
- Irritability
- Confusion
- Somnolence
- Coma

Diagnostic tests: adrenal gland stimulation tests, blood urea nitrogen (BUN) (high with dehydration), and urine cortisol levels (low).

Treatment for Addison disease: corticosteroid supplementation. Because corticosteroids help to mitigate the stress response, not having any can be very dangerous, so corticosteroid supplementation, especially in times of stress, is extremely important.

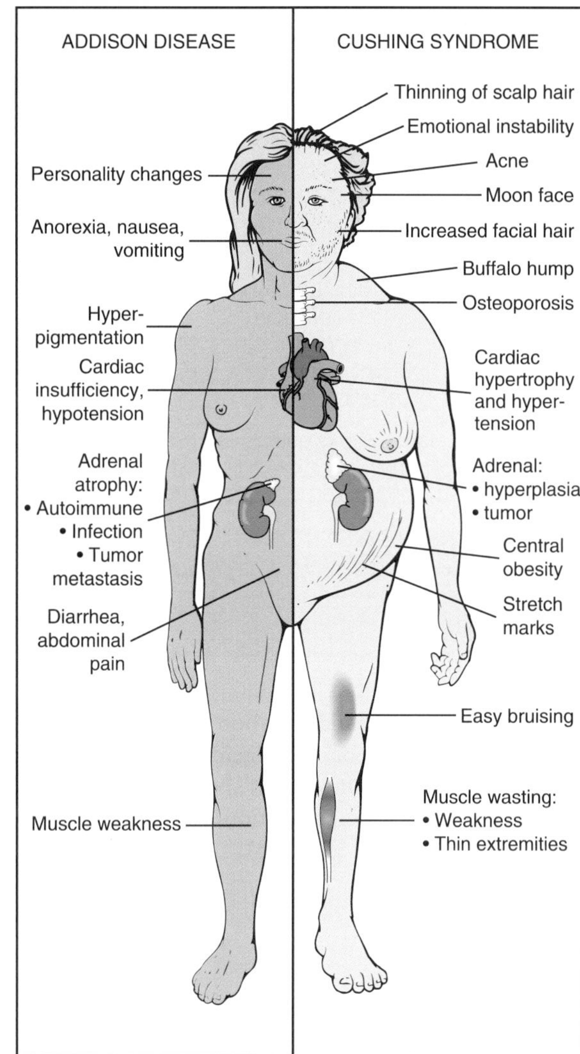

• **Fig. 10.3** Addison and Cushing symptoms. (From Salvo, S. G. (2022). *Mosby's pathology for massage professionals* (5th ed.). Elsevier. Fig. 7.9.)

Treatment for Addisonian crisis: fluid resuscitation (for hypotension), high-dose corticosteroid infusions, and addressing electrolyte and glucose imbalances

Cushing Syndrome/Disease

When there is oversecretion of corticosteroids, Cushing syndrome or Cushing disease can result. Cushing syndrome is an issue with the adrenal gland or hypothalamus. When there is a secondary disorder, such as an anterior pituitary tumor, it is called Cushing disease. Exogenous steroids, or steroids taken by mouth, may also cause Cushing syndrome (Table 10.4). When there is an excess of corticosteroids, it makes the liver less sensitive to insulin and blood sugar increases, resulting in hyperglycemia. Aldosterone levels also increase, causing sodium and water retention. Excess steroids also cause decreased inflammation and immune response and slower healing. Muscle atrophies because protein is catabolized and fat accumulates in the midsection, the back of the neck (buffalo hump), and around the clavicles. Due to extra aldosterone,

TABLE 10.4 Cushing Hormone Levels

Disorder	Causes	Hormone Levels
Primary (Cushing syndrome)	Adrenal tumor, excessive use of corticosteroid medication, gender affirming therapy	↑Steroid hormones ↓ACTH ↓CRH
Secondary (Cushing disease)	Issue with anterior pituitary, adenoma, paraneoplastic syndrome (cancer cells secreting ACTH)	↑Steroid hormones ↑ACTH ↓CRH
Tertiary (Cushing syndrome)	Issue with hypothalamus	↑Steroid hormones ↑ACTH ↑CRH

ACTH, Adrenocorticotrophic hormone; *CRH,* corticotropin-releasing hormone.

there is fluid retention. Fluid retention and fat also cause the face to become puffy (moon face). Steroids also cause the skin to be thinner, lose subcutaneous fat, and become more fragile due to decreased collagen production, causing bruising and stretch marks (striae) (see Fig. 10.3).

Symptoms:

- Hyperglycemia
- Edema
- Sodium and water retention
- Decreased immune response
- Muscle atrophy
- Visceral weight gain
- Fat pad on back of neck and clavicles
- Puffy face
- Bruising
- Stretch marks (striae)
- Hirsutism (for AFAB)
- Gynecomastia (for AMAB)

Diagnostic tests for Cushing syndrome/disease: serum levels of ACTH, cortisol, urine levels of cortisol, adrenal gland suppression tests, and MRI and CT scans for possible tumors

Treatment: the goal is to normalize secretion of hormones; the cause will need to be addressed; if it is a tumor, removal and hormonal supplementation for life will need to take place; if the cause is external steroid medication, the medication will need to be tapered down; this is so there is enough time for the adrenal glands and hypothalamus to start making hormones. When steroids are taken externally, production decreases, due to the negative feedback loop; stopping steroids suddenly will cause adrenal insufficiency and may cause adrenal crisis.

NOTE

Just like hypo- and hyperthyroidism, Addison disease and Cushing syndrome have opposite symptoms. If you know one, you know them both!

Diabetes Mellitus

The pancreas functions as both an endocrine gland and an exocrine gland, as it secretes hormones into the bloodstream and produces digestive enzymes that are released into the small intestine. Within the pancreas, the islets of Langerhans contain alpha, beta, and delta cells, which produce endocrine hormones. Alpha cells produce and secrete glucagon, beta cells produce and secrete insulin, and delta cells produce and secrete somatostatin. Diabetes mellitus is caused by a lack of insulin or insulin resistance.

Interestingly, in the first part of the 20th century, diabetes, mainly T2DM, was looked at as a "clean" disease, or a disease of the White and privileged population. It was considered a "good" disease, compared to other infectious diseases. However, in 1985, the Secretary of Health and Human Services, Margaret Heckler, released a landmark report called "Report of the Secretary's Task Force on Black and Minority Health." This report revealed that Black and minority populations had long suffered from diabetes that went undiagnosed and untreated. The report also revealed that the prevalence of diabetes was much higher in Black individuals than in White individuals, and much higher in Black AFAB than in White AFAB. Given these findings and the health disparity, the attitude toward diabetes shifted. Black individuals faced provider bias, social determinants of health (SDOH) were not taken into consideration, and they did not receive the same treatments for diabetes as White individuals. Diabetes also went from being known as a "privileged or good" disease to a "poor" or "bad" disease.

Type 1 Diabetes Mellitus

T1DM is an epigenetic autoimmune disease that attacks and destroys beta cells. It is triggered by viral illnesses, such as coxsackievirus, rotavirus, mumps, and cytomegalovirus. These are childhood diseases, and once the virus triggers the autoimmune reaction, the pancreatic beta cells are destroyed, leaving the patient insulinopenic. Typically, there is a long preclinical period before the disease is diagnosed. The usual age of diagnosis is between 10 and 14 years of age; however, diagnosis can sometimes occur when very young (2–3 years of age) or much older (30–40 years of age). By the time symptoms show, over 90% to 95% of the beta cells are destroyed, and the patient becomes severely hyperglycemic. Because this is an autoimmune disease, it is possible to test for insulin and islet cell autoantibodies to confirm T1DM.

Symptoms:

- The 3Ps—polydipsia, polyphagia, and polyuria
- Sudden weight loss
- Weakness
- Dehydration
- Blurry vision

Diagnostics: fasting plasma glucose level, oral glucose tolerance test, random plasma glucose, hemoglobin A1C, capillary blood glucose, urine test, and autoantibody testing (Table 10.5)

Treatment: insulin therapy, diet, fluids

TABLE 10.5 Serum Glucose Levels

	A1C (%)	Fasting Plasma Glucose (mg/dL)	Oral Glucose Tolerance Test (mg/dL)
Normal	5	70–99	≤139
Prediabetes	5.7–6.4	100–125	140–199
Diabetes	≥6.5	≥126	≥200

Severe T1DM can result in diabetic ketoacidosis (DKA). Because individuals with T1DM cannot uptake glucose into their cells, fat is used for fuel by breaking down into fatty acids, causing ketone bodies to form. This causes metabolic acidosis as well as severe hyperglycemia. This only occurs in individuals who can no longer produce insulin. It can be caused by new-onset T1DM, acute illness and infection, and not taking insulin. A common misconception is that insulin should not be taken during acute illness. However, due to the stress of the infection, the body releases cortisol, which results in increased blood glucose and can cause severe hyperglycemia. The onset of DKA is rapid.

Lab findings for DKA:

Serum glucose: 250 to 800 mg/dL

Arterial blood gas (ABG): pH 6.9 to 7.3

Metabolic panel: hyperkalemia >5 mg/dL, bicarbonate <15 mEq/L

Serum osmolality: >300 mOsm/kg

Urine: +urine ketones, +glucose

Symptoms for DKA:

- Abdominal pain
- Nausea and vomiting
- Weakness
- Lethargy
- Extreme dehydration
- Polyuria
- Polydipsia
- Fruity breath
- Kussmaul breathing
- Mental status changes, coma, seizures
- Arrhythmias, and cardiac arrest

Treatment: rehydration, insulin administration, and monitoring fluid electrolyte balance

Type 2 Diabetes Mellitus

Most people with diabetes have T2DM, which is an epigenetic disease caused by insulin resistance. Insulin resistance is caused by not having enough insulin receptors and lack of cellular response to insulin. Because of this, glucose is not taken into the cells and the client becomes hyperglycemic. Thinking back to Chapter 2, remember that T2DM is a multifactorial genetic disorder. This means that there is a genetic component to the disease, which is triggered by environmental conditions. Typically, T2DM is seen in adults over 30 years of age, although children who are overweight have been diagnosed with T2DM. T2DM is also associated with abdominal weight gain, physical inactivity, smoking, hypertension, and the SDOH. If an individual has a predisposition to T2DM, they have a higher risk of gestational diabetes.

T2DM starts with a genetic predisposition combined with environmental factors (SDOH, obesity, etc.). This results in insulin resistance and decreased glucose uptake. The pancreas, sensing the increased serum blood glucose, starts to frantically produce more insulin. This is called deranged insulin release. However, the beta cells cannot keep up, and eventually they start to die off. Meanwhile, receptors on the liver sense the overproduction of insulin, and as a result, the liver increases gluconeogenesis. This is the main cause of the hyperglycemia experienced in T2DM (Fig. 10.4). With T2DM, the individual has a gradual onset. They may go for years without symptoms or with very vague symptoms.

Common symptoms:

- Fatigue
- Recurrent infections (e.g., vaginal yeast infections)
- Slow wound healing

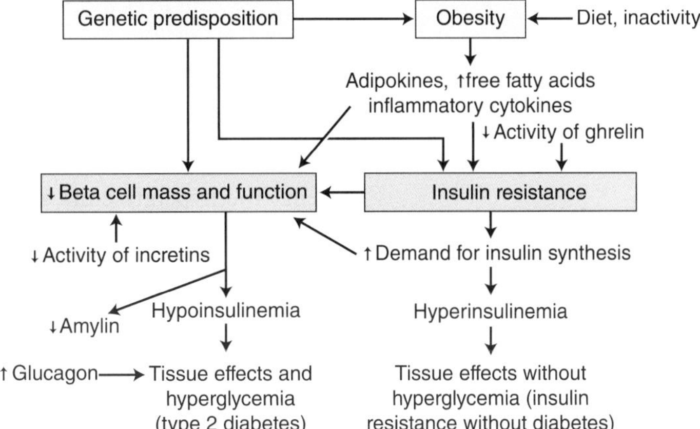

• **Fig. 10.4** Pathophysiological mechanism of type 2 diabetes mellitus. (From McCance, K. L. (2019). Cancer Epidemiology. In K. L. McCance, S. E. Huether, V. Brashers, & N. Rote (Eds.), Pathophysiology: The Biologic Basis for Disease in Adults and Children (8th ed). Elsevier.)

- Visual changes
- Clients may have manifestations of type 1 diabetes, such as polydipsia and polyuria as well

Eventually the hyperglycemia is so severe that it results in hyperglycemic hyperosmolar state (HHS).

Lab Findings for HHS:

Serum glucose: 600 to 1200 mg/dL
Serum osmolality: >350 mOsm/L
pH: normal 7.35 to 7.45
Urine: +glucose

As you can see, the serum lab values for glucose and osmolality are much higher than in T1DM. This is because HHS does not happen acutely. It has a very gradual, insidious onset. By the time symptoms appear, they are severe and require hospitalization. Also, because the individual with T2DM is still able to produce some insulin, they do not have to break down fat and ketone bodies do not form.

Symptoms are severe:

- Profound dehydration
- Electrolyte abnormalities
- Elevated BUN and creatinine
- Acute kidney failure
- Tachycardia
- Seizures
- Stroke
- Altered level of consciousness
- Paralysis
- Coma and death

Diagnostic studies: fasting plasma glucose level, oral glucose tolerance test, random plasma glucose, hemoglobin A1C, capillary blood glucose, urine test, and autoantibody testing

Treatment: is the same as DKA; rehydration, insulin administration, and monitoring fluid and electrolyte balance; mortality rate is much higher for HHS than for DKA

Hypoglycemia

Hypoglycemia is when serum blood sugar is low, less than 70 mg/dL. This can be caused by too much insulin or oral antidiabetic medications, too little food, and/or strenuous activity.

Symptoms:

- Mild: hunger
- Moderate: sweating, tremors, anxiety, palpitations, lightheadedness, paresthesia, headache, drowsiness, and poor coordination
- Severe: disoriented, seizures, lethargy, coma; can be mistaken for a stroke!

Hypoglycemic unawareness is seen mostly in children and elderly clients. This is when hypoglycemia is asymptomatic until severe. This can happen with habitually low blood sugars or autonomic neuropathy.

Diagnostic studies: fasting plasma glucose level, oral glucose tolerance test, random plasma glucose, hemoglobin A1C, capillary blood glucose, urine test

Treatment: give carbohydrates orally, if able. If unresponsive, glucagon injections or intravenous (IV) dextrose can be used

Complications From Diabetes

Somogyi Syndrome

Somogyi syndrome typically occurs with T1DM or insulin-dependent diabetes. A hypoglycemic episode occurs late at night (2 am) and the body compensates with increased growth hormone and cortisol secretion to cause rebound hyperglycemia. This is likely due to too much insulin prior to bedtime or not enough food. Cutting down on insulin or having a snack will mitigate this.

Dawn Phenomenon

Hormones are released early in the morning, decreasing glucose uptake and causing hyperglycemia. Dawn phenomenon occurs with both T1DM and T2DM.

Macroangiopathy

Macrovascular angiopathy is a disease of larger vessels and commonly affects individuals with T2DM and metabolic syndrome. This complication has the same risk factors as cardiac disease, such as obesity, hypertension, hyperlipidemia, hyperglycemia, and systemic inflammation. Macrovascular angiopathy can result in coronary artery disease, stroke, peripheral arterial disease, dilated cardiomyopathy, and heart failure (Fig. 10.5). Weight loss, smoking cessation, and medication may be utilized for management.

Microvascular Angiopathy

Microvascular angiopathy is small vessel damage caused by hyperglycemia and specific to diabetes, both type 1 and type 2. Hyperglycemia causes an inflammatory and immune response. There is an influx of innate and immune cells, and scarring, fibrosis, and clotting occur, causing narrowing and necrosis of the vessel. There is also a thickening of the basement membrane, which is the extracellular matrix separating different cells and tissues. Microvascular angiopathy causes injury to small vessels in the kidneys (diabetic glomerulosclerosis) (Fig. 10.6), eyes (retinopathy), and nervous system (neuropathy). Diabetic microvascular angiopathy is the primary cause of kidney failure and blindness.

Peripheral Neuropathy

Peripheral neuropathy occurs in 50% of clients with diabetes and affects the Schwann cells of peripheral nervous system. The hyperglycemia and inflammatory response cause vessel wall thickening of nutrient vessels (glial cells) that support neurons. They also cause damage to the myelin sheath, which results in decreased neuromuscular signals.

Somatic Neuropathy

Somatic neuropathy affects the hands and feet bilaterally. This type of neuropathy causes decreased perception of pain, temperature, and vibration. Because of decreased pain, injuries can result, and ulcers, necrosis, and amputation can result.

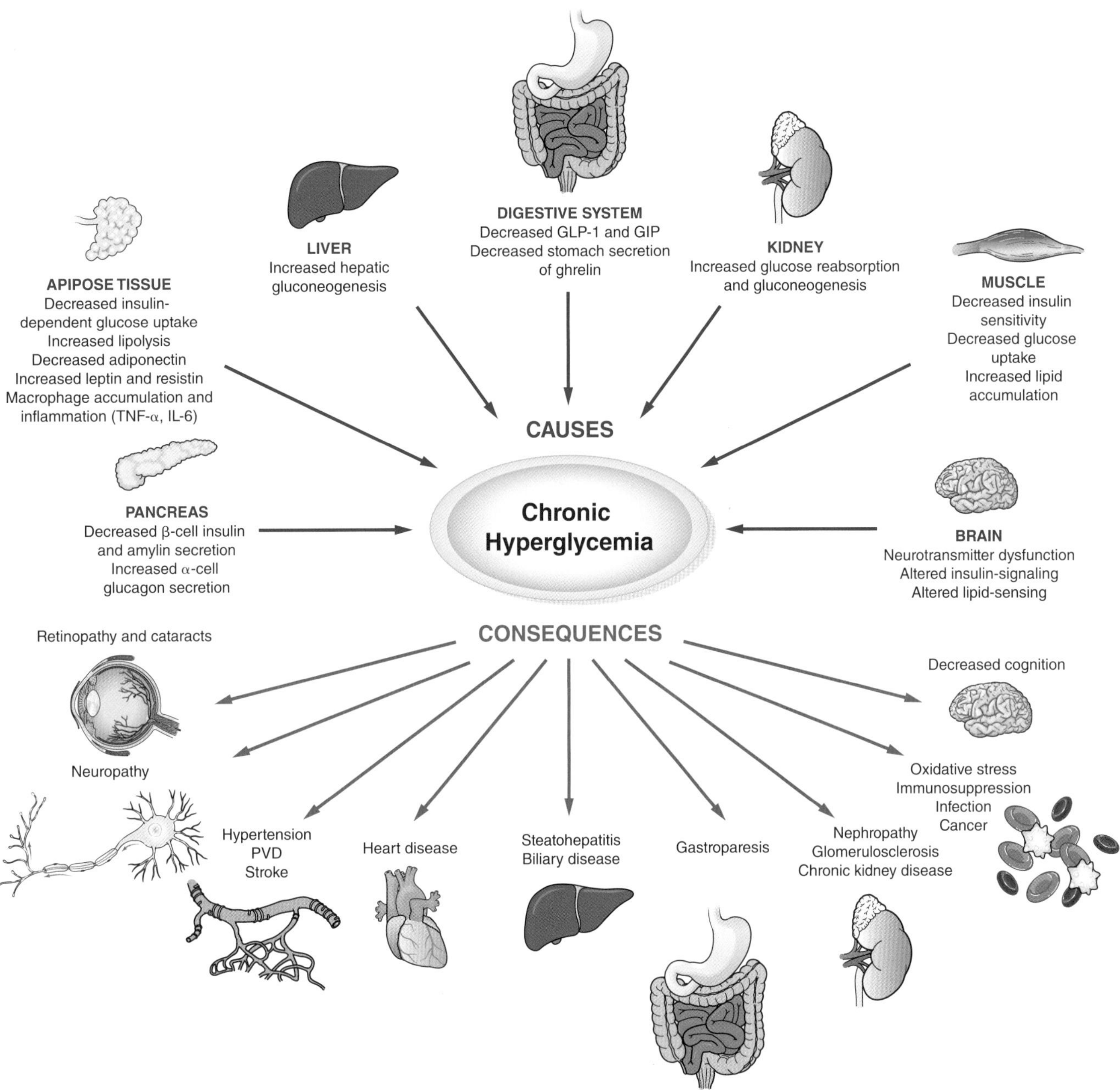

• **Fig. 10.5** Consequences from hyperglycemia. *GIP,* Gastric inhibitory peptide; *GLP-1,* glucagon-like peptide-1; *IL-6,* interleukin 6; *PVD,* peripheral vascular disease; *TNF-α,* tumor necrosis factor-alpha. (From Fig. 20.13 p. 462 UP, 7th edition.)

Autonomic Neuropathy

Autonomic neuropathy affects the sympathetic and parasympathetic nervous system. It is when there is damage to neurons that control automatic body functions, such as blood pressure, temperature, digestion, urination, and defecation. Gastroparesis, diarrhea, postural hypotension, syncope, erectile dysfunction, and neurogenic bladder can result.

Immune Dysfunction

Individuals with diabetes are far more susceptible to infections. This is because of macro- and microvascular angiopathies, which lead to poor circulation, and neuropathy. Having excess glucose in the blood creates a hospitable environment for bacteria. Innate and immune cell dysfunction also occurs with hyperglycemia.

Metabolic Syndrome

Instead of looking at insulin resistance on its own, research has shown that multiple factors (waist circumference, triglycerides, low high-density lipoprotein [HDL] cholesterol, blood pressure, and serum blood glucose levels) lead to metabolic syndrome.

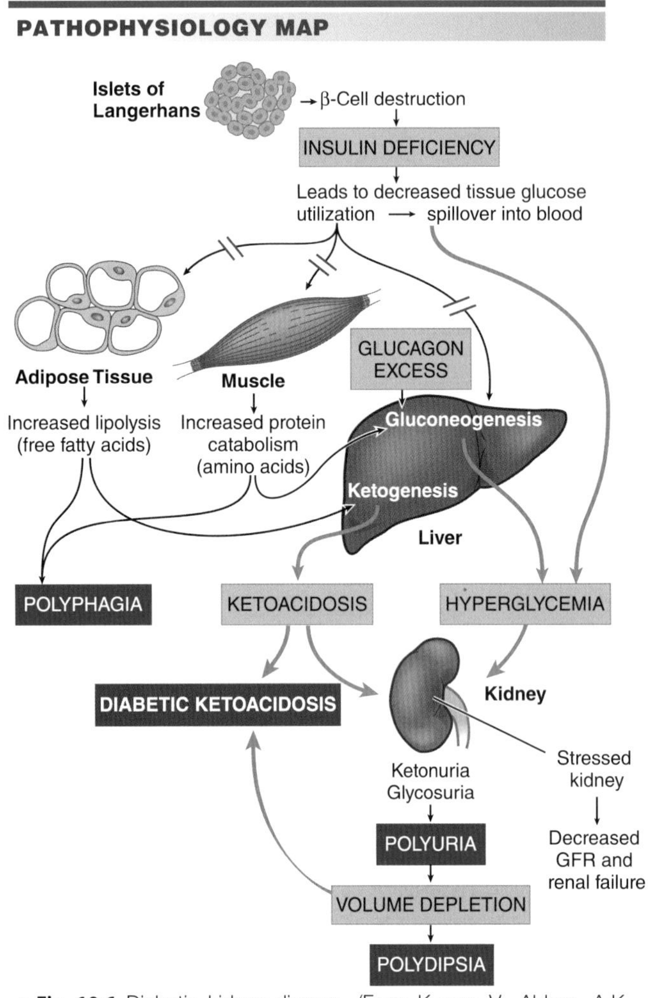

• **Fig. 10.6** Diabetic kidney disease. (From Kumar, V., Abbas, A.K., Fausto, N., et al. (2010). Disease of Immune System, 8th South Asia Edition, Elsevier Publication.)

Metabolic syndrome leads to increased risk of stroke, coronary artery disease, and type 2 diabetes mellitus. By looking at these factors together, it provides a more complete picture of client comorbidities and will allow you to assess multiple risks together (Fig. 10.7). Having three risk factors in the abnormal range would result in a diagnosis of metabolic syndrome.

Study Guide for Chapter 10

Make sure that you have your class notes and textbooks on hand to answer these questions. A concept map is included to help you to diagram and link disease concepts together.

1. Why does Addison disease occur? What is the pathophysiology? What are the causes? What are the clinical manifestations and complications?

____

____

____

____

2. Describe the pathophysiology behind Cushing syndrome. What is the difference between Cushing syndrome and Cushing disease? What are the signs and symptoms? What do you need to know about taking oral steroids?

____

____

____

____

The metabolic syndrome

Any three or more of the following five components

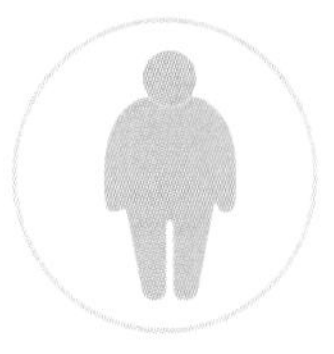

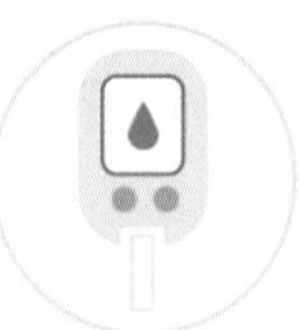

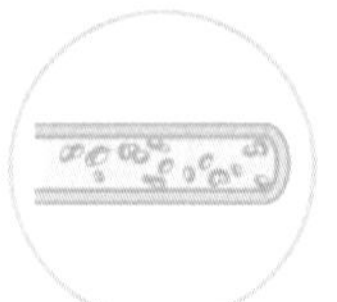

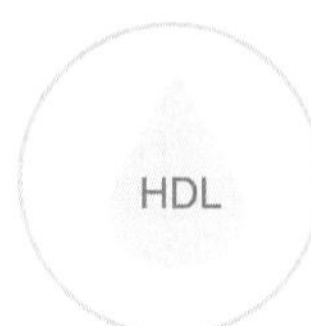

Abdominal obesity	Increased blood pressure	Elevated fasting blood sugar	High triglycerides	Low HDL cholesterol
Waist circumference: Men: > 102 cm Women: > 88 cm	130/85 mmHg or higher	>6.1 mmol/L (110 mg/dl)	>1.7 mmol/L (150 mg/dl)	Men: <1.03 mmol/L (40 mg/dl) Women: <1.30 mmol/L (50 mg/dl)

• **Fig. 10.7** Criteria for metabolic syndrome. *HDL*, High-density lipoprotein. (From Lamb, H. J. (2022). *Visceral and ectopic fat—Risk factors for type 2 diabetes, atherosclerosis, and cardiovascular disease* (1st ed.). Elsevier. Fig. 17.)

3. Describe the pathophysiology of hyper- and hypothyroidism. Outline the clinical manifestations and complications of each.

4. What is Graves disease and how does it occur? What are the hallmark characteristics? How would you diagnose it?

5. Describe thyroid storm. Why does it occur and what are the clinical manifestations?

6. What happens in myxedema coma? What is it a complication of?

7. Explain metabolic syndrome and the criteria to diagnose it.

8. Describe the pathophysiology behind type 1 and type 2 diabetes. How do they differ? What are the symptoms of each?

9. Describe DKA and hyperosmolar hyperglycemic syndrome. What is the difference between the two?

10. When does a person become hypoglycemic? Why? What kinds of symptoms accompany this?

11. What chronic complications are due to diabetes? Why do these complications occur?

12. What happens when there is a Somogyi effect? How does it differ from what happens in Dawn phenomenon?

13. What are the lab values and diagnostic tests for thyroid, adrenal cortex, diabetes, and metabolic syndrome?

STUDY TIPS

Endocrine disorders are perfect for T-charts!
Examples:

	Hypothyroidism	Hyperthyroidism
Cause?		
Pathophysiology?		
Symptoms?		

	Addison disease	Cushing syndrome
Cause?		
Pathophysiology?		
Symptoms?		

	T1DM	T2DM
Cause?		
Pathophysiology?		
Symptoms?		

T1DM, Type 1 diabetes mellitus; *T2DM,* type 2 diabetes mellitus.

Concept Map

Use this concept map to link each disease to its pathophysiology, diagnostics, causes, risk factors, complications, and clinical manifestations together. This way, you will be able to see the whole picture of the disease.

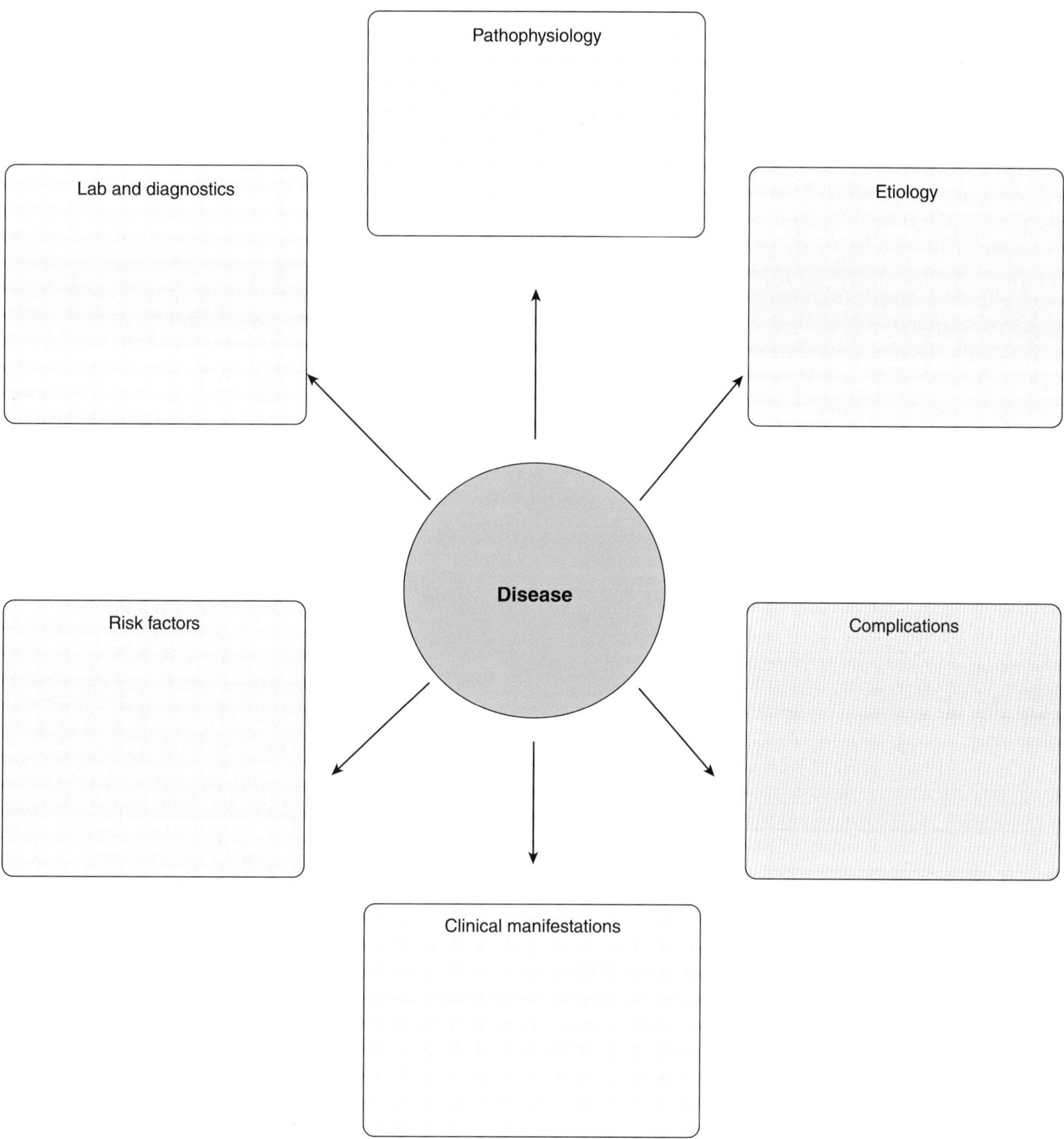

Case Studies for Chapter 10

Case Study 10.1

Allison, a 20-year-old Black cis-female (she/her), has a history of type 1 diabetes mellitus, which is well controlled. She is in her second year of college and extremely stressed about her exams. She starts to have palpitations and loses 10 pounds over a few weeks. She notices that her blood glucose levels are higher than usual, and she needs to use more insulin. She goes to her provider.

Vital Signs	Assessments	Labs
BP: 150/90 mm Hg HR: 124 beats per minute Temp: 99.9°F RR: 20 breaths/minute O_2 sat: 99% on room air Height: 5′9″ Weight: 115 pounds	Client uses she/her pronouns Appears thin, jittery, diaphoretic States that she has been losing weight and losing hair States that she feels like her heart is racing	Serum glucose: 200 mg/dL BUN: 220 mg/dL Creatinine: 1.1 mg/dL Free T4: 49 mcg/dL TSH: 0.2 mIU/L Hct: 45% Hgb: 17 g/dL

Looking at Allison's report:

1. What condition do you think she has? What indicates this?

2. How did she get this condition? Explain the pathophysiology.

3. What are some of the severe complications of this condition?

Allison has her thyroid removed and starts to take hormone supplements (levothyroxine). Ten years go by, and Allison comes to see her provider for her yearly physical exam. She tells her provider that she often feels slow and sluggish, has been gaining weight, and feels cold all the time.

4. How would you explain Allison's condition now?

5. How could you verify this?

6. What are the complications of this condition?

BP, Blood pressure; *BUN*, blood urea nitrogen; *Hct*, hematocrit; *HR*, heart rate; *O_2 sat*, oxygen saturation; *RR*, respiratory rate; *T4*, thyroxine; *Temp*, temperature; *TSH*, thyrotropin-stimulating hormone.

Case Study 10.2

Tara, a 45-year-old White trans-female (they/them), comes to the health clinic because they have been feeling weak, tired, and shaky for the past few weeks. They are thin and state that they have no appetite and have been losing weight. The provider notices that Tara's skin looks dry and chapped. Tara states that their medical history includes rheumatoid arthritis and mitral valve prolapse.

1. What diagnostic tests might the provider run to help diagnose Tara?

The provider diagnoses Tara with a gastrointestinal virus, and sends them home with orders to rest, hydrate, and try to eat a bland diet.

A week later, Tara is brought to the hospital by ambulance. They are vomiting, have diarrhea, and are extremely weak, confused, and dehydrated. When medics check their blood sugar, it is 40 mg/dL.

2. What would you diagnose Tara with? Explain the pathophysiology of the disease.

3. What tests would verify this?

4. How would this condition be treated?

Case Study 10.3

Kalyani, a 54-year-old Indian American cis-female (she/her), developed kidney failure and received a kidney transplant 3 years ago. She is taking prednisone (an oral steroid) and other immunosuppressants to avoid organ rejection. On her most recent visit, her report showed the following:

Vital Signs	Assessment	Labs
BP: 165/92 mm Hg RR: 18 breaths/minute HR: 80 beats per minute Temp: 97.8°F O_2 sat: 98% on room air Height: 5′3″ Weight: 165 pounds	Client uses she/her pronouns Client appears in good spirits Face appears puffy, seems to have gained weight in abdominal area since last visit Noticed a few bruises on arms and legs. Client states that she gets bruised every time she bumps up against anything. Denies any abuse.	Serum glucose: 280 mg/dL BUN: 20 mg/dL Creatinine: 1.2 Free T4: 10 mcg/dL TSH: 0.4 mIU/L Hct: 36% Hg: 13 g/dL K: 3.6 mg/dL Na: 140 mg/dL Ca: 9.5 mg/dL Mg: 1.4 mg/dL

Looking at the report:

1. What condition would you diagnose Kalyani with? Why?

2. Is this a primary, secondary, or tertiary condition?

3. As her nurse, what teaching would you do regarding her antirejection medication?

BP, Blood pressure; *BUN,* blood urea nitrogen; *Hct,* hematocrit; *HR,* heart rate; *O_2 sat,* oxygen saturation; *RR,* respiratory rate; *T4,* thyroxine; *Temp,* temperature; *TSH,* thyrotropin-stimulating hormone.

Case Study 10.4

Dario is a 32-year-old Latinx cis-male (he/him). He is brought to the emergency room with nausea, vomiting, and confusion. Police saw him near the town center walking unsteadily and stopped him. They found that he was confused, and they smelled alcohol on his breath. They brought him to the emergency room for further assessment. Upon arrival, he is nauseated, vomiting, and only alert to person and place. You are his nurse. When you go to assess him, you find that his skin is hot to touch, he has a medical alert bracelet on, and his breath smells fruity. When you ask him about his alcohol use, he denies drinking alcohol.

1. What do you suspect is happening to Dario? Explain.

2. Why would the police think that Dario had been drinking alcohol?

3. What lab findings would you expect with this condition?

4. Is this a medical emergency? Why or why not? How would this be treated?

Case Study 10.5

Trevor is a Black 60-year-old cis-male who appears to be in good health. He is athletic, eats well, is happily married with two children, and lives in a nice neighborhood. He does not smoke or drink. He arrives for his yearly physical exam.

Vital Signs	Assessment	Labs
BP: 166/98 mm Hg HR: 72 beats/minute RR: 16 breaths/minute O_2 sat: 99% on room air Height: 6′2″ Weight: 198 pounds	Client uses he/him pronouns Client appears healthy, no complaints States that he occasionally has headaches and dizziness when getting out of bed	Serum glucose: 170 mg/dL HgA1C: 6.3 Triglycerides: 210 mg/dL HDL: 32 mg/dL BUN: 10 mg/dL Creatinine: 0.8 Hct: 42% Hg: 17 g/dL K: 4.0 mg/dL Na: 138 mg/dL Ca: 9.2 mg/dL Mg: 1.8 mg/dL

1. The provider looks at the report and has some concerns. What do you think that the provider is concerned about?

2. What might be a potential diagnosis for Trevor? Explain using the results above.

The provider decides to monitor Trevor and schedules him for follow-up labs and a checkup in 3 months. Three months later:

Vital Signs	Assessment	Labs
BP: 182/100 mm Hg HR: 74 beats/minute RR: 18 breaths/minute O_2 sat: 99% on room air Height: 6′2″ Weight: 194 pounds	Client appears healthy States that he has had more frequent headaches and has had some episodes of blurry vision	Serum glucose: 244 mg/dL HgA1C:10 mmol/mol Triglycerides: 222 mg/dL HDL: 34 mg/dL BUN: 20 mg/dL Creatinine: 1.0 Hct: 43% Hg: 17 g/dL K: 4.2 mg/dL Na: 140 mg/dL Ca: 9.5 mg/dL Mg: 1.8 mg/dL

3. What would you diagnose Trevor with? Provide rationale(s).

4. The provider talks to Trevor about a condition called metabolic syndrome. When the provider leaves, Trevor turns to you, his nurse. He is visibly upset. He says, "I work hard to be healthy, to provide a safe and loving home for my family, and now I have this syndrome? I don't even understand what it is and what it has to do with my diagnosis!" What would you say to Trevor?

5. What are the complications that could result from Trevor's condition?

BP, Blood pressure; *BUN,* blood urea nitrogen; *Hct,* hematocrit; *HDL,* high-density lipoprotein; *HgA1C,* hemoglobin A1C; *HR,* heart rate; *O_2 sat,* oxygen saturation; *RR,* respiratory rate; *T4,* thyroxine; *Temp,* temperature.

11 Gastrointestinal Disorders

Gastroesophageal Reflux

Before starting this chapter, make sure you review the gastrointestinal system! Gastroesophageal reflux disease (GERD) occurs when there is mucosal layer damage in the esophagus due to persistent reflux of gastric contents into the lower esophagus. Typically, symptoms occur after eating, as the lower esophageal sphincter (LES) spontaneously relaxes.

- It is the most common gastroesophageal condition
- More common with assigned females at birth and older adults

Risk factors

- Chocolate, caffeine, fatty foods, and alcohol relax the LES
- Antidepressants also relax the sphincter
- Obesity
- Pregnancy (progesterone, pressure)
- Nicotine

Causes

- Weak LES allowing gastric reflux into esophagus
- Hiatal hernia putting pressure on LES causing incompetence (Fig. 11.1)
- Impaired esophageal motility and peristalsis
- Delayed gastric emptying increasing pressure in stomach; this causes LES incompetence

Results in (esophageal)

- Inflammatory response
- Erosion
- Ulcers
- Fibrosis
- Stricture

Symptoms

- Heartburn
- Noncardiac chest pain
- Water brash
- Coughing
- Hoarseness
- Sore throat
- Lump in throat
- Pain with swallowing
- Difficulty swallowing
- Regurgitation

Complications

- Esophagitis
- Strictures
- Asthma, bronchitis, aspiration pneumonia
- Chronic sinusitis
- Dental erosions
- Barrett's esophagus

Diagnosis

- History and physical exam
- Endoscopy
- Barium swallow
- pH study
- Esophageal manometry

Treatment

- Medication that decreases stomach acid (H2 receptor antagonists, antacids, proton pump inhibitors)
- Diet
- Lifestyle modifications
- Positioning (do not lie down after a meal for 4–5 hours, do not bend over for long periods of time)

Barrett's Esophagus

Barrett's esophagus refers to esophageal precancerous finding and often occurs with chronic GERD. The esophageal squamous epithelium is replaced by metaplastic intestinal epithelium.

- More common with GERD
- Middle-aged individuals, assigned males at birth
- Asymptomatic
- Slow growing
- Diagnosed with endoscopy
- Monitored every 3 to 5 years with endoscopy

Achalasia

Achalasia is a genetic, autoimmune, or secondary disorder where the esophageal innervation is affected (Chagas disease, sarcoidosis, Addison disease, neurofibromatosis). The esophagus cannot perform peristalsis to move the food bolus down to the LES. The LES is also affected, staying tightly contracted. The food bolus cannot move into the stomach and causes dilation and inflammation of the esophagus.

Complications

- Ulceration
- Aspiration
- Risk of esophageal cancer

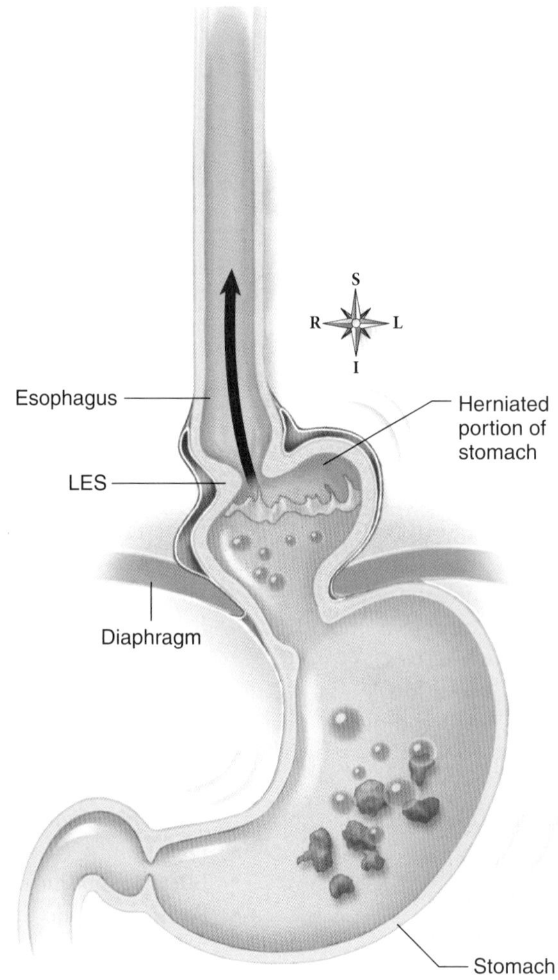

• **Fig. 11.1** Hiatal hernia. *LES,* Lower esophageal sphincter. (From Patton, K. T., Bell, F. B., Thompson, T., & Williamson, P. L. (2023). *The human body in health & disease* (8th ed.). Elsevier. Fig. 18.14.)

Diagnosis: endoscopy
Treatment: monitoring, surgery

Gastritis

Gastritis occurs in the stomach when there is a breach in the gastric mucosal barrier. The stomach, to protect itself from the acid and pepsin, has tight cell junctions and a lipid layer, which is coated with mucus. This mucus production is facilitated by prostaglandins. (Think back to Chapter 1.) That's why taking medications, like nonsteroidal anti-inflammatory drugs (NSAIDs), can cause gastritis and ulcerations. These medications block production of prostaglandins. Once this breach occurs, the stomach tissue is unprotected and begins to digest itself. Inflammation occurs and there is swelling, bleeding, and stomach pain.

Acute Gastritis

Acute gastritis is self-limited and typically heals in a few days. With this, the superficial layer of the stomach, the gastric mucosa, sloughs off and there is gastric bleed. Acute gastritis occurs most commonly because of:

- NSAIDs
- Alcohol
- Steroids
- Chemotherapy
- Radiation
- Bacterial toxins

Symptoms

- Heartburn
- Gastric distress
- Nausea and vomiting
- Blood in vomit or stool

Chronic Gastritis

Chronic gastritis occurs from bacterial infection of the stomach (*Helicobacter pylori*), autoimmune disease, or chemical gastropathy. With this condition, there is no bleeding or ulcerations. The gastric mucosal layer becomes thin and degenerates with chronic inflammatory changes.

Often it is asymptomatic, with atrophy of the stomach epithelium.

H. pylori is the most common cause of chronic gastritis. This is often contracted in childhood, through the fecal-oral route in areas with less access to sanitation and clean water. It is a Gram-negative bacterium, which colonizes the gastric mucosa. The bacterium can live in this environment because it secretes an enzyme called urease. Urease converts urea to ammonia, creating a basic environment in the stomach. As a result the antrum and body of the stomach are chronically inflamed.

Symptoms
- Initial: abdominal pain and nausea
- Later: becomes asymptomatic

Autoimmune gastritis is the most severe form of chronic gastritis. Autoantibodies destroy parietal cells and intrinsic factor (causing decreased hydrochloric acid [HCl] secretion and B_{12} uptake). This causes more gastrin to be secreted from the stomach and small intestine, as gastrin stimulates HCl secretion. This increased HCl production causes inflammation and ulcers. Chemical gastropathy occurs when small intestine secretions leak back into the stomach. This contains pancreatic enzymes and bile, which inflames and damages the stomach lining.

Complications: peptic ulcer disease (PUD), gastric cancer

Diagnostic tests: urea breath test, antibody titer, stool sample

Treatment: antibiotics, proton pump inhibitor

Peptic Ulcer Disease

PUD occurs when ulcers or lesions develop in the stomach (15%), duodenum (80%), and esophagus (5%). These ulcers can penetrate one layer or multiple layers of the stomach, with scarring and erosion (Fig. 11.2). This is mostly due to H. *pylori* and NSAIDs

Risk factors
- NSAIDs
- Smoking
- Genetics
- Age
- Assigned male at birth
- Chronic disease

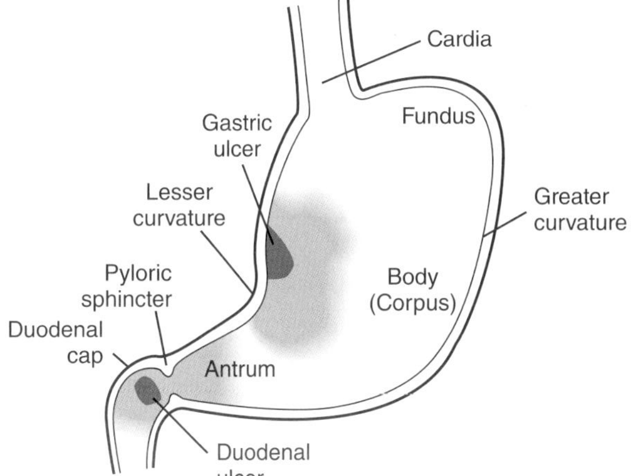

• **Fig. 11.2** Peptic ulcers. (From Ignatavicius D.D. & Bayne M.V. (1991). Medical-surgical nursing. WB Saunders.)

Symptoms
- Burning gnawing, cramping pain that radiates to back
- With gastric ulcers, pain with eating (increased secretions cause irritation)
- With duodenal ulcers, pain between meals or at night (bicarbonate is released with chyme, neutralizes, and decreases pain); pain is alleviated by food

Diagnosis: labs, endoscopy, barium swallow

Complications:
- Gastrointestinal (GI) bleeding
- Hemorrhage
- Perforation → peritonitis
- Fistula
- Obstruction of pyloric valve (pyloric stenosis) due to scarring and edema

Treatment: lifestyle changes, antibiotics, medications decreasing stomach acidity

Appendicitis

Inflammation and obstruction of appendix by a fecalith (hardened fecal matter) cause appendicitis. This is a common surgical emergency and typically is seen in younger adults (20–30 years). With inflammation and swelling, perfusion decreases, and the area becomes hypoxic.

Hypoxia → abscess → gangrene → peritonitis

Symptoms
- Periumbilical pain that progresses to right lower quadrant (McBurney point)
- High white blood cell count
- Low-grade fever
- Loss of appetite, nausea, vomiting
- Rebound tenderness and guarding
- Right leg flexed for comfort

Diagnosis: history and physical, ultrasound, computed tomography (CT) scan

Treatment: IV antibiotics and surgery

Diverticular Disease

Diverticulosis is caused by constipation and straining, which increases intraluminal pressure and causes partial herniation of the signmoid colon. Diverticula are pouches of mucosa that bulge because of the weakness in the colonic mucosa (Fig. 11.3)

Risk factors
- Low fiber diet
- Lack of exercise
- Constipation

When the diverticula become inflamed, diverticulosis becomes diverticulitis.

Inflammation → bleeding → abscess → perforation

Symptoms
- Left lower quadrant pain and tenderness
- Low-grade fever
- Obstruction and constipation
- Nausea and vomiting
- Increased white blood cell production

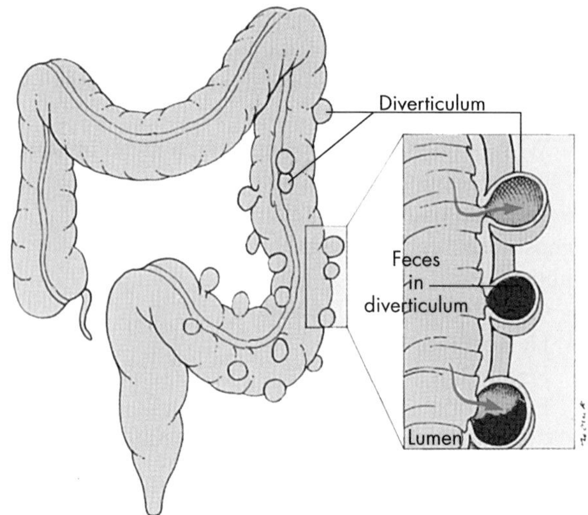

• **Fig. 11.3** Diverticular disease. (From Wilk, M. J. *Sorrentino's Canadian textbook for the support worker* (5th ed.). Elsevier. Fig. 33.21.)

Complications
- Fistulas
- Obstruction
- Perforation
- Peritonitis

Diagnosis: history and physical, ultrasound, CT scan

Treatment

For diverticulosis: fiber, fluids, and exercise

For diverticulitis: bowel rest, intravenous (IV) fluids and antibiotics, surgery

Peritonitis

Peritonitis is an inflammation of the peritoneum.

Primary cause: ascites (fluid shift to peritoneum)

Secondary cause: abdominal organ leakage, perforation, rupture, or trauma

Hallmark symptoms: rigid board-like abdomen, rebound tenderness

Other symptoms
- Severe abdominal pain and distension
- Fever
- Nausea and vomiting
- Paralytic ileus and constipation

Complications
- Sepsis
- Shock

Diagnosis
- History and physical
- X-ray
- CT scan
- Analysis of peritoneal fluid

Treatment
- Nothing by mouth (NPO)
- Nasogastric tube to decompress the stomach and prevent distention, ascites and pain
- IV fluids and IV antibiotics administered
- IV narcotics for pain management

Bowel Obstruction

Bowel obstructions occur when fluids/solids/gas are unable to pass. Most obstructions occur in the small bowel (80%). The rest occur in the large bowel (20%). The higher the obstruction, the more severe it is. Obstructions can be either mechanical or nonmechanical and either complete or partial blockages (Fig. 11.4).

- Small bowel obstruction: rapid onset, vomiting, severe abdominal pain, may pass feces for short time
- Large bowel obstruction: gradual onset, no vomiting, low-grade cramping pain, constipation

Mechanical bowel obstructions cause a physical blockage. Examples would be:
- Surgical adhesions
- Hernias
- Tumors or polyps
- Intussusception
- Volvulus
- Diverticulitis
- Fecal impaction

Diagnosis
- Hyperactive bowel sounds above obstruction, absent or hypoactive bowel sounds below obstruction
- Pain is crampy and colicky
- Visible on x-ray, CT scan

Nonmechanical obstructions are caused by disease or medications.
- Paralytic ileus—anesthesia, medications, peritonitis
- Intestinal pseudo-obstruction—spinal cord injury, diabetes mellitus, hypothyroidism
- Mesenteric vascular obstruction (bowel ischemia)—atherosclerosis, clotting, emboli

Diagnosis
- Bowel sounds are absent
- Pain is continuous
- Visible on x-ray, CT scan

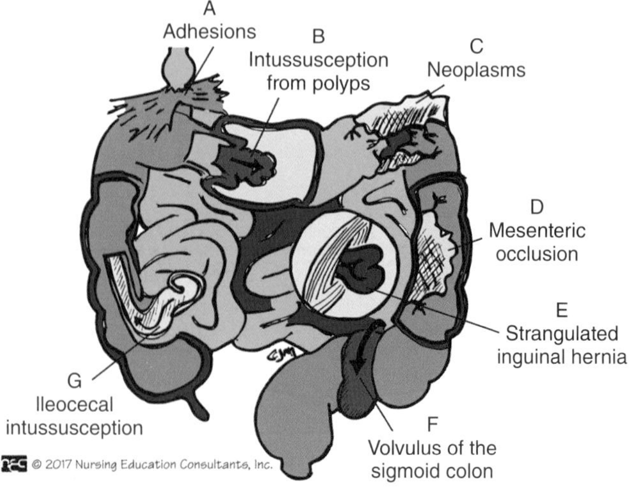

• **Fig. 11.4** Bowel obstructions. (Zerwekh, J., Garneau, A., & Zerwekh, T. (2025). Mosby's medical-surgical notecards (1st ed.). Elsevier.)

Symptoms

- Gas, fluid, and solids accumulate and cause the obstruction to move up the GI tract.
- The pressure in the bowels increases, pushing fluid into the peritoneum.
- Blood volume decreases and perfusion to the bowel decreases, causing ischemia.

Ischemia → gangrene → bowel perforation → peritonitis

Complications: sepsis, dehydration, hypovolemic shock

Treatment: nasogastric tube for gastric decompression, IV antibiotics, NPO, IV pain management

Gastrointestinal Bleeding

Gastrointestinal bleeding is a symptom, not a disease. When there is bleeding in the GI tract, the blood volume decreases, causing hypotension, low cardiac output, and tachycardia. As the bowels are not a vital organ, perfusion will shift away from them causing bowel ischemia. As blood loss increases, urine output decreases. Ultimately, there will be a lack of perfusion to the brain and heart, causing mental status changes, angina, and heart failure.

Upper Gastrointestinal Bleeding (esophagus → duodenum)

Causes: esophageal varices, Mallory-Weiss tears

Symptoms

- Bright, red, hematemesis
- Coffee-ground emesis
- Melena

Lower Gastrointestinal Bleeding (jejunum → rectum)

Causes: polyps, tumors, diverticulitis, inflammatory bowel disease, hemorrhoids

Symptoms

- Hematochezia
- Melena

Diagnostics: test for occult bleeding, endoscopy, colonoscopy

Treatment: identify the source of bleeding, transfusions, IV fluids

Inflammatory Bowel Disease

Crohn disease and ulcerative colitis are known as inflammatory bowel disease. These are chronic, recurring inflammations of the GI tract. The exact cause is unknown. There are aspects of autoimmune disease, epigenetics, dysfunction of GI epithelial cell dysfunction, and disruption of the gut microbiome. Intestinal tissue is constantly inflamed and damaged.

NOTE

Inflammatory bowel disease was thought to be genetically more prevalent in individuals who are White and Ashkenazi Jews. However, it has been found that marginalized and minority populations are underdiagnosed or are not diagnosed until the disease is advanced, due to disparities in care.

Ulcerative colitis is the inflammation of the superficial, mucosal layer of the colon.

- Small polyps, papillae
- From rectum, continuous progression up colon
- Does not involve all bowel layers
- Does not involve small bowel
- Increased risk of colorectal cancer associated with it
- Exacerbations and remissions (triggered by stress, infections)
- Weight loss
- Abdominal pain, bloody diarrhea → hemorrhage
- Tenesmus (painful urge to defecate)

Crohn disease is an inflammation of all bowel layers.

- Cobblestone appearance
- Lesions can occur anywhere from the mouth to anus
- Does not have to progress continuously
- Skip lesions
- Fistulas and abscesses → perforation → peritonitis
- Scarring of the bowel lumen → narrowing → bowel obstruction
- Nutritional deficiencies due to malabsorption
- Weight loss

Due to the autoimmune nature of this disease, you may see extraintestinal symptoms such as: fever, arthritis, ankylosing spondylitis, anemia, skin lesions, and cholangitis.

Diagnosis: endoscopy, colonoscopy, CT scan, lab work (complete blood count [CBC], erythrocyte sedimentation rate [ESR], C-reactive protein [CRP], B_{12}, vitamin D, comprehensive metabolic panel [CMP], stool cultures)

Treatment: bowel rest, lifestyle changes, diet changes, correct malnutrition, immunosuppressants, steroids, anti-inflammatories, antibiotics for any infection, and pain management; may need bowel surgery, colostomy, ileostomy

Colon Cancer

Colorectal cancer is the second leading cause of cancer deaths (Fig. 11.5).

Risk factors

- Genetics (familial adenomatous polyposis, Lynch syndrome)

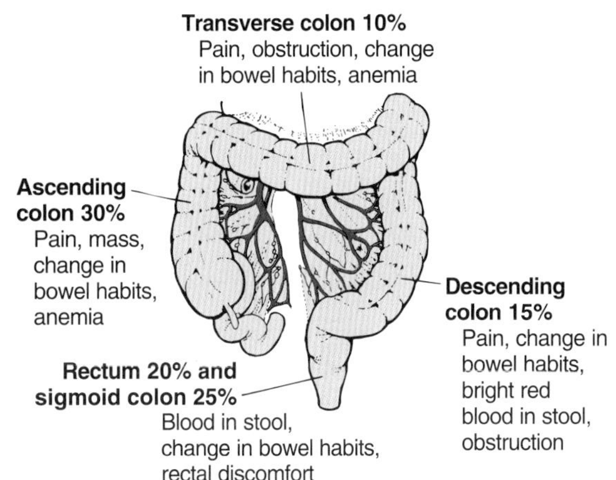

• **Fig. 11.5** Signs and symptoms of colorectal cancer. (Heuther S.E., et al. (2019). Understanding Pathophysiology. (7th ed.). Elsevier.)

- Age
- History of ovarian, uterine, GI cancer
- Ulcerative colitis
- PUD
- Smoking
- Alcohol
- Obesity
- Diet high in red meat, processed foods

Symptoms
- Change in bowel habits
- Blood in stool
- Anemia
- Perforation/obstruction
- Rectal pain

Diagnostics: colonoscopy, CT scan, magnetic resonance imaging (MRI), ultrasound

Treatment: surgery, chemotherapy, radiation

Prevention: colonoscopy every 10 years starting at 45 years of age

Diarrhea

Diarrhea is defined as the frequent passage of loose, often liquid stools. It can be due to acute or chronic causes. Infants and older adults are particularly susceptible to diarrhea because of fluid loss and electrolyte disturbances.

> **NOTE**
>
> With climate change and rising temperatures, bacterial and viral diarrheal diseases are becoming more common, especially with young children. Increasing temperatures help to create a more hospitable environment for pathogens to spread. Globally, diarrhea is the fifth leading cause of death in children. Natural disasters, such as earthquakes, hurricanes, and typhoons, as well as wars and conflicts, can exacerbate diarrheal illness by contaminating the water supply (e.g., contamination with sewage, lack of clean water and sanitation). Diarrheal disease can happen both in flood conditions and in drought conditions. In flood conditions, diarrheal pathogens can spread through contact with contaminated water. In drought conditions, water is limited, hygiene is often not possible, and pathogens are more concentrated in the water, all of which would lead to diarrheal illness. Oral rehydration therapy and WASH (water, adequate sanitation, hygiene) are techniques being used globally to reduce mortality from diarrheal illness.

Acute (<2 weeks)

Pathophysiology: disruption of intestinal absorption and secretion, dehydration, acidosis

Noninflammatory (*Vibrio cholerae, Escherichia coli, Giardia lamblia*)
- Watery, large volume
- Nonbloody stool
- Nausea/vomiting
- Cramping
- Bloating

Pathophysiology: disruption of intestinal absorption and secretion, dehydration, acidosis

Inflammatory disease (*Salmonella, Clostridium difficile*)
- Fever
- Small volume
- Bloody diarrhea
- Lower abdominal pain
- Urgency
- Fecal leukocytes

Pathophysiology: invasion of intestinal cells and inflammation by pathogens

Chronic (≥4 weeks)

Causes: lactase deficiency, bacterial overgrowth, indiscriminate laxative use, inflammatory bowel disease, parasites, viruses

Diagnostics

History and physical, lab work, thyroid function, celiac sprue testing, stool studies, radiographic studies, colonoscopy

Treatment

Oral rehydration therapy, antidiarrheals (after 24–48 hours), antibiotics (only if bacterial), IV fluids, time

Constipation

Constipation has varying definitions. Typically, stools are hard, infrequent, and individuals with constipation often have less than three stools a week.

Common primary causes: failure to respond to urge, not enough fluid/fiber, abdominal and pelvic weakness, and hemorrhoids

Secondary causes: Hirschsprung disease, cancer, spinal cord injury, hypothyroidism, Parkinson disease, celiac disease, multiple sclerosis, irritable bowel disorder, and medication (opioids)

Diagnostics: history and physical

Treatment: laxatives, suppositories, enema, disimpaction

Complication: fecal impaction, rectoceles, large bowel obstruction

Prevention: fluid and fiber

Study Guide for Chapter 11

Make sure that you have your class notes and textbooks on hand to answer these questions. A concept map is included to help you to diagram and link disease concepts together.

1. Why does GERD happen? What is the pathophysiology behind GERD? What are the signs and symptoms?

____

____

____

____

2. What are the major causes of acute gastritis? What are the major causes of chronic gastritis? How are they different? What are the signs and symptoms of each?

____

____

____

____

3. How does PUD develop? Describe the ulcers and the complications of PUD. What is the difference between a duodenal ulcer and a gastric ulcer?

4. What causes diverticulitis? Explain the pathophysiology. What are the clinical manifestations?

5. How does *H. pylori* colonize the stomach mucosa? Describe the pathophysiology. How does it thrive in this environment?

6. What are the signs and symptoms of *H. pylori* infections? What are the complications?

7. What are the different kinds of bowel obstructions? What are the causes of each?

8. What are the signs and symptoms of a bowel obstruction? What are the complications?

9. Know all the structures of the GI tract (mouth, pharyngoesophageal sphincter, esophagus, etc.). What protects the esophagus? The stomach? The bowel?

10. What occurs in peritonitis? Describe the pathophysiology. Why does infection spread quickly in the peritoneum? What protective factors does the peritoneum have?

11. Describe the pathophysiology behind appendicitis. What are the signs and symptoms? What are the complications?

12. What is Barrett's esophagus and what does it cause?

13. Outline the differences and similarities between ulcerative colitis and Crohn disease. What are the manifestations and complications of each?

14. How and when would you screen for colon cancer? What are the causes/risks?

____

____

15. What are the different types of diarrhea and what causes each type?

____

____

____

____

16. Describe the different types of constipation and the causes of each type.

____

____

____

____

STUDY TIPS

Think about the symptoms that come with gastrointestinal disease logically.

- With abdominal diseases, abdominal pain, nausea, and vomiting are common symptoms.
- With gastrointestinal (GI) disease, if there is a rupture or perforation, peritonitis is always a complication and concern.
- T-chart example:

	Ulcerative colitis	Crohn disease
Cause?		
Pathophysiology?		
Symptoms?		

Concept Map

Use this concept map to link each disease to its pathophysiology, diagnostics, causes, risk factors, complications, and clinical manifestations together. This way, you will be able to see the whole picture of the disease.

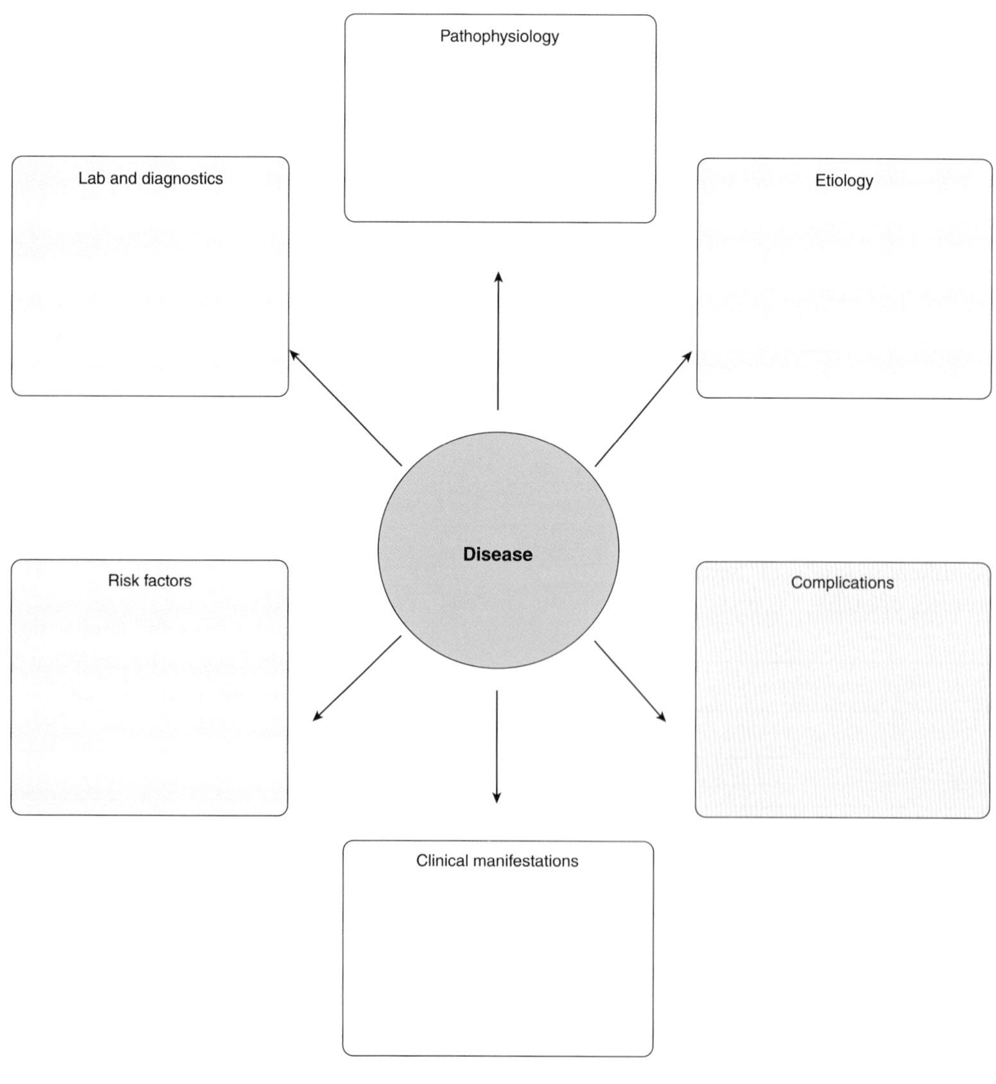

Case Studies for Chapter 11

Case Study 11.1

Doreen is a 51-year-old Filipina cis-female (she/her). She is an avid tennis player, but she has developed tennis elbow (lateral epicondylitis) from years of playing. She goes to an urgent care provider, who prescribes physical therapy and ibuprofen, 800 mg every 8 hours with food as needed. Doreen takes ibuprofen every 8 hours for 1 week. At the start of the second week, she starts to get nauseated and experiences burning epigastric pain.

1. What is the reason behind Doreen's pain?

2. What would you diagnose her with?

3. How can she treat the pain?

Doreen continues to take ibuprofen with food intermittently for her joint pain. After a few months, she notices that she has severe cramping abdominal pain that wakes her out of a sound sleep. She finds that drinking a warm glass of milk helps with the pain.

4. Has her condition progressed? Why or why not?

5. What are the risks with this condition?

Doreen's abdominal pain continues to get worse. She starts to run a high fever and is taken to the emergency room by ambulance. When the nurse examines her, the nurse notices that Doreen is guarding, and her abdomen is rigid. When the nurse auscultates her abdomen, the nurse cannot hear bowel sounds.

6. What has happened to Doreen? Explain the pathophysiology.

Case Study 11.2

Ryan is a 25-year-old White trans-male (he/him). He starts feeling sick with abdominal pain and a low-grade fever, and hopes it is just a passing virus. By the next day, the pain is worse and has migrated to his lower right abdomen. Ryan is taken to the emergency room by his fiancé Jay. When the nurse examines him, they find rebound tenderness, guarding, and a fever. Ryan's labs show his white blood cells to be 16,000/L.

1. What condition/disease does Ryan have? Explain the pathophysiology.

2. What are the hallmark symptoms of this condition/disease?

Ryan has a CT scan, and it confirms appendicitis. An hour later, Ryan suddenly feels better and wants to leave. Jay asks the nurse to disconnect Ryan's IV so that they can leave.

3. Is this the right decision? Why or why not?

Case Study 11.3

Krishna is healthy 72-year-old Indian American cis-female (she/her). She has a history of hypertension, type 2 diabetes mellitus, depression, and gastroesophageal reflux, which are all well-managed with medication. She arrives for her scheduled colonoscopy and tells the nurse her only complaint is that she is occasionally bloated and constipated. She gets the colonoscopy with no issues. Afterwards, the provider tells Krishna that she has diverticulosis.

1. Krishna is worried and asks, "Is this serious? How did I get this?" What would you tell her?

A year later, Krishna starts experiencing persistent lower left quadrant abdominal pain and has an abdominal computed tomography (CT) scan. The scan shows that Krishna has diverticulitis.

2. What is the difference between diverticulosis and diverticulitis?

3. Krishna asks if she try to eat more fiber. What would you tell her?

4. What is the treatment for diverticulitis?

Case Study 11.4

Rose is an 18-year-old White cis-female (she/her) who has come to the clinic to be seen for recurring abdominal pain and new-onset diarrhea. She denies any nausea or vomiting. Vital signs are all stable.

1. What labs would you expect to be ordered to find out the cause of these symptoms?

2. What are two differential diagnoses?

The provider starts Rose on antibiotics and the symptoms resolve. However, 6 weeks later, Rose is admitted to the hospital for severe lower abdominal pain, nausea, vomiting, and diarrhea. She states that the cramping pain and diarrhea have been intermittent for the last 2 weeks and that she has lost 8 pounds. A colonoscopy shows ulcerations in the ileum, duodenum, and rectum.

3. What do these findings indicate?

4. What complications would you be worried about?

5. Is this condition curable? What can be done?

Case Study 11.5

Raquel is a Latinx nonbinary individual (they/them). They have end-stage endometrial cancer and are on hospice services. The nurse examines Raquel, hears bowel sounds in all quadrants, and asks when their last bowel movement was. Raquel states that the last bowel movement was 2 days ago.

1. Does this mean that Raquel is constipated?

2. What suggestions would you make to Raquel?

The hospice nurse comes back 2 days later. Raquel still has not had a bowel movement, has abdominal distension and dull lower abdominal pain. The nurse hears hypoactive bowel sounds on the left. The nurse is concerned about a possible obstruction.

3. Why is the nurse concerned about obstruction? What would cause this?

4. Would increasing fluids and fiber help at this stage? Why or why not?

Case Study 11.6

Rawan is a 2-year-old girl who has recently been evacuated from Syria, along with her parents. Her parents have brought her to an international health station to be evaluated. Rawan has been losing weight, has been vomiting and has had watery diarrhea, and appears listless. You are part of an international team providing health care.

Vital Signs	Assessment
HR: 158 beats per minute	Eyes and cheeks look sunken
RR: 36 breaths/minute	Pulse is rapid and weak
Temperature: 99°F	Child has rapid and shallow breaths
O_2 sat: 98% on room air	Child appears listless, cry is weak

HR, Heart rate; *O_2 sat,* oxygen saturation; *RR,* respiratory rate.

1. What five questions would you ask Rawan's parents to find out what the cause of her illness is?

Rawan's parents tell you that their situation in Damascus was very difficult. Due to war and repeated bombings, it was difficult for them to get adequate food and water.

2. What do you think Rawan's diagnosis may be? Why?

3. What would you be most concerned about? Why?

4. Rawan's parents are very upset. They feel that they caused her illness. What would you tell them?

5. How would you treat this illness?

12 Disorders of Liver, Gallbladder, and Pancreas

Liver Disorders

To understand what happens when there is liver disease, you first must understand what the liver does. The liver removes toxins and bacteria, stores vitamins (A, D, E, K, and B_{12}), produces most of the body's proteins and clotting factors, conjugates bilirubin and produces bile to help absorb fats, performs glycogenolysis, and converts ammonia to urea so that it can be excreted through the urine. Bilirubin is a by-product of the breakdown of red blood cells and hemoglobin. It is usually recycled into bile or excreted in the feces, giving fecal matter that brown color. When the liver is diseased, bile production is impacted. The bile made by the hepatocytes starts to accumulate. The bile channels (canaliculi) are plugged up and rupture. This causes a backup of bile which causes necrosis of the hepatocytes. Eventually, the bile leaks into the blood. This is called cholestasis (Fig. 12.1).

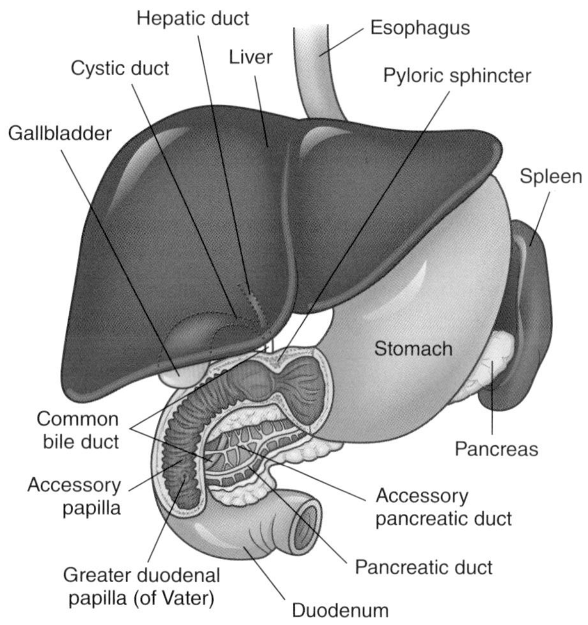

• **Fig. 12.1** Liver, gallbladder, pancreas. (McCance K.L., & Huether S.E. (2018). Pathophysiology: the biologic basis for disease in adults and children. Elsevier Health Sciences.)

Diagnosis

To diagnose liver disease, you would look at the following:

- History and physical
- Alkaline phosphatase (ALP)
- Aspartate aminotransferase (AST)
- Alanine aminotransferase (ALT)

These three tests are called liver function tests (LFTs) and would be elevated. You would also look at:

- serum bilirubin (0.1–1.2 mg/dL)—increases with disease
- albumin (3.5–5.0 g/dL)—decreases with disease
- coagulation factors—decrease with disease
- clotting times—prothrombin time (PT), partial thromboplastin time (PTT) increase with disease

Ultrasounds, computed tomography (CT) scans, magnetic resonance imaging (MRI), and liver biopsies can also identify disease.

Liver disease has distinct signs and symptoms:

- Dark urine—due to accumulation of bilirubin in the blood
- Light clay–colored stool—due to lack of bile in stool
- Anorexia, nausea, vomiting—due to ascites, poor digestion
- Malaise
- Fatigue
- Pruritus—intense itching due to buildup of bile salts
- Jaundice—due to accumulation of bilirubin in the blood; there are three types of jaundice: prehepatic (damage to red blood cells before the liver), intrahepatic (disease within the liver), and posthepatic (blockage to the flow of bile).

Hepatitis

Viral hepatitis is one of the most common diseases of the liver. The virus causes inflammation, sometimes chronic inflammation, and damage to the hepatocytes. With the inflammation, macrophages (Kupffer cells) infiltrate the liver and there is Kupffer cell hyperplasia. There is vascular damage and hepatocyte death. With chronic disease, there is scarring, cirrhosis, and liver failure.

Hepatitis A—transmitted orally and through feces. It occurs in areas with water and sanitation issues. It is self-limiting and patients become immune for life. It is preventable with hepatitis A vaccine.

Hepatitis B—transmitted sexually, perinatally, and through blood and blood products. Hepatitis B can become chronic and lead to liver failure and liver cancer. It is preventable with hepatitis B vaccine.

Hepatitis C—transmitted through blood and blood products. Few people clear the virus; most have chronic disease, resulting in cirrhosis, liver failure, and liver cancer. There is no vaccine; however, there are antiviral medications.

With acute viral hepatitis, there are three phases:

- Prodromal—vague symptoms; muscle aches, joint pain, nausea, vomiting, loss of appetite, fever, diarrhea, abdominal pain
- Icteric—jaundice, severe itching, hepatomegaly
- Convalescent—return to baseline within 2 to 3 weeks

Treatment and prevention include vaccines and antiviral medications.

Acute Fulminant Hepatitis

Acute fulminant hepatitis is rare. It usually occurs with viral/bacterial/fungal infection, severe hepatitis A, alcoholic hepatitis, and acetaminophen toxicity and progresses quickly, resulting in liver failure within days to weeks. There is a systemic inflammatory response and can result in disseminated intravascular coagulation. Hepatic encephalopathy and hepatorenal syndrome develop rapidly. Mortality rate is very high, and the only cure is a liver transplant.

Liver Cirrhosis

Liver cirrhosis occurs as the damage to the liver progresses. The liver tissue gets scarred and fibrous. The liver and spleen become enlarged; there is right upper quadrant (RUQ) abdominal pain and weight loss. Most symptoms and complications arise from portal hypertension. Portal hypertension occurs when there is abnormally high blood pressure in the portal venous system. This happens as the vessels gets scarred and narrowed with liver inflammation and disease (Fig. 12.2).

- Prehepatic—before the liver (splenic or portal vein clot)
- Intrahepatic—in the liver (cirrhosis)
- Posthepatic—after the liver → back to the heart (hepatic vein clot, heart failure)

Portal hypertension can result in the following.

- Ascites—occurs from increased peritoneal vessel pressure causing fluid shift to the peritoneal space and abdominal distension
- Varices, caput medusae, and hemorrhoids—collateral veins develop, bypassing the liver. These veins are thin, twisting, and fragile, and rupture easily, causing hemorrhaging.

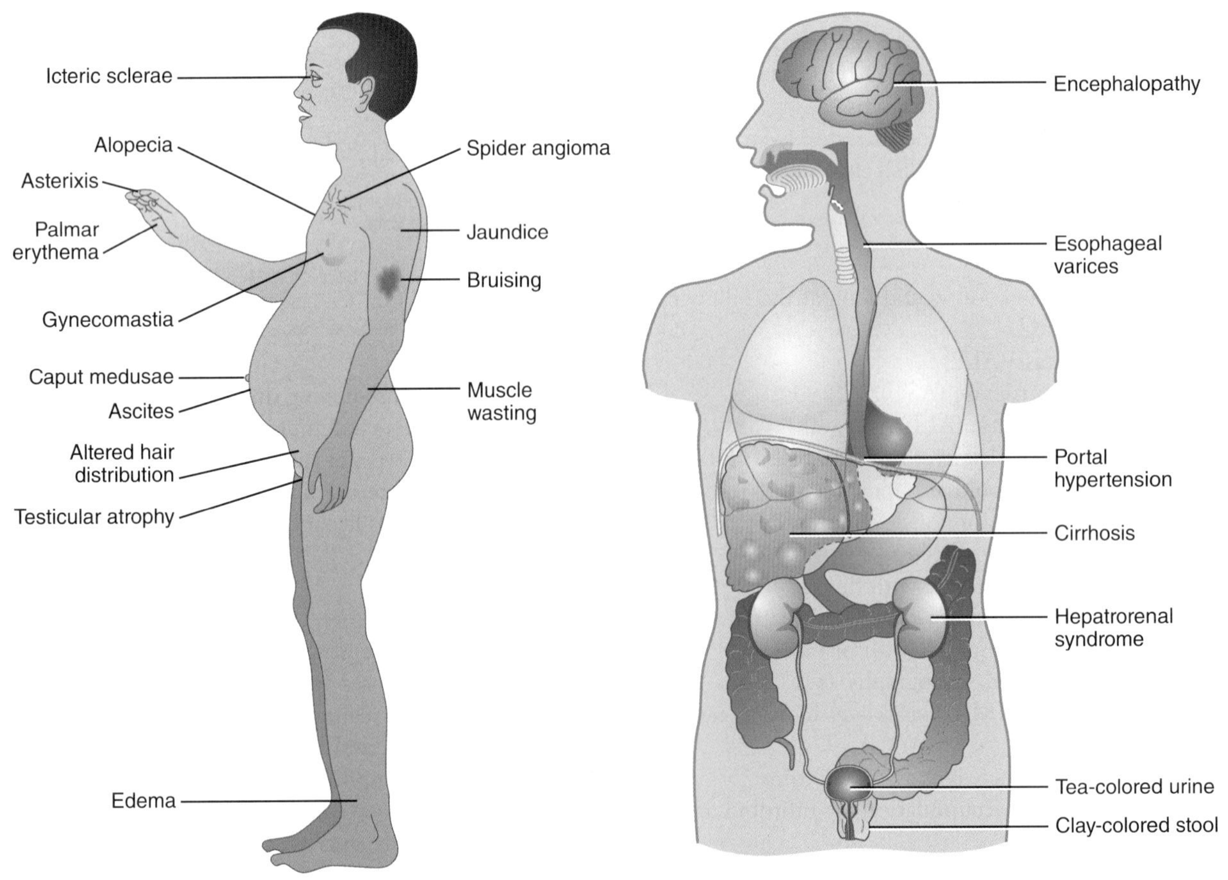

• **Fig. 12.2** Manifestations of cirrhosis. (Mahan L.K., & Escott-Stump S. (2012). Krause's Food, Nutrition, & Diet Therapy. (13th ed.). Saunders.)

- Splenomegaly—enlargement of the spleen, resulting in destruction of red blood cells (red pulp), white blood cells (WBCs/white pulp), and sequestering of platelets (the spleen stores platelets)
- Hepatorenal syndrome
  - Cause unknown
  - Portal system vasodilates, renal system vasoconstricts
  - Perfusion to kidney decreases
  - Oliguria and azotemia result, as creatinine and blood urea nitrogen (BUN) increase.
  - Kidney failure occurs.
- Hepatic encephalopathy—occurs with the shunting of ammonia and toxins into the blood
  - Caused by toxins and excess ammonia from bleeding or excess protein
  - Excess ammonia is typically converted to urea by the liver and excreted through urine
  - Increased ammonia and narcotics can affect neurotransmitters
  - Confusion, poor hygiene, memory loss, and personality changes may result
  - In later stages, asterixis (flapping hand tremor), stupor, seizures, decerebrate posturing, coma may result.

Liver Failure

End-stage liver failure occurs when over 80% of the liver is destroyed.

Symptoms
- Fetor hepaticus—musty breath
- Anemia, thrombocytopenia, leukopenia
- Lack of clotting factor, albumin, fat-soluble vitamins, and B_{12} → bleeding
- Skin disorders, itching (due to bile buildup)
- Lack of enzymes to break down steroid hormones → excess aldosterone and sex hormones → fluid retention, ascites, gynecomastia
- Increased bilirubin in blood → jaundice, fatty stools
- Increased ammonia → encephalopathy

Treatment: lactulose (decreases ammonia levels), diuretics, paracentesis, liver transplant

Gallbladder Disorders

The gallbladder stores the bile that the liver makes. Cholecystokinin and motilin are hormones that regulate bile and pancreatic enzyme release into the small intestine (Fig. 12.3).

Cholelithiasis

Cholelithiasis is the development of gallstones and sludge in the gallbladder and bile ducts. Most of the time these stones are made of cholesterol (80%) or bilirubin/calcium (20%). Stasis of bile causes these stones to form. Gallstone formation is caused by bile that is saturated with cholesterol. Supersaturated bile → forms crystals → microstone

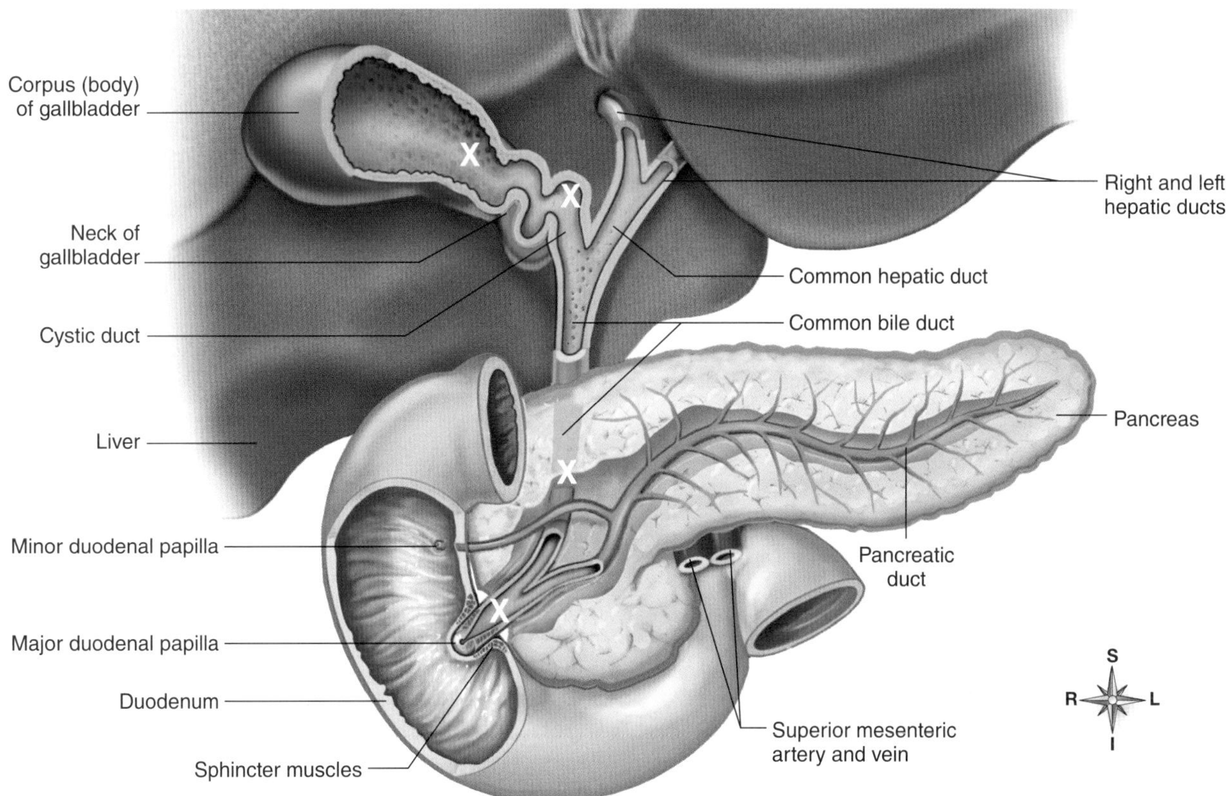

• **Fig. 12.3** Gallbladder and pancreas. (From Patton K.T., & Thibodeau G.A. (2018). The human body in health & disease. (7th ed.). Elsevier.)

→ macrostone. Small stones cause colic and pain as they pass through the bile ducts. Large stones (>8 mm) can obstruct the cystic or common ducts (Fig. 12.4).

Risk factors

- Obesity
- Assigned female at birth (AFAB)
- Genetics
- Diet
- Age
- Malabsorption

Symptoms

- RUQ pain referred to back or right shoulder
- Jaundice
- Heartburn
- Flatulence
- Epigastric pain
- Intolerance of rich, spicy, or fatty foods

Diagnosis

- History and physical
- Complete blood count
- Blood cultures
- LFTs
- Ultrasound
- CT scan
- Endoscopic retrograde cholangiopancreatography (ERCP)

Treatment: medications, laparoscopic surgery

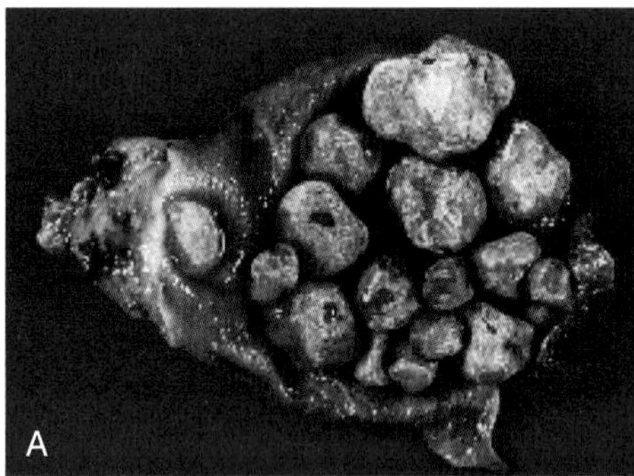

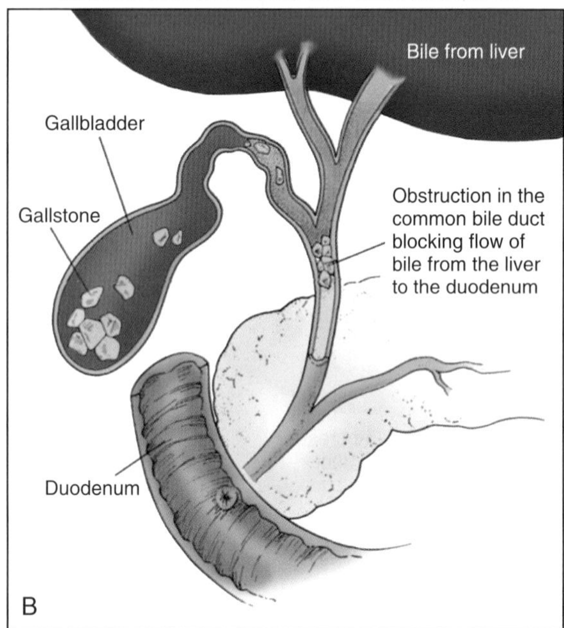

• **Fig. 12.4** (A) Gallstones and (B) Cholelithiasis. (A. From Shiland, B. J. (2022). *Mastering healthcare terminology* (7th ed.). Mosby. Fig. 5.17; B. From McIntosh, S. N. (2022). *Williams' basic nutrition and diet therapy* (16th ed.). Elsevier. Fig. 22.5.)

Cholecystitis

Acute calculous cholecystitis is the inflammation of the gallbladder caused by the blockage of a gallbladder duct by a stone. Acute acalculous cholecystitis is inflammation of the gallbladder due to illness/infection/injury of the gall bladder, leading to biliary stasis. It is not caused by a stone. Stasis → ischemia → necrosis → perfusion. Both conditions can advance to chronic cholecystitis, which has vague symptoms. The gallbladder wall is thick and scarred from constant irritation of gallstones.

Diagnosis

- History and physical
- Complete blood count
- Blood cultures
- LFTs
- Ultrasound
- CT scan
- ERCP

Symptoms

- RUQ and epigastric pain
- Fever
- Loss of appetite
- Nausea and vomiting

Treatment: often resolves within 7 to 10 days, may need laparoscopic surgery

Choledocholithiasis and Cholangitis

Choledocholithiasis is the blockage of the common duct with a gallstone. Depending on where the stone is, it can also block the pancreatic duct, causing pancreatitis.

Symptoms

- RUQ pain
- Chills
- Fever
- Jaundice
- Bilirubinemia

Cholangitis is the inflammation and infection of an obstructed common bile duct. Symptoms are known as Charcot triad (jaundice, fever, RUQ pain).

Acute suppurative cholangitis is a medical emergency. The infection has become purulent and can lead to septic shock.

Symptoms

- Reynolds pentad (includes: jaundice, fever, RUQ pain)
- Altered mental status
- Hypotension

Diagnosis

- History and physical
- Complete blood count

- Blood cultures
- LFTs
- Ultrasound
- CT scan
- ERCP

Treatment: ERCP decompression, biliary stents, gallbladder removal, laparoscopic surgery, intravenous (IV) fluids and antibiotics

Pancreatic Disorders

The pancreas has an exocrine function, releasing pancreatic enzymes into the pancreatic duct, which connects to the common duct and small intestine.

Acute Pancreatitis

Acute pancreatitis is an inflammatory process that occurs with chronic alcohol use and pancreatic duct obstruction. The inflammation stimulates pancreatic enzyme secretion. Trypsin activates all the other pancreatic enzymes (chymotrypsin, amylase, and lipase) and causes autodigestion of the pancreas.

Risk factors

- Alcohol use (most common)
- Gallstones (most common)
- Infections
- Autoimmune disease
- Hyperlipidemia
- Cystic fibrosis

Symptoms

- Severe left upper quadrant (LUQ) epigastric pain radiating to chest, back, or flank
- Fever
- Systemic inflammation → septic shock and acute respiratory distress syndrome!
- Eventually, hypoxia and necrosis can occur → perforation → peritonitis

Diagnostics

- History and physical
- Labs
  - High serum amylase and lipase
  - High WBC
  - High C-reactive protein
  - Elevated glucose
  - Elevated bilirubin
- Abdominal ultrasound
- Abdominal CT scan
- ERCP

Treatment: nothing by mouth (NPO), pancreas rest, hospitalization, IV antibiotics and fluid, pain management, nasogastric (NG) tube decompression

Chronic Pancreatitis

Chronic pancreatitis is progressive destruction of the pancreas, often due to alcohol use disorder or obstruction of the pancreatic duct (gallstones). With chronic inflammation, strictures, scarring, and cysts develop.

Symptoms

- Similar to acute pancreatitis, not as severe
- Persistent LUQ pain
- Insulinopenia
- Weight loss
- Fatty stools
- Malabsorption

Complications: diabetes mellitus, pancreatic cancer

Treatment: same as acute

Study Guide for Chapter 12

Make sure that you have your class notes and textbooks on hand to answer these questions. A concept map is included to help you to diagram and link disease concepts together.

1. Describe the structure and function of the liver.

____
____
____
____

2. What are the general symptoms of liver disease? Why do they occur?

____
____
____
____

3. Why does jaundice occur in liver disease? What happens?

____
____
____
____

4. How are the different types of viral hepatitis transmitted (A, B, C)? Can you prevent hepatitis? How? Is hepatitis acute or chronic?

____
____
____
____

5. Describe the signs and symptoms of each phase of viral hepatitis (prodromal, icteric, and convalescent).

6. What is portal hypertension? When does it happen? Describe the signs and symptoms.

7. What are the prehepatic, intrahepatic, and posthepatic causes of portal hypertension?

8. Explain the pathophysiology and clinical manifestations of the following:
   - Ascites
   - Esophageal varices
   - Hepatorenal syndrome
   - Hepatic encephalopathy

9. What is cirrhosis? When does it happen?

10. When does liver failure occur? What are the signs and symptoms of liver failure?

11. Why does acute cholecystitis occur? What are the clinical manifestations of cholecystitis?

12. What is the difference between acute cholecystitis and chronic cholecystitis?

13. What is cholangitis? What happens when there is suppurative cholangitis?

14. Describe the pathophysiology and risk factors for cholelithiasis. What are the clinical manifestations? What are the different types of gallstones?

15. What happens when someone has acute pancreatitis? Describe the pathophysiology of pancreatitis and clinical manifestations (acute vs. chronic).

16. What are the lab results you need to consider with these diseases?

Concept Map

Use this concept map to link each disease to its pathophysiology, diagnostics, causes, risk factors, complications, and clinical manifestations together. This way, you will be able to see the whole picture of the disease.

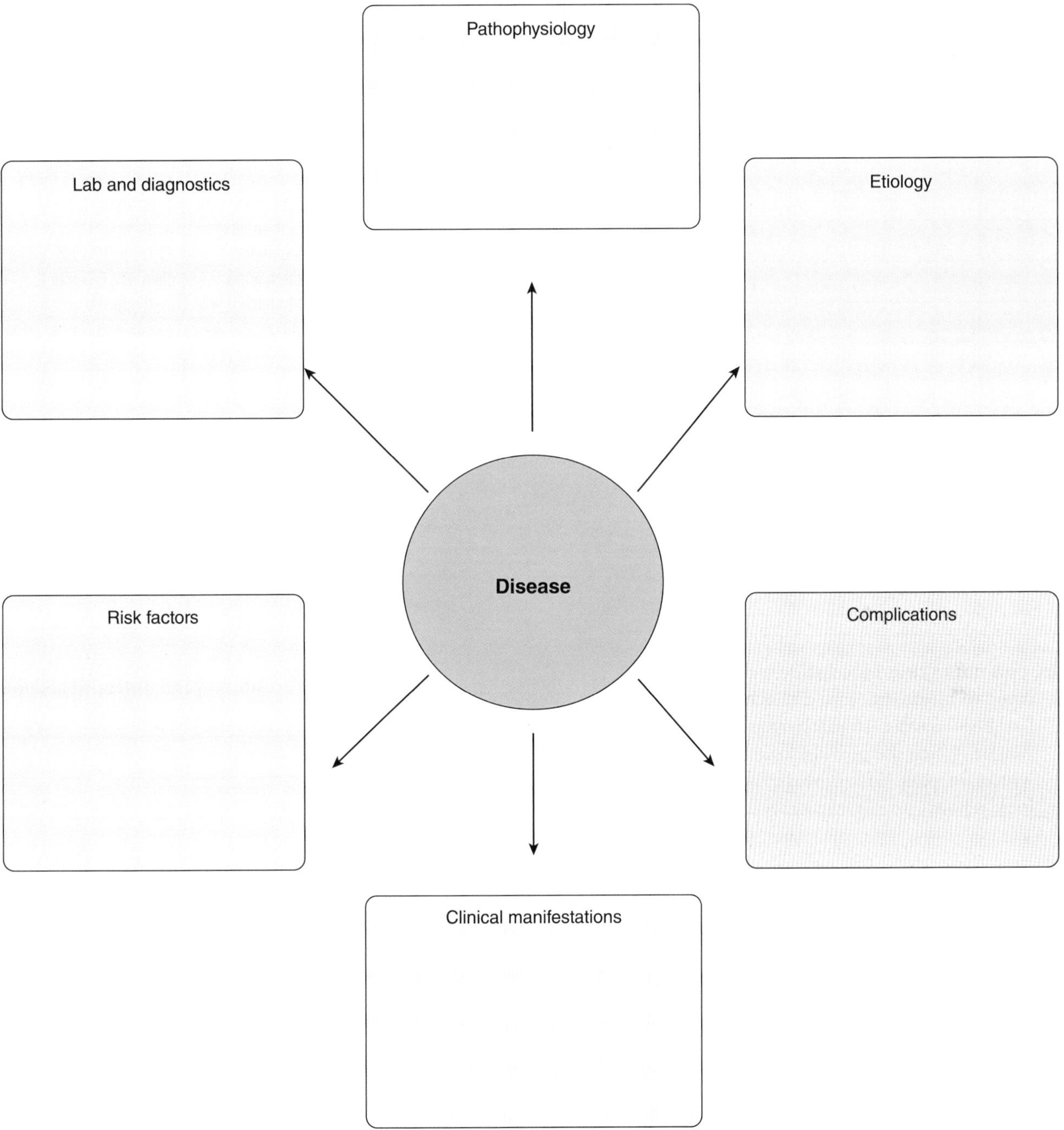

Case Studies for Chapter 12

Make sure that you have your class notes and textbooks on hand to answer these questions.

Case Study 12.1

Joe is a generally healthy 63-year-old cis-male (he/him) with no health complaints. He states that his past medical history includes hypertension, anxiety, and substance use disorder. He is taking two medications: lisinopril and methadone. During a routine physical, he is screened for hepatitis C. The test has come back positive.

1. Joe is extremely upset. He says, "I haven't touched drugs in 35 years! I've been faithful to my wife! How did I get this?" How would you answer him?

2. Joe states that he does not want to take medication for something that has no symptoms and is not affecting his lifestyle. Is this the right decision? Explain.

Joe opts not to treat his condition. Five years later, he has come to his provider for a checkup and states that he has been having stomach trouble and been losing weight. When the provider palpates his abdomen, Joe winces in pain. His provider notices that Joe's eyes look yellow.

3. Are Joe's symptoms indicative of hepatitis C? Explain the pathophysiology of these symptoms.

4. Is hepatitis C treatable? How?

Case Study 12.2

Milo is a 25-year-old nonbinary individual (they/them) who was brought to the emergency room by ambulance with confusion, abdominal pain, and lethargy. Patient denies any past medical history, but electronic medical records show that they were hospitalized for COVID-19 1 month ago.

Vital Signs	Assessment	Labs
BP: 162/94 mm Hg RR: 18 breaths/minute HR: 126 beats/minute Temperature: 101°F O_2 sat: 95%	Client uses they/them pronouns Client oriented to person and place, complaining of RUQ abdominal pain, nausea, diarrhea, and loss of appetite Client's sclera is observed to have a yellowish tinge and abdomen is distended	WBC: 9000/L (normal) Hct: 35% (slightly low) Hgb: 12 mg/dL (slightly low) BUN: 32 mg/dL (high) Creatinine: 1.7 mg/dL (high) LFTs: >300 IU/L (high) Bilirubin: 6.9 mg/dL (high) Albumin: 3.0 g/dL (low)

1. What do you think is happening to Milo? What may have led to this condition?

2. What is causing Milo's confusion and distended abdomen?

3. Why would Milo's condition cause diarrhea and jaundice?

4. Are there other labs that are abnormal? Explain why.

Milo is admitted to the ICU. They initially start to improve, but on day 3 of admission, they become drowsy and lethargic, severely jaundiced, and oliguric.

Labs
Hct: 30% (low) Hgb: 10 mg/dL (low) BUN: 300 mg/dL (high) Creatinine: 4.2 mg/dL (high) LFTs: >10,000 IU/L (high) Bilirubin: 10 mg/dL (high) Albumin: 2.4 g/dL (low) Ammonia: 124 micromol/L (high) Prothrombin time: 30 seconds (high)

5. Why has Milo's condition changed?

6. Use the labs to explain the pathophysiology of Milo's symptoms.

Milo suddenly starts to vomit blood and the urine coming out of their Foley catheter appears to contain blood.

7. Why would Milo start to bleed?

BP, Blood pressure; *BUN,* blood urea nitrogen; *Hct,* hematocrit; *Hgb,* hemoglobin; *HR,* heart rate; *ICU,* intensive care unit; *LFTs,* liver function tests; *O_2 sat,* oxygen saturation; *RR,* respiratory rate; *RUQ,* right upper quadrant; *WBC,* white blood cell.

Case Study 12.3

Champane is a 41-year-old Black cis-female (she/her) with a history of gallstones. She arrives at the urgent care with a low-grade fever (101°F). RUQ pain and yellowing of sclera.

1. What would you suspect as a diagnosis? Why?

Champane is transferred to the emergency room, where she receives an abdominal CT scan. The scan showed that she has multiple gallstones that were blocking the bile duct. Champane was admitted to the medical floor and scheduled for an ERCP with gallstone removal. While the nurse was assessing her on the floor, Champane started to become anxious and stated that she was in a lot of pain. The nurse said that Champane would just have to wait for pain medications to be ordered.

2. Was the nurse correct in asking Champane to wait for pain medications? Why or why not?

When the night nurse came in to assess Champane, they noticed that she was agitated and appeared delirious. Vital signs were BP: 80/62 mm Hg, HR: 134 beats/minute, Temp: 102°F, RR: 24 breaths/minute, O_2 sat: 97%. The rapid response team was called, and Champane was transferred to the ICU.

3. Why would Champane's condition be considered a medical emergency?

4. What diagnosis would you give Champane? How would this be treated?

BP, Blood pressure; *CT,* computed tomography; *ERCP,* endoscopic retrograde cholangiopancreatography; *HR,* heart rate; *ICU,* intensive care unit; *O_2 sat,* oxygen saturation; *RR,* respiratory rate; *Temp,* temperature.

Case Study 12.4

Blue is an 18-year-old Puebloan cis-female (she/her) diagnosed with cystic fibrosis, who lives in a remote Pueblo First Nations community in northeastern Arizona. She is followed by a care team from the Indian Health Service. Blue's mother has been brought her to the health center for severe epigastric pain that radiates to her back.

Vital Signs	Assessment	Labs
BP: 130/97 mm Hg RR: 28 breaths/ minute HR: 118 beats/ minute O_2 sat: 94% Temperature: 100.6°F	Client uses she/her pronouns Client is doubled over in pain, nauseated, and diaphoretic Pain started suddenly 24 hours ago On exam, epigastric tenderness, radiating to back	WBC: 2000/L CRP: 300 mg/L Serum amylase: 200 U/L Serum lipase: 182 U/L

1. Looking at the assessment data, what would you suspect Blue's diagnosis is? Why?

2. How can you diagnose Blue's condition?

3. Is this connected to Blue's cystic fibrosis diagnosis? If so, explain the connection.

4. What complications would you be concerned about?

BP, Blood pressure; *CRP,* C-reactive protein; *HR,* heart rate; *O_2 sat,* oxygen saturation; *RR,* respiratory rate; *WBC,* white blood cell.

13

Neurological Disorders Part 1

In this chapter, we will be discussing spinal cord injury (SCI), brain injury, and meningitis. SCI can cause damage to both motor and sensory nerves. Complete transections will result in complete loss of function below the level of injury. Consequences of spinal cord and brain injury are devastating to clients and families and have huge impacts socially and economically, as well as physically. Caregiver burden is also high with these types of injuries.

Spinal Cord Injuries

- Trauma/penetrating wounds
- Spinal fractures
- Spinal dislocations
- Primary injury
  - Happens at the time of injury
  - Irreversible
  - Hemorrhage and edema → necrosis
  - Secondary injury results
- Secondary injury
  - More hemorrhaging, edema, vascular damage
  - Injury progresses above and below level of injury

Spinal Shock

- Spinal shock happens immediately after spinal injury and is temporary
- Flaccid paralysis below level of injury
- Absence of sensation below injury
- Loss of bowel and bladder

Neurogenic Shock

- Inhibition of the sympathetic nervous system (SNS) below injury
- Activation or parasympathetic nervous system (PNS) above injury
- Vasodilation → hypotension
- Bradycardia
- Hypothermia
- Lasts 3 to 4 days; can be longer

Level of injury determines the level of impairment.

- Cervical injury—quadriplegia
  - C4 and above—loss of respiratory function
- Thoracic, lumbar, sacral—paraplegia

With SCI, the autonomic nervous system is disrupted, the SNS is dysfunctional and cannot oppose PNS.

- Vasovagal response
  - Cause: suctioning, position change
  - If vagal nerve is stimulated:
    - bradycardia → cardiac output → hypotension → asystole
  - Need anticholinergic drugs to reverse

Autonomic Dysreflexia

- Communication between hypothalamus and SNS below level of injury is lost (Fig. 13.1)
- Symptoms occur in people with T6 injuries or higher after spinal shock resolves
- Triggered by discomfort at T6 and below
- Causes
  - Full bladder
  - Full rectum or fecal impaction
  - Tight clothes
  - Pressure ulcers
- Exaggerated PNS symptoms above injury
  - Vasodilation
  - High blood pressure
  - Profuse sweating
  - Bradycardia↑
  - Headache↑
  - Distended jugular veins
- Exaggerated SNS symptoms below injury
  - Vasoconstriction
  - Paleness
  - Coolness
  - Piloerection
  - No sweating
- Injuries at C4 or higher affect respiratory system

Intracranial Pressure

- Pressure inside skull
- Cerebral perfusion pressure (CPP) = mean arterial pressure (MAP) − intracranial pressure (ICP)
  - Normal CPP: 70 to 100 mm Hg
  - ↓CPP → ↓perfusion → hypoxia → neuronal necrosis

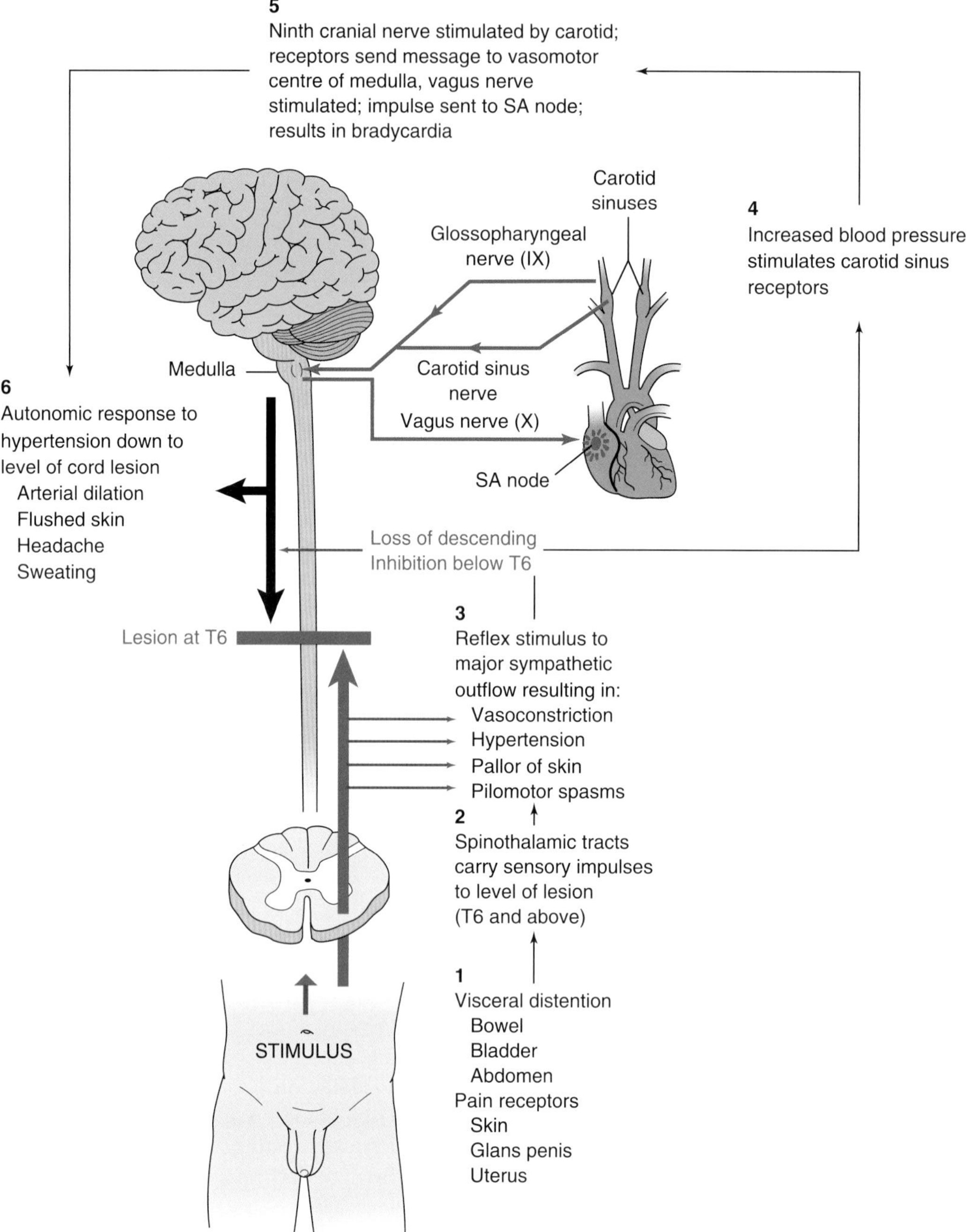

• **Fig. 13.1** Autonomic dysreflexia pathway. *SA*, Sinoatrial. (From Rudy E.B. (1984). Advanced neurological and neurosurgical nursing. Mosby.)

- Early signs: confusion
- Late signs: stupor and coma
- Brain tissue (80%), blood (10%), cerebrospinal fluid (CSF) (10%)
  - Monro-Kelly doctrine—if one compartment increases, then other one or two of the other compartments must decrease
- Normal ICP: 0 to 15 mm Hg
- Increased ICP: greater than 20 mm Hg
- Causes of increased ICP
  - Brain tumors
  - Bleeding in brain
  - Inflammation → edema
  - CSF drainage obstructed
  - Vasodilation
  - Increased metabolism (fever, pain, anxiety)
- Compensation
  - Brain herniation (Fig. 13.2)
  - CSF absorption or decreased production of CSF
  - Venous compression
- Volume-pressure compliance—brain is less compliant to pressure as volume increases

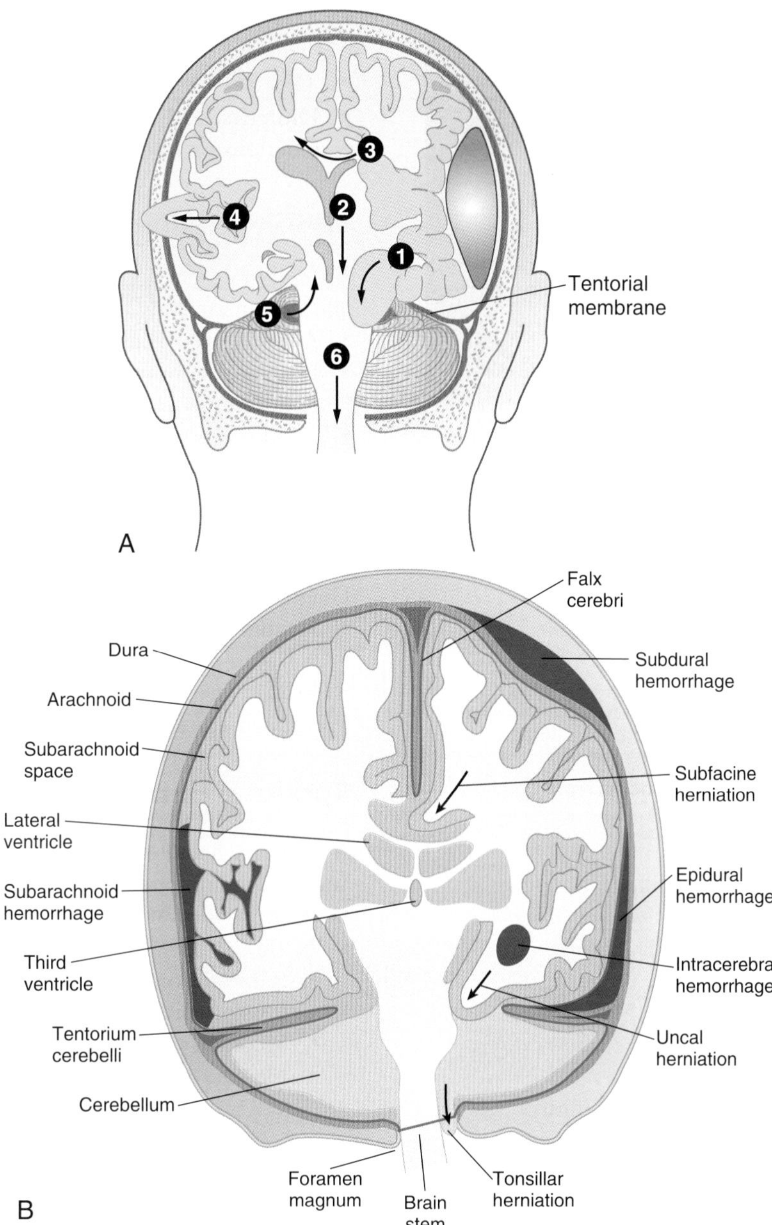

• **Fig. 13.2** (A) Pathways of brain herniation. 1, Uncal; 2, central; 3, cingulate, 4, transcalvarial; 5, upward cerebellar 6, tonsillar. (B) Causes of brain herniation. (From A. Power-Kean, K., Zettel, S., El-Hussein, M. T., Huether, S. E., & McCance, K. L. (2022). *Huether and McCance's understanding pathophysiology, Canadian edition* (2nd ed.). Elsevier. Fig. 15.10; B. From Herring, W. (2023). *Learning Radiology: Recognizing the basics* (5th ed.). Elsevier. Fig. 26.8.)

- Herniation can happen from hemisphere to hemisphere or downward into foramen magnum

Symptoms

- Early
  - Decreased level of consciousness
  - Headache
  - Projectile vomiting
  - Abnormal eye movement, pupillary changes, papilledema
- Late
  - Cushing triad—abnormal respirations, bradycardia, widening pulse pressure
  - Posturing
    - Decorticate
    - Decerebrate
  - Seizures
  - Bulging fontanels and high-pitched cry (infants)

Traumatic Brain Injury

Traumatic brain injury (TBI) can be caused by any kind of head injury. It may result in a skull fracture, hemorrhaging, or brain injury.

- Blunt force trauma
  - Causes brain to accelerate and hit skull
  - Coup-contrecoup injury (whiplash)

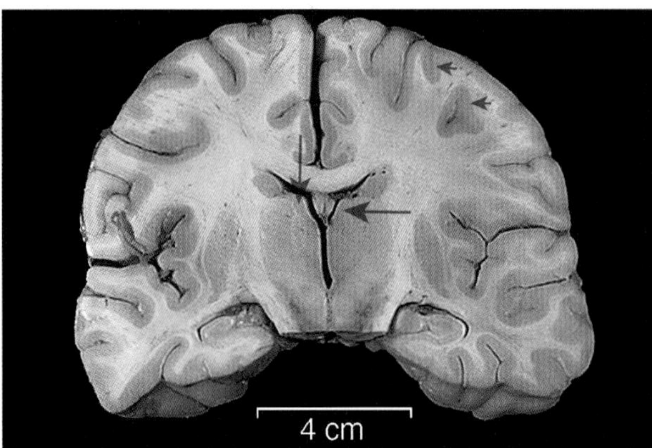

• **Fig. 13.3** Brain edema resulting in subfalcine herniation (midline shift). (From Klatt E.C. (2010). Robbins and Cotran atlas of pathology. (2nd ed.). Saunders.)

  - Contusion and hematoma
- Common causes
  - Motor vehicle accidents
  - Biking accidents
  - Falls
  - Military injuries
  - Sports injuries
- Primary injury
  - Immediate injury (contusion, hemorrhage)
  - Focal lesions (concussion)
- Secondary injury
  - Caused by edema, brain swelling (Fig. 13.3)
  - Inflammation, infection
  - Results in ↓ CPP, brain hypoxia, and ischemia

Concussions

- Mechanical force
- Diffuse, short-term injury, no physical injury
- Loss of consciousness, amnesia, irritability, poor concentration
- Second impact syndrome
- Multiple concussions → chronic traumatic encephalopathy (CTE)
  - Buildup of tau protein in neurons
  - Loss of function, dementia, psychosis

Diagnosis: History and physical, head CT scan, MRI

Treatment: time, rest, and non-contact activities until the symptoms have resolved.

Contusion

- Direct force, skull fracture
- Focal bruising or laceration of brain tissue
- Severe secondary injury
  - Edema
  - ↑ ICP
  - Herniation

Diagnosis
- History and physical exam
- Computed tomography (CT) scan
- Magnetic resonance imaging (MRI)

Treatment
- Time
- Diuretics, such as mannitol
- Craniotomy to drain blood

Epidural Hematoma

An epidural hematoma is a hemorrhage between the skull and dura mater (Fig. 13.4).
- Arterial bleed—fast
- Hematoma compresses the brain
  - Accumulating blood → brain herniation → death
- Head injury followed by brief period of unconsciousness followed by lucid period
- Rapid decompensation after lucid period
- Coma
- Ipsilateral pupillary changes

Diagnosis
- History and physical exam
- CT scan
- MRI

Treatment: craniotomy to drain blood

Subdural Hematoma

A subdural hematoma is a venous bleed between the dura and arachnoid mater.
- Venous—slower
- Acute
  - Rapid decompensation
  - Loss of consciousness with no lucid period
  - Secondary edema → ↑ICP
  - Hematoma needs to be drained

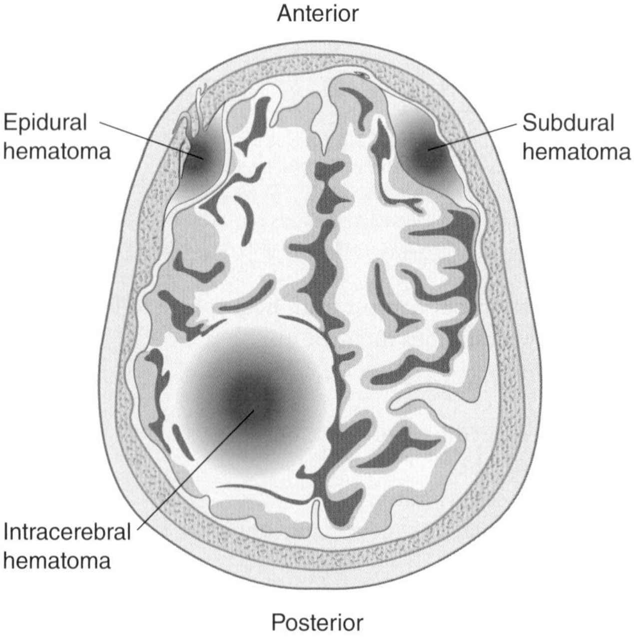

Anterior

Epidural hematoma

Subdural hematoma

Intracerebral hematoma

Posterior

• **Fig. 13.4** Types of brain hematomas. (From Heuther, S.E., & McCance, K.L. (2019). Understanding Pathophysiology. Elsevier.)

- Subacute
  - 2 to 10 days after injury
  - Initial improvement, then deterioration
  - Hematoma needs to be drained
- Chronic
  - Weeks after injury
  - Common in elderly, especially on blood thinners
  - Loss of consciousness, headache, apathy

Diagnosis
- History and physical exam
- CT scan
- MRI

Treatment: time, surgery, craniotomy

Meningitis

Meningitis is an inflammation of the meninges, or membranes that covers the brain and spinal cord.
- Pia mater, arachnoid, subarachnoid space
- Caused by bacteria (purulent) or viruses
  - *Streptococcus pneumoniae*
  - *Neisseria meningitidis*
  - Enteroviruses

Risk factors
- Basilar skull fracture
- Otitis media
- Sinusitis
- Sepsis
- Close quarters, such as dorms

Symptoms
- Headache
- Photophobia
- Fever
- Vomiting
- Nuchal rigidity
- Petechial rash
- Kernig sign
- Brudzinski sign

Diagnosis
- History and physical exam
- Lumbar puncture (after increased ICP ruled out)
  - If CSF is cloudy, it is a bacterial infection
- Droplet precautions: face mask, isolation

Treatment
- Antibiotics (if viral, stop after bacterial has been ruled out)
- Supportive care if viral (self-limiting)

Study Guide for Chapter 13

Make sure that you have your class notes and textbooks on hand to answer these questions. A concept map is included to help you to diagram and link disease concepts together.

1. What is SCI? How does it occur?

2. What is spinal shock? How does it manifest? What is the difference between spinal shock and neurogenic shock?

3. What is the difference between the primary vs secondary SCI? What leads to each one?

4. What motor-sensory function would you expect to see in a person with an SCI at C3, T7, or L1 level? Which one would require a ventilatory support—why?

5. Explain the vasovagal response. Why is it a concern in SCI patients?

6. What is autonomic dysreflexia? What leads to it and why does it occur? What are the signs and symptoms?

7. What is the Monro-Kellie doctrine? What happens if ICP or MAP increase?

8. What are possible causes and factors leading to an increased ICP? Which conditions contribute to the vasodilation of cerebral blood vessels?

9. What is CPP and what factors influence it? What are the early and late clinical manifestations of a decreased CPP?

10. What is compliance and how does it change with the volume increase? What happens when the ICP compensatory mechanisms have reached their limit? What clinical manifestations would alert you to that?

11. What are the late manifestations of an increased ICP? Explain what leads to them.

12. What are the stages of brain pathology development after a TBI? What happens in each stage?

13. What is the difference between contusion and concussion? Which one is more dangerous? What are the complications of each?

14. What is the difference between epidural and subdural hematoma? Which one occurs more rapidly? Why?

15. What are the signs and symptoms of an epidural hematoma? What is the biggest complication?

16. What are the different classifications of subdural hematomas? What are the symptoms of each?

17. What is meningitis? What causes it? Which one is more severe, viral or bacterial?

18. What are the clinical manifestations of meningitis?

Concept Map

Use this concept map to link each disease to its pathophysiology, diagnostics, causes, risk factors, complications, and clinical manifestations together. This way, you will be able to see the whole picture of the disease

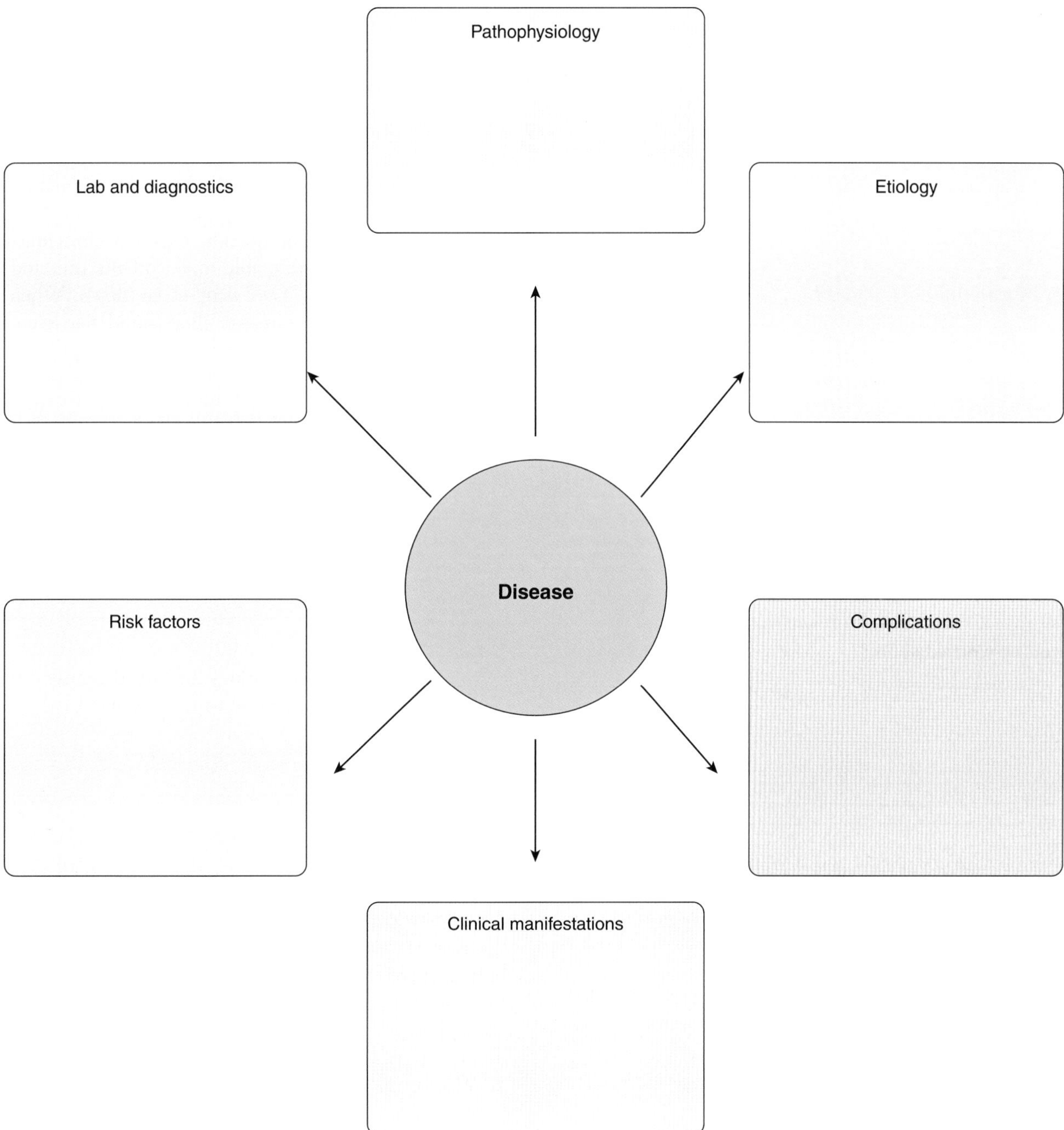

Case Studies for Chapter 13

Case Study 13.1

Rosa is a 35-year-old Latinx cis-female (she/her), who is an architect. She was inspecting work on a three-story building, when she fell from the ladder and landed on her back. Her coworkers rushed to her side and found her conscious. However, she was extremely anxious, stating, "I can't feel my legs, I can't feel my legs!"

1. Why can't Rosa feel her legs? What other symptoms of this condition would you look for?

2. Is this condition permanent?

Rosa was rushed to the hospital by ambulance. After an emergency MRI, it is determined that Rosa has sustained an irreversible C6 injury.

3. With a C6 spinal injury, what complication(s) would you be worried about?

Rosa is now paraplegic and is wheelchair-bound. She is admitted to rehab and has worked with physical and occupational therapy to go back to work with accommodations. One day, her nurse notices that Rosa is sweating and flushed.

Assessment: vital signs: BP: 184/98 mm Hg, RR: 26 breaths/minute, HR: 42 beats per minute, O_2 sat: 97% on room air

4. What is happening to Rosa?

5. What symptoms justify your answer?

BP, Blood pressure; *HR,* heart rate; *O_2 sat,* oxygen saturation; *MRI,* magnetic resonance imaging; *RR,* respiratory rate.

Case Study 13.2

Geo, a 28-year-old nonbinary individual (he/they/them), is skiing with his partner. As he was skiing, he skidded off the path and hit a tree. When his partner got to him, Geo was briefly unconscious, but quickly regained consciousness. Geo and his partner were able to ski off the trail and get back to their lodgings. Geo went to lay down. When his partner came to wake him up, they found that Geo was unconscious.

1. What would you suspect? Is this an emergency? Why or why not?

2. Explain the pathophysiology of the diagnosis. What complication would you be worried about?

Case Study 13.3

Lee is an 18-year-old cis male (he/him) who is on the varsity football team at his high school. During a football game, Lee was hit in the head and lost consciousness. He regained consciousness quickly and wanted to go back into the game. The coach let him back into the game.

1. Was this the right decision? Why or why not?

After the game, Lee felt nauseated and started to vomit. He complained of a severe headache. His parents took him to the emergency room, where he received a head computed tomography (CT) scan. He was diagnosed with a concussion. He comes in for a follow-up appointment at his pediatric provider's office.

2. Lee asks, "Can I go back to playing football next week? We have a big game!" What would you say?

3. Lee tells you that he is having difficulty focusing in class and getting through assignments. Are these normal symptoms of concussion?

Case Study 13.4

At a local college, Lizzie, a White cis-female (she/her) has been complaining of headaches, fever and chills, and neck and back pain. Health services sent Lizzie to the local emergency room to be evaluated. When she arrives at the emergency room, the triage nurse assesses her.

Vital Signs	Assessment
BP: 110/60 mm Hg RR: 20 breaths/minute HR: 110 beats per minute O_2 sat: 98% on room air Temperature: 101.2°F	Client uses she/her pronouns Client has fever and chills, states that her eyes hurt "from the lights" Complaining of neck and back pain. Appears lethargic States that she vomited twice +Kernig sign

1. If you were the triage nurse, what would you do next? Why?

Lizzie is taken back to a room. The provider comes in to assess. Labs are drawn. After a head CT scan, a lumbar puncture is done.

Labs
WBC: 22,000/mm^3 (high) D-dimer: 3600 ng/mL (high) PLT: 50,000 mm^3 (low) PTT: 45 seconds CSF: cloudy, yellow Blood and CSF cultures pending

2. Why is a head CT scan done prior to the lumbar puncture?

3. What do Lizzie's lab results and assessments tell you? Explain the pathophysiology.

BP, Blood pressure; *CT,* computed tomography; *CSF,* cerebrospinal fluid; *HR,* heart rate; *O_2 sat,* oxygen saturation; *PLT,* platelet; *PTT,* partial thromboplastin time; *RR,* respiratory rate; *WBC,* white blood cell.

14 Neurological Disorders Part 2

Myasthenia Gravis

Myasthenia gravis (MG) is an acquired autoimmune disease where antibodies bind to acetylcholine receptors, blocking them. Eventually, the receptors are destroyed. Acetylcholine is a neurotransmitter that causes neuromuscular excitability. Without it, neuromuscular impulses cannot occur, and muscle weakness results.

MG is a disease with remissions and exacerbations. People who have other autoimmune diseases, such as type 1 diabetes mellitus, lupus, and rheumatoid arthritis, are susceptible to MG. Individuals with a thymus tumor, a thymoma, are also at high risk for MG. When the thymoma is removed, individuals often go into remission. Stress, pregnancy, cold, and infection can trigger an MG exacerbation (Fig. 14.1).

Symptoms are descending, starting from the eyes and can be unilateral or bilateral.

- Ptosis (eyelid droop)
- Diplopia (double vision)
- Muscle weakness
- Chewing/swallowing dysfunction
- May affect respiratory muscles
- Respiratory arrest
- Paralysis
- May proceed downward to extremities

Diagnosis

- History and physical
- Labs—autoantibody titer

Treatment: thymectomy, steroids, immunosuppressants

Guillain-Barre Syndrome

Guillain-Barre syndrome (GBS) is an immune-mediated ascending neuromuscular disorder. It is triggered by a viral illness. Molecular mimicry causes the viral antigen to resemble the neural antigen. These antibodies attack the myelin and neuronal axons. It can result in motor or motor and sensory effects. GBS attacks the peripheral nerves and attacks the longest axons first. It progresses symmetrically and ascends from the legs up. Most patients make a full recovery. It is rare for GBS to reoccur.

Symptoms

- Paresthesia in hands and feet
- Muscle weakness
- Absent deep tendon reflexes
- Respiratory failure

Diagnosis

- History and physical
- Antibody titer

Treatment: intravenous (IV) immune globulin, plasmapheresis

Parkinson Disease

Parkinson disease is an epigenetic disease believed to be caused by a lack of dopamine, as there is a loss of dopamine-producing neurons in the substantia nigra and basal ganglia. Causes for this are thought to be environmental and genetic. Secondary parkinsonism can be caused by pesticides, Agent Orange, brain damage, and antipsychotics. It is typically diagnosed later in life but can have an early onset. Death of the dopamine-producing neurons is thought to be caused by oxidative stress and mitochondrial dysfunction. Dopamine is an inhibitory neurotransmitter, which means that muscles are not able to relax and stay contracted, causing spasms. Another issue that happens with Parkinson disease is that alpha-synuclein protein, which is normally found in neurons, is abnormally formed, and accumulates in the neuron-forming Lewy bodies. This can lead to Lewy body dementia, which happens to 25% of patients with Parkinson disease.

Hallmark symptoms (Fig. 14.2)

- Tremor
- Bradykinesia
- Rigidity
- Postural instability and falls

Other symptoms

- Autonomic neuropathy
- Fatigue
- Pain
- Anxiety and depression
- Insomnia
- Dementia
- Excessive saliva and sweating

Diagnosis

- History and physical
- Diagnosis by exclusion

Treatment: deep brain stimulation, synthetic dopamine, interdisciplinary care

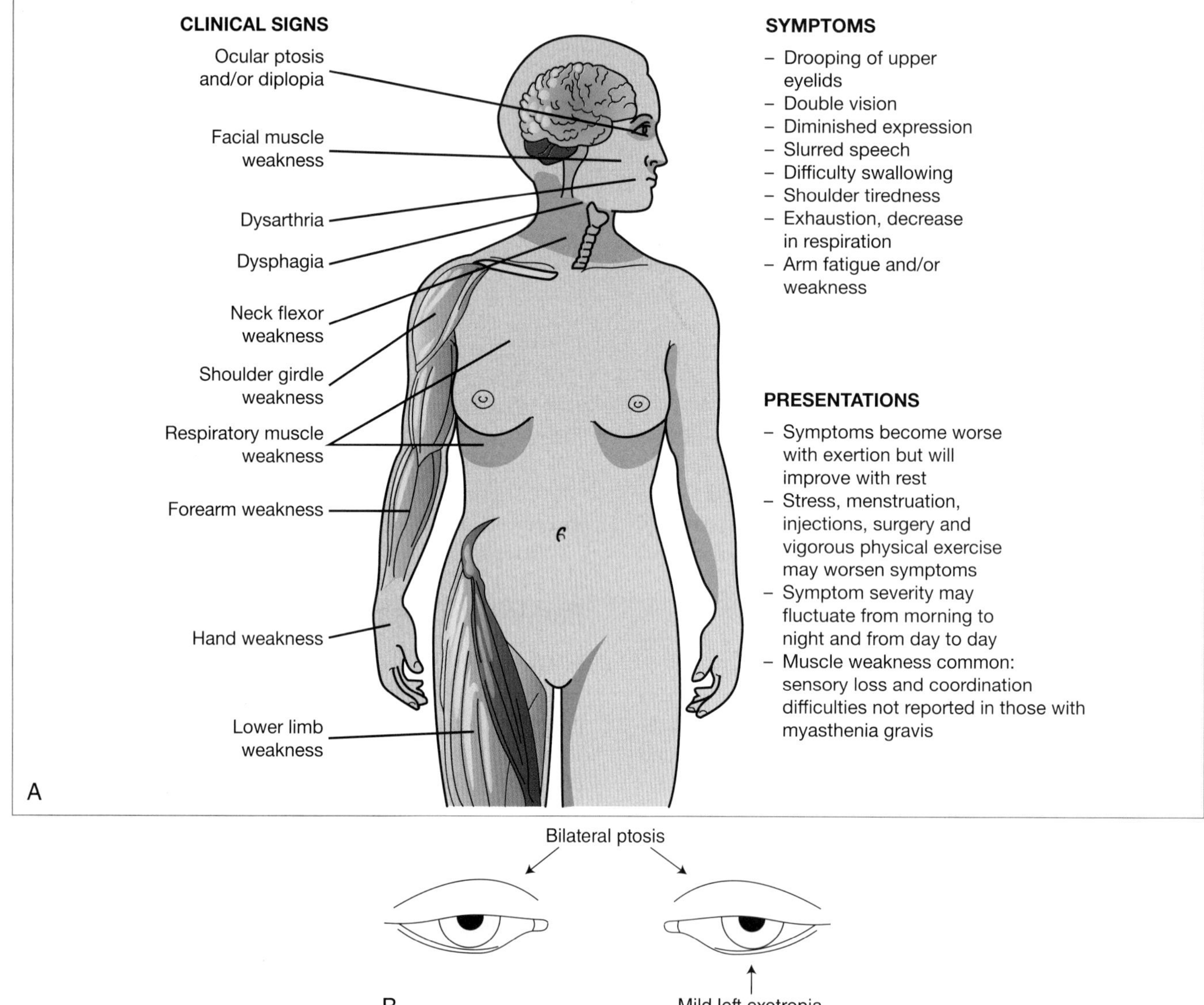

• **Fig. 14.1** (A and B) Clinical manifestatons of myasthenia gravis. (A. From Knights, K., Rowland, A., Darroch, S., Bushell, M. (2023). *Pharmacology for health professionals* (6th ed.). Elsevier. Fig. 24.3; B. From Ferri, F. F. (2022). *Ferri's clinical advisor* 2023 (1st ed.). Elsevier. Fig. 1.)

Multiple Sclerosis

Multiple sclerosis is also an epigenetic disease that is still not well understood. The triggers are thought to be stress, viral illness (Epstein-Barr virus), amount of sunlight, and vitamin D levels. It is typically not an inherited disease, but there can be a genetic predisposition, as well as environmental factors like smoking. Individuals who have autoimmune disease are more susceptible. Multiple sclerosis has widely been thought to affect White individuals of European descent in countries in the northern hemisphere. However, recent studies have shown that more people of color are being diagnosed with MS than previously expected. Black individuals have been found to have a more aggressive form of MS, with different symptoms, and greater disability. However, this may be because of later diagnosis and difference in the access to care.

With MS, inflammation and immune reactions occur. Self-reactive T and B cells cross the blood-brain barrier. The T and B cells recognize the myelin covering the axons and oligodendrocytes as antigens and destroy them. The lack of myelin and myelin-producing cells causes neuronal death and brain atrophy. This affects both white and gray matter (Fig. 14.3).

Types of MS (Table 14.1)

- Relapsing-remitting (most common)
- Secondary progressive
- Primary progressive
- Progressive relapsing

Symptoms

- Clumsiness
- Paresthesia
- Lhermitte syndrome
- Optic neuritis

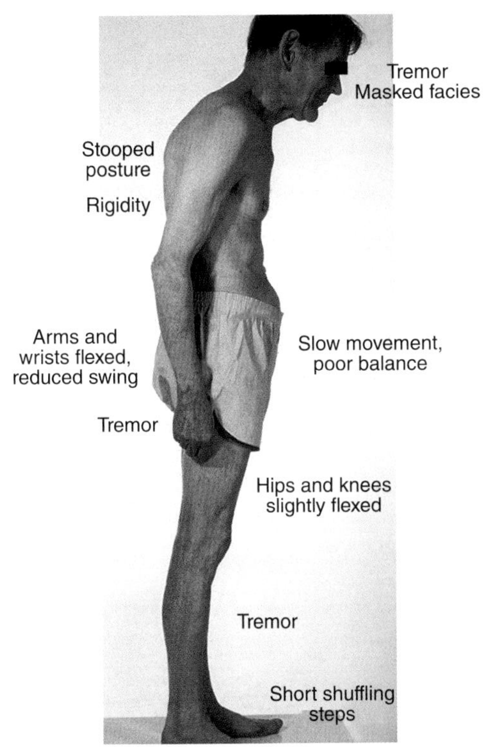

• **Fig. 14.2** Parkinson disease symptoms. (From Perkin D.G. (2002). Mosby's color atlas and text of neurology (2nd ed.). Mosby.)

- Spasms
- Intention tremors
- Constipation
- Bladder retention
- Anxiety
- Depression
- Pain
- Fatigue
- Inability to tolerate extreme temperatures

Diagnosis
- History and physical
- Magnetic resonance imaging (MRI)
- Diagnosis by exclusion
- Lumbar puncture—myelin antibodies

Treatment: symptom management, steroids, immunosuppressants, vitamin D

Ischemic Stroke

Ischemic strokes happen when there is a sudden blockage to a cerebral artery (usually the middle cerebral artery). This causes acute ischemia and oxygen deprivation to the brain. Symptoms depend on where in the brain the stroke occurred (Table 14.2). The area of infarction/occlusion becomes inflamed, edematous, and necrotic. The area of necrosis is

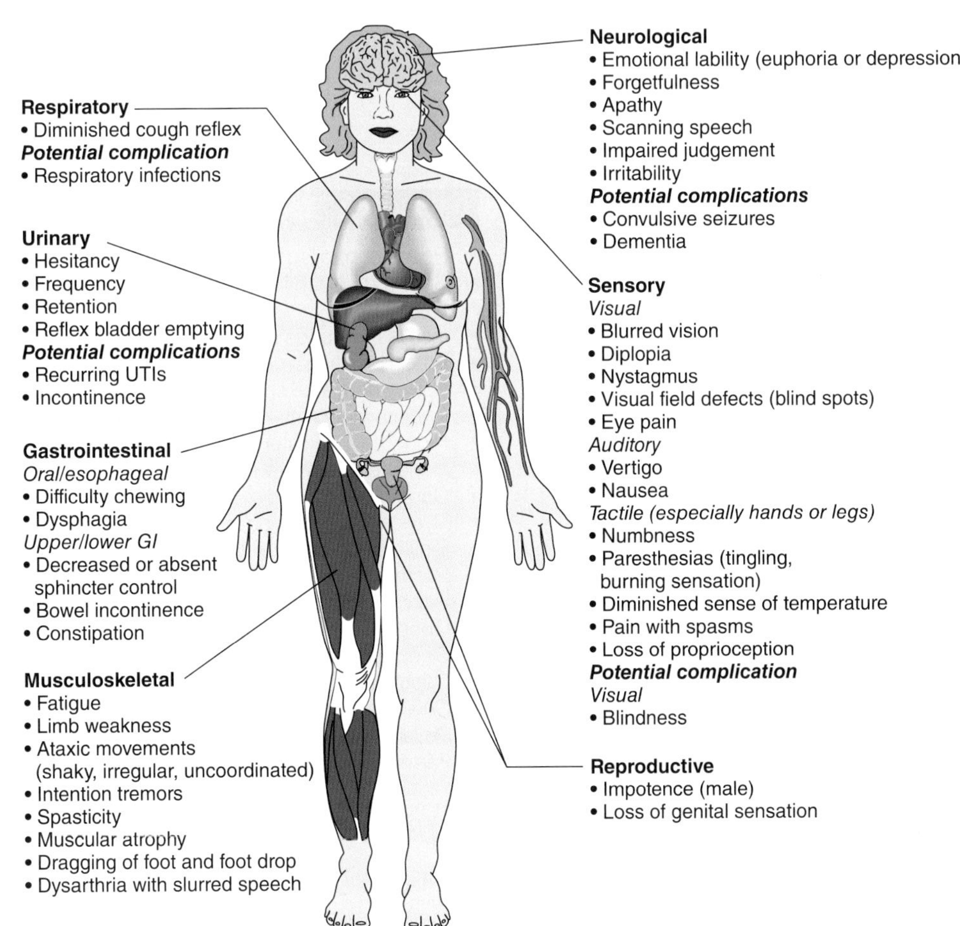

• **Fig. 14.3** Neural degeneration of multiple sclerosis. *GI,* Gastrointestinal; *UTI,* urinary tract infection. (From Lemone, P. T., Burke, K. M., & Bauldoff, G. (2011). Medical-surgical nursing: Critical thinking in patient care (7th ed.), Pearson Education, Inc, 9780134868189.)

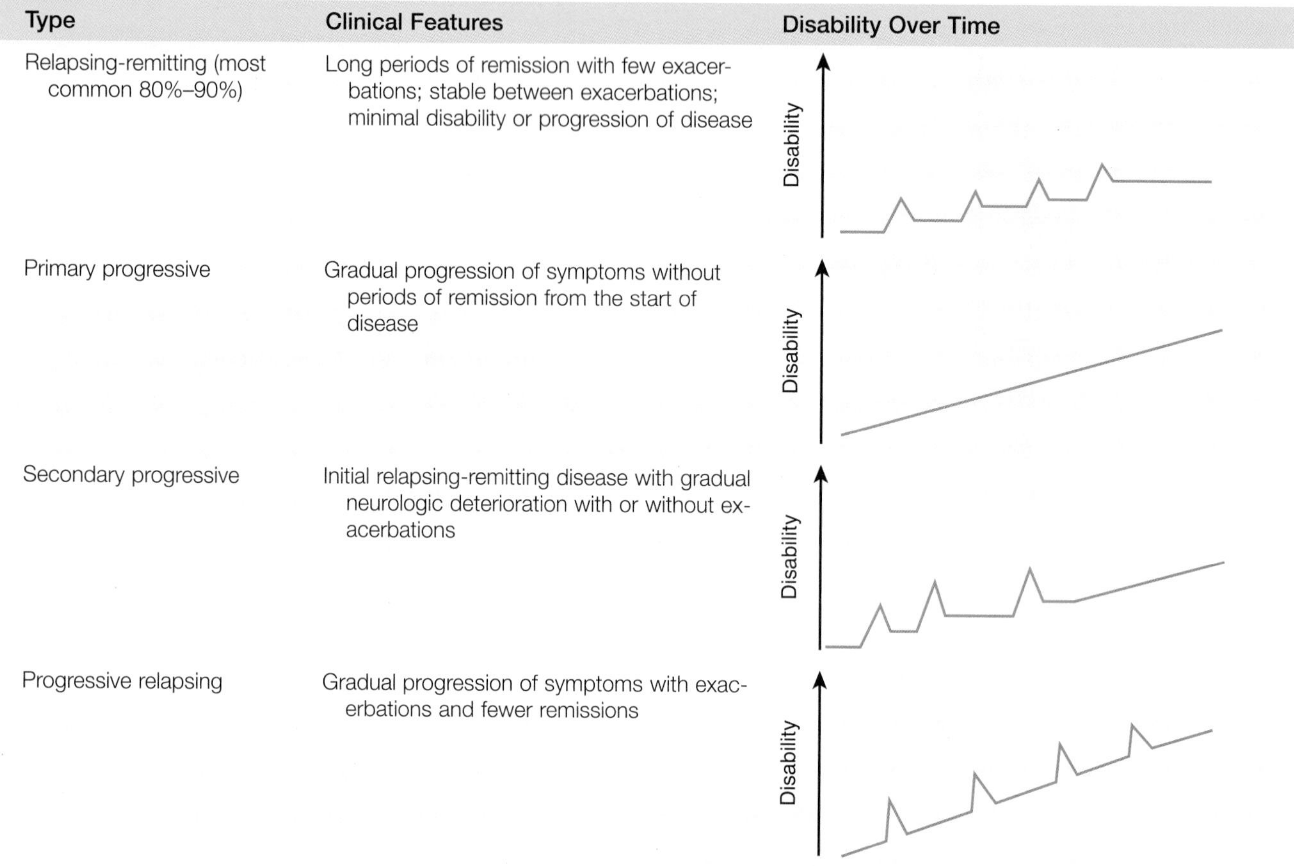

TABLE 14.1 Types of Multiple Sclerosis

Type	Clinical Features	Disability Over Time
Relapsing-remitting (most common 80%–90%)	Long periods of remission with few exacerbations; stable between exacerbations; minimal disability or progression of disease	Disability
Primary progressive	Gradual progression of symptoms without periods of remission from the start of disease	Disability
Secondary progressive	Initial relapsing-remitting disease with gradual neurologic deterioration with or without exacerbations	Disability
Progressive relapsing	Gradual progression of symptoms with exacerbations and fewer remissions	Disability

TABLE 14.2 Symptoms of Right-and Left-Sided Strokes

Left Brain Damage	Right Brain Damage
Motor deficits on the right	Motor deficits on the left
Right-sided hemiplegia	Left-sided hemiplegia
Receptive/expressive aphasia[a] • Inability to comprehend • Inability to formulate words	Left-sided neglect
Impaired right/left discrimination	Spatial-perceptual deficits
Aware of deficits, depression, anxiety	Tends to deny/minimize problems
Cautious, slow performance	Impulsive, safety problems
Mood swings	Impaired judgment

[a]Some 85% of left-handed individuals are also left-brain dominant.

• BOX 14.1 Risk Factors for Stroke

- Poorly controlled or uncontrolled arterial hypertension
- Smoking, which increases the risk of stroke by two to four times
- Insulin resistance and diabetes mellitus
- Atrial fibrillation
- Polycythemia (excess red blood cells) and thrombocythemia (excess platelets)
- High total cholesterol or low high-density lipoprotein (HDL) cholesterol, elevated lipoprotein-a
- Congestive heart disease and peripheral vascular disease
- Hyperhomocysteinemia
- Sickle cell disease
- Postmenopausal hormone therapy
- High sodium intake >2300 mg; low potassium intake <4700 mg
- Obesity
- Sleep apnea
- Depression
- *Chlamydia pneumoniae* infection
- Physical inactivity
- Family history of ischemic stroke

called the central core. The hypoxic area around the central core is called the penumbra. It is important to reperfuse the cerebral artery as soon as possible so that the penumbra does not become necrotic and so brain tissue and function is spared. Eventually, the area will heal, and scarring and a cavity will result.

Risk factors (Box 14.1)

- Atherosclerosis
- Hypertension
- Type 2 diabetes mellitus
- Visceral/abdominal fat

- Genetics
- Smoking
- Stress
- Hypercoagulability

NOTE

In most textbooks, you will see that the risk of stroke is stated to be twice as high for Black individuals than for White individuals. However, this is only part of the story. Remember that race is not biological, nor is it genetic. You need to look at the social determinants of health and equity. Do both Black and White clients have the same access to care? The same access to good jobs, education, and safe neighborhoods? Do they receive equitable treatment from providers? Statistically, Black clients who have strokes have much higher mortality rates than White clients with stroke, which suggests a disparity in care.

Types of ischemic strokes
- Thrombotic—clot from atherosclerosis
- Embolic—clot that has traveled (e.g., deep vein thrombosis [DVT], endocarditis, atrial fibrillation)
- Lacunar—small vessels in deep brain tissue

Diagnosis
- Computed tomography (CT) scan (to differentiate between ischemic and hemorrhagic stroke)
- MRI
- Carotid ultrasound
- Echocardiogram
- Cardiac monitoring
- Lab work: serum blood glucose (hypoglycemia can mimic stroke), HbA1c, lipid levels

Treatments: tissue plasminogen activator, thrombectomy, craniotomy

Transient Ischemic Attack

A transient ischemic attack can be a precursor to an ischemic stroke. There is a temporary blockage to a cerebral artery and a loss of perfusion to the brain, caused by a partial occlusion (atherosclerosis). The client will have stroke-like symptoms that resolve on its own within 24 hours.

Hemorrhagic Stroke

Hemorrhagic strokes occur most commonly due to hypertension, aneurysms, and anticoagulation medications. Secondary causes are from traumatic brain injury and ischemic stroke that has become hemorrhagic due to injury. Bleeding causes vasospasm leading to tissue ischemia. This causes inflammation and edema, and stroke symptoms.

Increased intracranial pressure (ICP) rises → Cushing triad → herniation and death

Types of bleeds

Intracerebral
- Gradual onset (minutes to days)
- Can happen at rest
- Often caused by hypertension
- Headache/nausea/vomiting
- Decreased level of consciousness
- Stroke symptoms (dependent on location)

Subarachnoid
- Sudden onset
- Happens with exertion
- Can be caused by ruptured aneurysms
- Thunderclap headache ("worst headache of my life")
- Neck pain
- Photophobia
- Nausea/vomiting/dizziness
- Possible loss of consciousness
- Silent killer!

Diagnosis
- History and physical
- CT scan
- MRI
- Cardiac monitoring

Treatment: surgery, craniotomy, mannitol (diuretic)

Alzheimer Dementia

Alzheimer disease is a progressive epigenetic disease that affects memory and behavior. Early onset (30–60 years) Alzheimer dementia is caused by chromosome 1, 14, and 21 mutations. These mutations are thought to increase beta-amyloid mutations. Late-onset Alzheimer disease is much more common, with mutations to chromosome 19 and chromosome 17. Chromosome 19 mutations affect the beta-amyloid protein clearance, causing the protein to accumulate outside the neurons in neuritic plaques. Chromosome 17 mutation causes tau proteins to accumulate inside the neurons, causing neurofibrillary tangles. These plaques and tangles cause neuronal death and brain atrophy. Alzheimer disease affects the limbic system and cortex of the brain (Fig. 14.4).

Risks
- Age
- Family history
- Environment

Stages
- Initial: short-term memory deficit, word finding difficulty
- Middle: difficulty with activities of daily living (ADLs), poor insight, aphasia
- Late: complete memory loss, global aphasia, motor deficits, bedbound, difficulty swallowing

Diagnosis
- History and physical
- Brain imaging
- Diagnosis of exclusion

Treatment: there is no cure; interdisciplinary care and symptom management

Vascular Dementia

Vascular dementia is caused by impaired blood flow (atherosclerosis, hypoxia, bleeding) in the brain, resulting in vascular changes. Atherosclerotic plaques cause hypoperfusion and tissue ischemia. The risk factors are the same as for cardiovascular disease. Although most dementia is

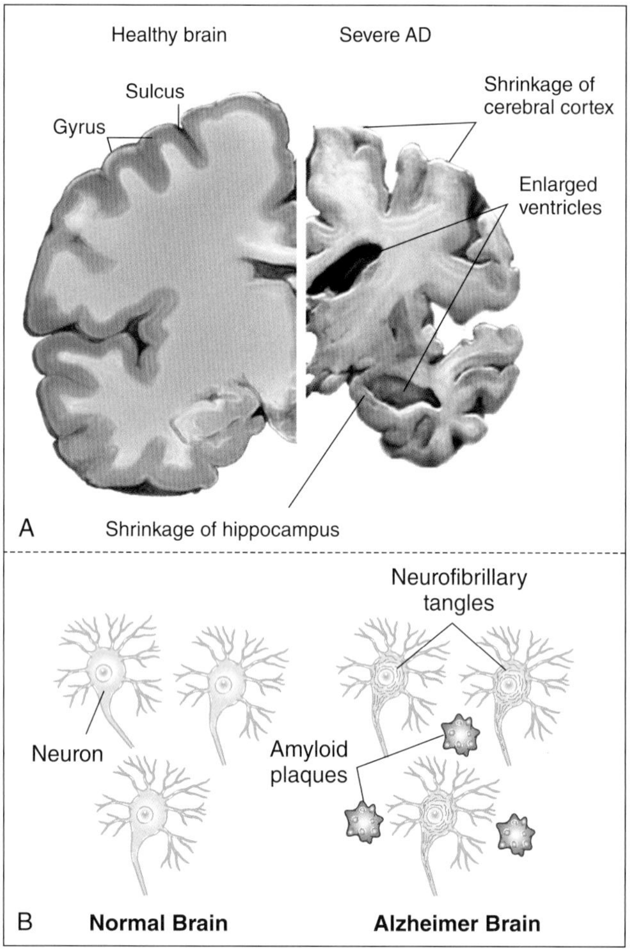

• **Fig. 14.4** Common findings in Alzheimer disease. *AD,* Atopic dermatitis. (A. From National Institute on Aging Scientific Images: Brain images. Available at https://www.nia.nih.gov/health/alzheimers-disease-fact-sheet#changes; B. From Huether, S.E., Kathryn L. McCance, K.L. (2020). Understanding Pathophysiology (7th ed.). Mosby. Fig. 16.8.)

diagnosed as Alzheimer disease (60–80 years), it is likely that vascular dementia is underdiagnosed and that most dementia is mixed dementia, meaning both Alzheimer and vascular dementia.

Risk factors

- Hyperlipidemia
- Hypertension
- High body mass index (BMI)
- Smoking
- Age
- Myocardial infarction/stroke
- Type 2 diabetes mellitus
- Assigned male at birth/postmenopausal assigned female at birth

Diagnosis

- History and physical
- Brain imaging
- Diagnosis by exclusion

Treatment: no cure; prevention is key (weight loss, smoking cessation, management of hyperlipidemia, hyperglycemia, and hypertension)

Study Guide for Chapter 14

Make sure that you have your class notes and textbooks on hand to answer these questions. A concept map is included to help you to diagram and link disease concepts together.

1. What happens in MG? Describe the role of acetylcholine and the neuromuscular junction in this disease.

2. What are the hallmark clinical manifestations of MG? When does muscle weakness occur?

3. What is myasthenic crisis? When does this happen and what are the symptoms?

4. What is the pathophysiology of GBS? How does it progress?

5. What is the pathophysiology behind Parkinson disease? What part of the brain undergoes degeneration? Which neurons are lost?

6. What are the cardinal signs of Parkinson disease? What are the nonmotor symptoms?

7. What type of disease is multiple sclerosis? What causes the disease? Describe the damage to the neurons.

8. Outline the four categories of multiple sclerosis. What are some of the symptoms?

9. What is a transient ischemic stroke?

10. What is the difference between a thrombotic and an embolic stroke? Describe the pathophysiology.

11. What are the differences between right-sided and left-sided ischemic strokes? What are the different clinical manifestations of each?

12. How is a hemorrhagic stroke different from an ischemic stroke? Outline the causes and manifestations.

13. What is the difference between an intraparenchymal, subdural, and subarachnoid stroke? Outline the causes and manifestations.

14. What are some of the causes/risk factors for Alzheimer disease?

15. What roles do the neuritic plaques and neurofibrillary tangles play in Alzheimer disease?

16. Differentiate between the symptoms of initial, early, middle, late, and end stages of Alzheimer disease.

17. What causes vascular dementia? Can it be prevented? How are the clinical manifestations different from Alzheimer disease?

Concept Map

Use this concept map to link each disease to its pathophysiology, diagnostics, causes, risk factors, complications, and clinical manifestations together. This way, you will be able to see the whole picture of the disease.

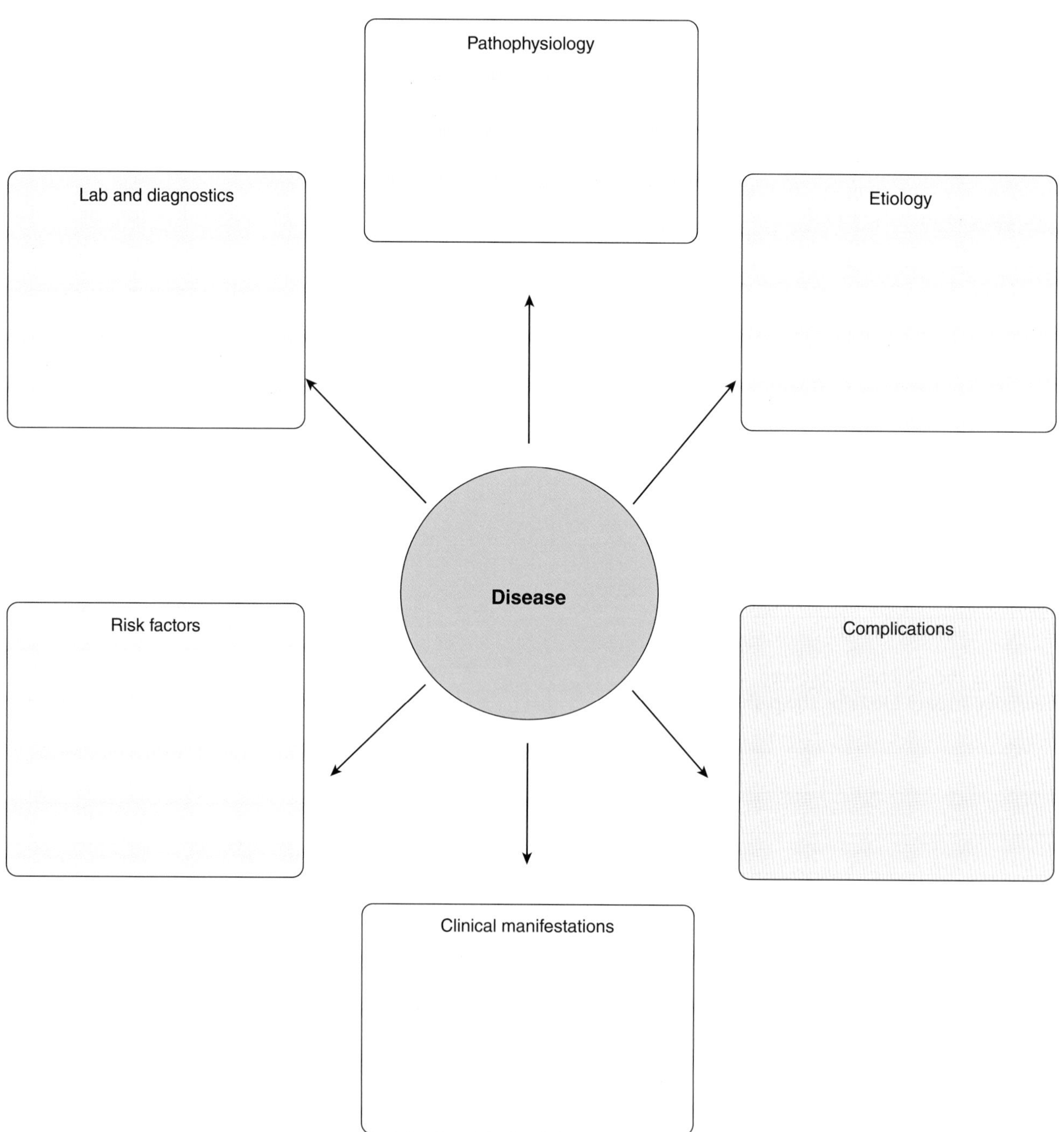

Case Studies for Chapter 14

Case Study 14.1

Cassandra is a 35-year-old Black cis-female (she/her) who noticed that she had double vision and some right-sided facial numbness and tingling (paresthesia). She went to see her provider, who assessed her and ordered some lab work.

Vital Signs	Assessment	Labs
BP:132/90 mm Hg HR: 86 beats per minute RR: 18 breaths/ minute O_2 sat: 98% on room air Temperature: 98°F Weight: 138 pounds Height: 5′6″	Client uses she/her pronouns Client states that she smokes "a couple of cigarettes a day," more if stressed States that she is a jogger and eats healthy States that she started feeling some facial tingling 3 weeks ago after she had a viral illness; she had double vision for a few hours 2 days ago, which prompted her to seek care	WBC: 12,000/L Hgb: 14 g/dL Hct: 40% Creatinine: 1.0 mg/dL BUN: 18 mg/dL ESR: 45 mm/hour (high) CRP: 20 mg/L (high) Serum glucose: 117 mg/dL HgA1c: 5.6% K: 3.5 mEq/dL Na: 140 mEq/dL Ca: 9.4 mEq/dL Mg: 1.8 mEq/dL LDL: 100 g/dL HDL: 55 g/dL

1. Looking at these results, what would you suspect is causing Cassandra's symptoms? Which results support your diagnosis?

____

____

____

____

The provider orders a head CT scan for Cassandra, which is inconclusive. The provider told her that she probably had a transient ischemic attack and told her to reduce her stress.

2. Does Cassandra have risk factors for a stroke? If so, what are they?

____

____

____

____

Cassandra's symptoms start to worsen over the next few months. She starts to experience severe fatigue and loss of balance. She is referred to a neurology provider, who scheduled an MRI. The MRI findings showed that Cassandra had lesions in her brain stem and left brain. After looking at the MRI, the provider wants her to come in for a lumbar puncture.

3. What does the MRI suggest that Cassandra has?

____

____

____

____

4. Cassandra tells the nurse that she does not want a lumbar puncture because she is afraid that she will be paralyzed. What would you say to her? Why is a lumbar puncture important?

____

____

____

____

Cassandra's lumbar puncture results show oligoclonal bands, elevated levels of IgG, and slightly elevated levels of protein in her cerebrospinal fluid.

5. Have these findings confirmed your diagnosis? Explain the pathophysiology of the diagnosis.

____

____

____

____

Cassandra is upset with her diagnosis. She says, "I thought only White people got this disease! Why did my provider tell me that I had a stroke and was too stressed out?"

6. How would you respond?

____

____

____

____

BP, Blood pressure; *BUN,* blood urea nitrogen; *CRP,* C-reactive protein; *CT,* computed tomography; *ESR,* erythrocyte sedimentation rate; *Hct,* hematocrit; *HDL,* high-density lipoprotein; *HR,* heart rate; *IgG,* immunoglobulin G; *LDL,* low-density lipoprotein; *MRI,* magnetic resonance imaging; *O_2 sat,* oxygen saturation; *RR,* respiratory rate; *WBC,* white blood cell.

Case Study 14.2

Tony is a 33-year-old nonbinary Cherokee individual (they/them) who has just lost their job and are dealing with depression. They are getting ready for an interview when they notice that their left eyelid is drooping. They have no other symptoms or discomfort, so they decide to ignore it and go to the interview. When they get home, their partner notices their left eye and comments on it, but Tony just shrugs it off. A few days later, Tony is talking with their partner when their partner notices that Tony is starting to slur their words. Tony also says that they are having some numbness to the left side of their face. Their partner thinks it may be Bell's palsy but urges Tony to get it checked out. Tony then goes to the emergency room.

Vital Signs	Assessment	Diagnostics
BP: 142/82 mm Hg HR: 78 beats/minute RR: 18 breaths/minute O_2 sat: 99% on room air Temperature: 99°F	Client uses they/them pronouns Client has a notable left-sided facial droop and ptosis, has some slurring of words Upper and lower extremities have equal bilateral strength within normal range Reports stress, viral illness 2 weeks ago. Has history of Addison disease	ECG normal sinus rhythm Head CT normal Labs pending

Tony is diagnosed with Bell's palsy and discharged home. The following week, Tony's symptoms grow worse, and the numbness and tingling start to affect their chewing and swallowing function. Panicked, Tony calls an ambulance and goes back to the emergency room.

1. What diagnosis do Tony's symptoms suggest? What findings might confirm this?

____

____

____

____

2. Explain the pathophysiology of the disease? What may have triggered it?

____

____

____

____

3. The provider orders a chest CT. Why would the provider order this?

____

____

____

____

4. Can this disease be cured? Why or why not?

____

____

____

____

CT, Computed tomography.

Case Study 14.3

Radhika is a 70-year-old Asian cis-female (she/her) who was just diagnosed with Parkinson disease 5 years ago. She lives with her husband, Shyam (he/him), who is her caretaker. A visiting nurse has arrived to check in on Radhika.

1. Shyam tells the nurse that no one in the family has a history of Parkinson disease. He asks how Radhika could have gotten the disease. What can the visiting nurse say?

____

____

____

____

2. What is the pathophysiology behind Parkinson disease? Explain the mechanism.

____

____

____

____

Radhika continues to decline and starts to have frequent falls and become more confused.

3. Explain the reason for her falls and confusion.

____

____

____

____

4. What can be done for Parkinson disease? Is it curable?

Case Study 14.4

Rose is an 89-year-old White trans-female (she/her) who lives at an assisted living facility. She has a history of hypertension, type 2 diabetes, hyperlipidemia, and transient ischemic attack X2. She has a family history of hypertension and Alzheimer disease. When her aide came to help her out of bed, she found Rose listing to the right, drooling, and unable to speak. Rose was rushed to the hospital by ambulance for a possible stroke.

1. On arrival, Rose had a fingerstick glucose done and IV placed before being rushed off to get a head CT scan. What is the rationale for these actions?

2. What may have caused Rose's stroke? Explain how Rose's risk factors may have contributed.

Rose's head CT is within normal limits.

3. Does this mean that Rose did not have a stroke? Explain.

4. What is the priority in treating a client with a stroke? Explain.

5. Will Rose fully recover function? Why or why not?

Rose, after receiving treatment and going to a skilled nursing facility to regain function, has returned to the assisted nursing facility. Her aide has noticed that Rose is increasingly confused, incontinent, agitated, and moody. Rose used to love crossword puzzles, but now her aide notices that she cannot concentrate long enough to complete them.

6. Is this Alzheimer disease? What are the structural changes associated with Alzheimer disease? Explain the pathophysiology.

7. Could these cognitive changes be due to her stroke? Explain.

CT, Computed tomography.

15 Musculoskeletal Disorders

Cartilage, Ligaments, Tendons, and Joints

Let's start with the building blocks of the musculoskeletal system.(Cartilage is connective tissue, made up of chondrocytes, and it is not vascular. The perichondrium is a vascular sheath, which covers most cartilage and supplies nutrients. Cartilage helps with skeletal resilience, flexibility, and support (Fig. 15.1).

Types of cartilage:

- Elastic (ear)
- Fibrocartilage (vertebral disks)
- Hyaline (nose, ribs)

Ligaments connect bones to one another (anterior cruciate ligament [ACL] behind knee). Tendons connect skeletal muscles to bone (Achilles tendon). Bursae are small synovial sacs cushioning tendons. Tendon sheaths are tube-like bursae wrapped around tendons (Figs. 15.1 and 15.2).

Joints

There are three different types of joints:

- Synarthroses
  - Immobile (skull)

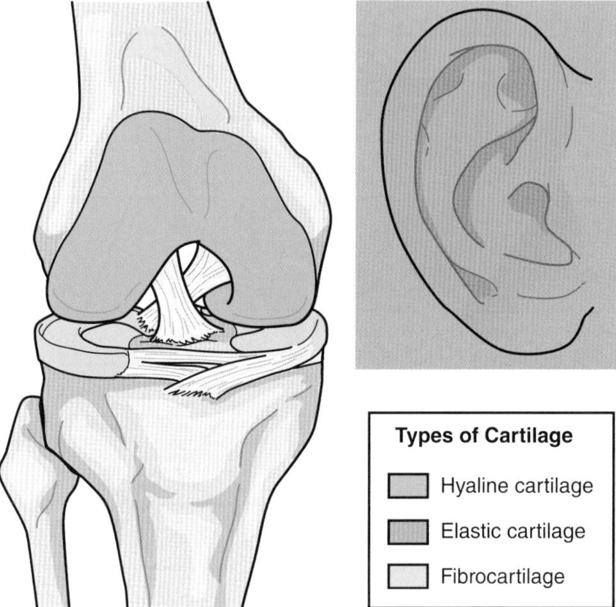

• **Fig. 15.1** Cartilage.

- Amphiarthroses
  - Slightly mobile
  - Pubic symphysis and pelvic girdle
- Diarthroses
  - Freely movable
  - Hip, shoulder, knees

Bone

Bone is a vascular connective tissue. Bones are made up of bone cells, collagen fibers, proteins, inorganic mineral salts, nerves, blood vessels, bone marrow, cartilage and endosteum, and periosteum. Laminar bone consists of cylinder-shaped osteons parallel to the long axis. Woven bone is weaker, it is poorly organized, and often results from injury or disease.

Bone structure:

- Epiphysis—end
- Diaphysis—shaft
  - Contains red marrow (produces blood cells and platelets)
  - Contains yellow marrow (fat)
- Metaphysis—widening before epiphysis
- Cortical bone (85%)—dense, hard, outer layer
- Cancellous bone (15%)—trabecular, flexible, contains bone marrow

Bones function in many different ways. Bones contribute to body shape, support, and movement. The skeleton serves to protect the rest of the body. The marrow inside the bones produces red blood cells, white blood cells, and platelets. Yellow marrow stores fat. Bones also act as buffers for acid-base balance. Finally, bone is made up of calcium and phosphate. There is a dynamic equilibrium between storing calcium and phosphate in bone and releasing calcium and phospate into the blood, increasing serum levels.

The periosteum, endosteum, and perichondrium are membranes that line the bone and aid in bone growth. The periosteum is a thin fibrous sheath that covers the bone. It supplies bone with blood, neurons, and bone cells. It is an insertion point for muscles, tendons, and ligaments. The endosteum is a membrane that lines the center of the bone where marrow is located. It is crucial in the deposition of calcium into the matrix as well as the resorption of calcium into the blood. The perichondrium covers the cartilage at the ends of your bones (Fig. 15.3).

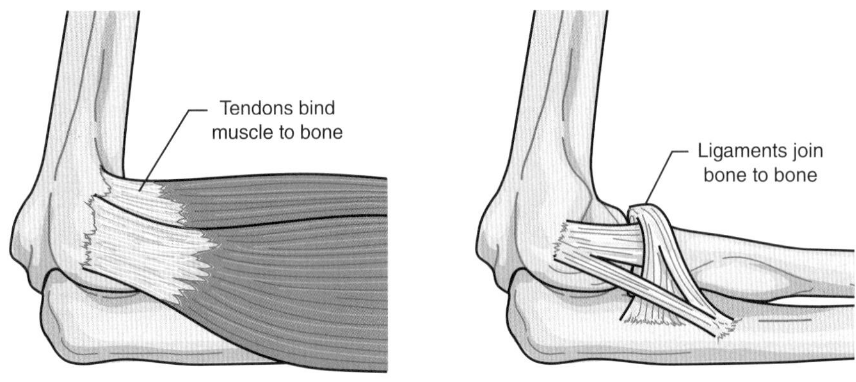

• **Fig. 15.2** Tendon vs. ligament.

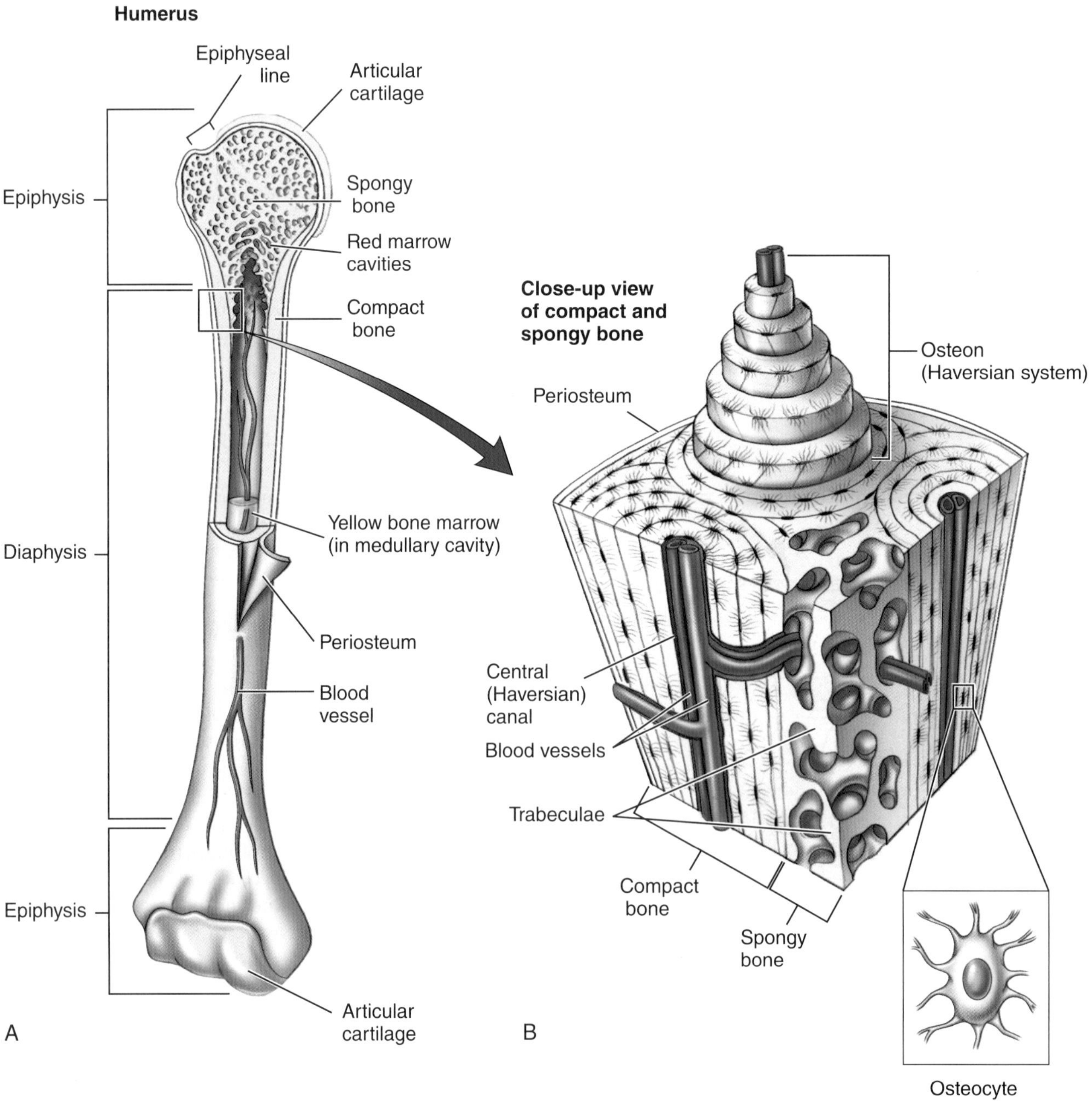

• **Fig. 15.3** Structure and anatomy of the bone. (From Fig 19.1- Massage therapy (9780323878159).)

Bone cells consist of:

- osteogenic cells
- osteoblasts
- osteocytes
- osteoclasts

Osteogenic cells are undifferentiated stem cells. These cells replicate and have high mitotic activity. These cells are found in the periosteum and osteum and differentiate into osteoblasts. Osteoblasts form new bone. These cells have an active and resting state and do not divide or replicate. They are activated by parathyroid hormone (PTH). Osteoblasts produce collagen, secrete bone matrix and alkaline phosphatase, and release a protein called the receptor activator of nuclear factor kappa beta ligand (RANKL), which aids in bone homeostasis. The osteoblasts are regulated by PTH, calcitonin, and vitamin D.

Osteocytes are transformed osteoblasts. These are mature osteoblasts that are trapped in the matrix secreted by osteoblasts. They connect with other osteocytes by long cytoplasmic processes that extend through tunnels called canaliculi. These cells maintain bone homeostasis, signal when there is bone injury, help to break down bone, and synthesize matrix.

Osteoclasts stem from monocytes and macrophages and are multinucleated. The bone marrow cells release cytokines to cause monocytes and macrophages to differentiate into osteoclasts. These cells help to break down bones. Calcitonin acts on osteoclasts to inhibit their activity and to increase bone production.

To maintain bone homeostasis, osteoblasts secrete the RANKL protein. This protein activates a receptor called RANK, which activates osteoclasts. Osteoprotegerin (OPG) is produced by bone marrow cells and osteoblasts. OPG binds to RANKL and protects bone from resorption. OPG, RANKL, and RANK keep the dynamic equilibrium between the bone and blood (Fig. 15.4).

When there is an injury to the bone, osteoclasts break down the damaged bone. Osteoblasts then form new bone matter.

Bone repair has five states:

- Hematoma formation
- Fibrocartilage/procallus formation
- Soft tissue callus formation
- Ossification
- Remodeling (Fig. 15.5)

Skeletal Injury, Infection, Breakdown

Types of musculoskeletal injuries:

- Contusion—bruise
- Hematoma—blood pools under skin
- Strain—injury or tear to muscle or tendon
- Sprain—injury/stretch/tear to ligaments around joint

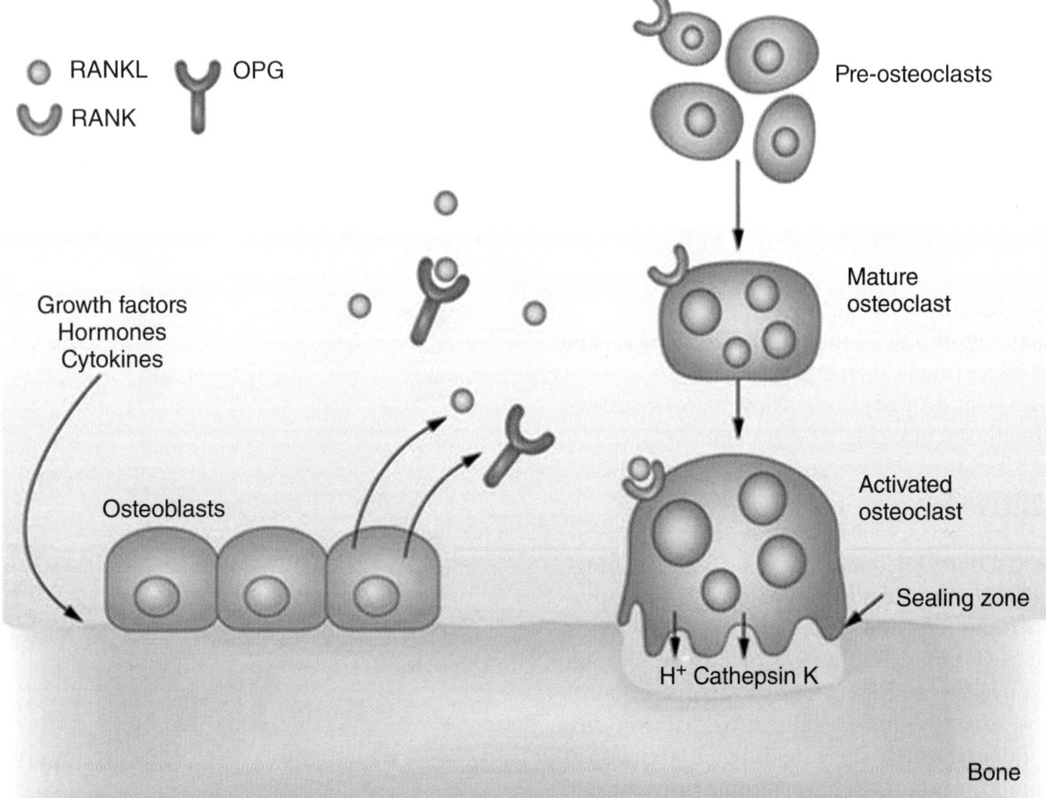

• **Fig. 15.4** Bone growth and breakdown. (From https://www.researchgate.net/publication/269577071_Biology_of_Receptor_Activator_of_Nuclear_Factor_Kappa-B_Ligand_RANKL_and_Osteoprotegerin_OPG_in_Periodontal_Health_and_Disease_-A_Review.)

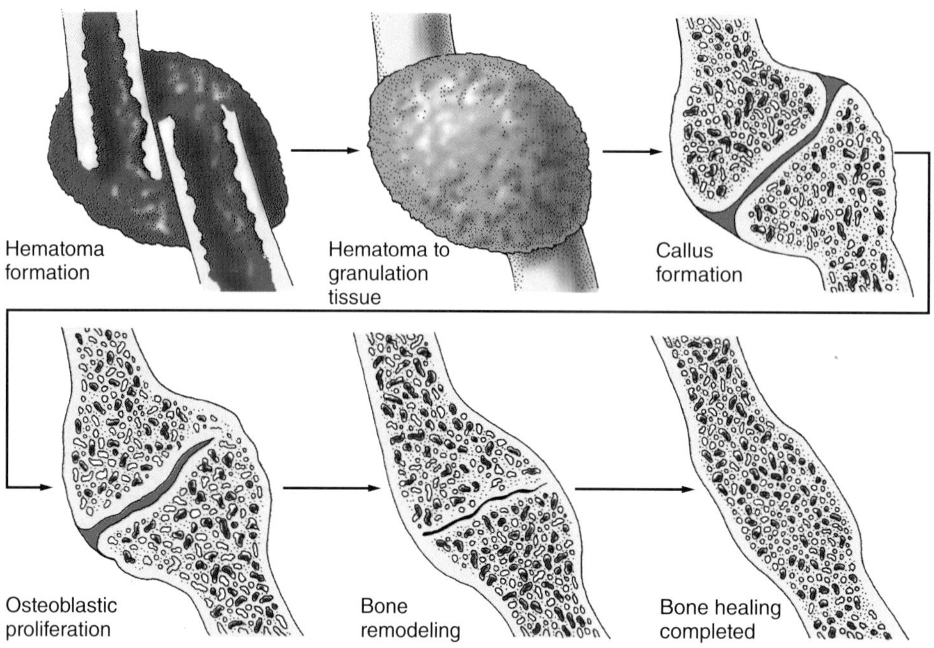

• **Fig. 15.5** Stages of bone repair. (From Medical Surgical Nursing-Concepts for Clinical Judgment and Collaborative Care, 11e, 9780323878265, Fig. 44.2.)

- Dislocation—separation of bones where they meet at the joint
- Subluxation—partial dislocation (Fig. 15.6)

Fractures are a break in the continuity of bone. In children, you will often see tibial, clavicular, and humoral fractures. Older individuals often sustain femur, humoral, vertebral, and pelvic fractures. Hip fractures are associated with osteoporosis and have a high morbidity rate. Complications include:

- malunion—healing with deformity
- delayed union—healing takes longer than normal
- nonunion—the bones do not fuse and the healing process stops
- skin injury—fracture blisters
- compartment syndrome—muscle, nerve injury, and swelling in fascia (medical emergency)
- fat embolism—fat droplets from yellow marrow released into blood with fracture (Fig. 15.7)

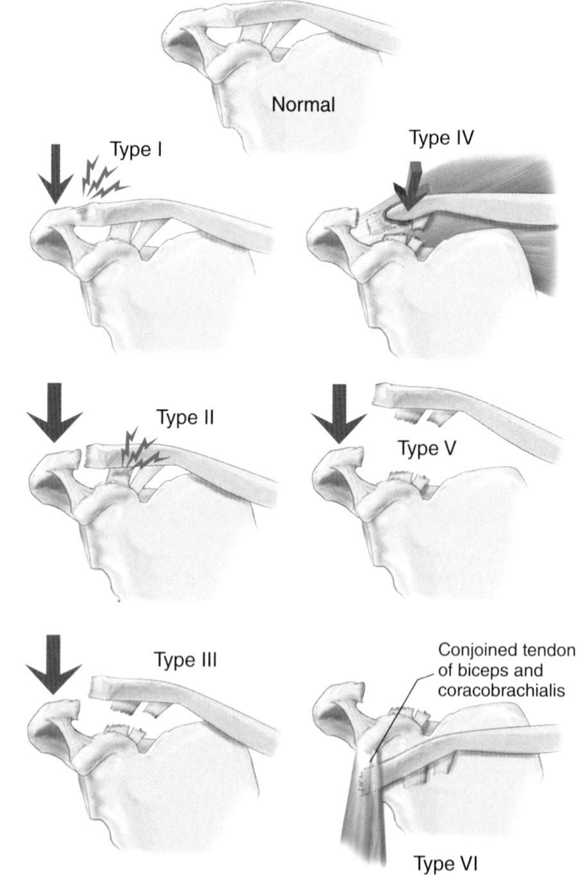

• **Fig. 15.6** Types of shoulder dislocations. (From Rockwood, C.A. Jr, Williams, G.R. Jr., & Young, D.C. (2004). Disorders of the acromioclavicular joint. In: Rockwood, C.A. Jr, Matsen, F.A. III, Wirth, M.A., et al. (eds.). The Shoulder. (3rd ed.). Elsevier.).

Osteomyelitis

Osteomyelitis is a bone infection caused by bacteria, fungi, parasites, or viruses. The most common cause is acute pyogenic staphylococcus infection. This can be caused by direct penetration by a wound, open fracture, or surgery. Chronic pyogenic osteomyelitis can be secondary to an open wound. Hematogenous osteomyelitis is caused by bacteria that travel to the bone through the bloodstream. Individuals who are immunocompromised, have chronic infections, or have substance use disorder are at risk for these infections.

Development of osteomyelitis:

- Invasion of pathogen

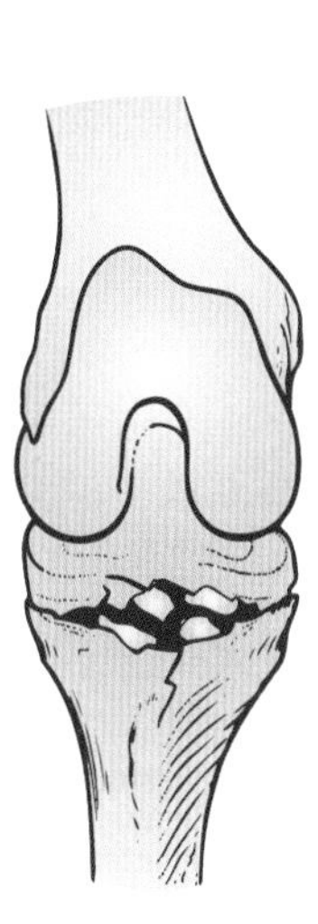
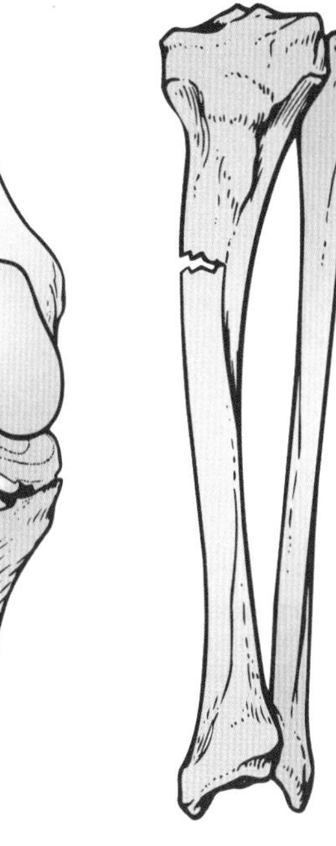
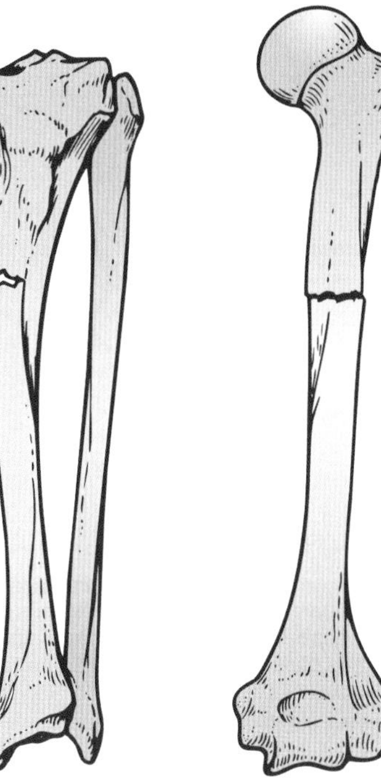
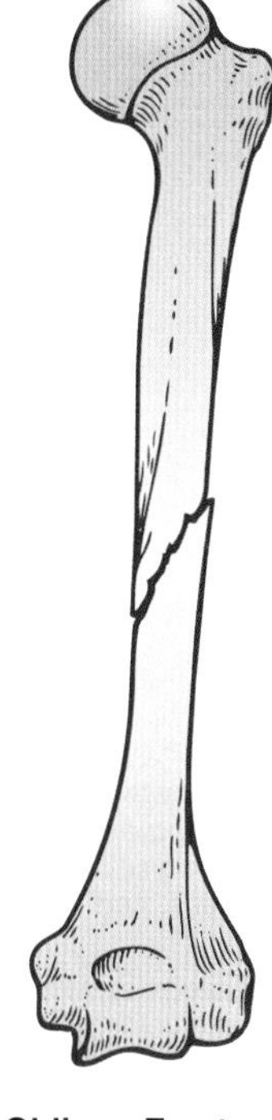
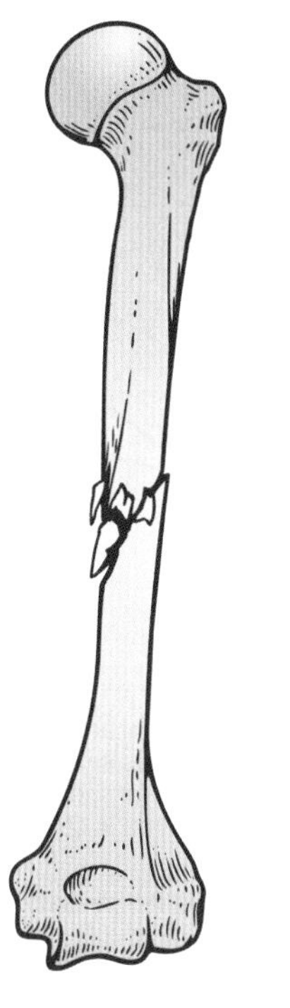
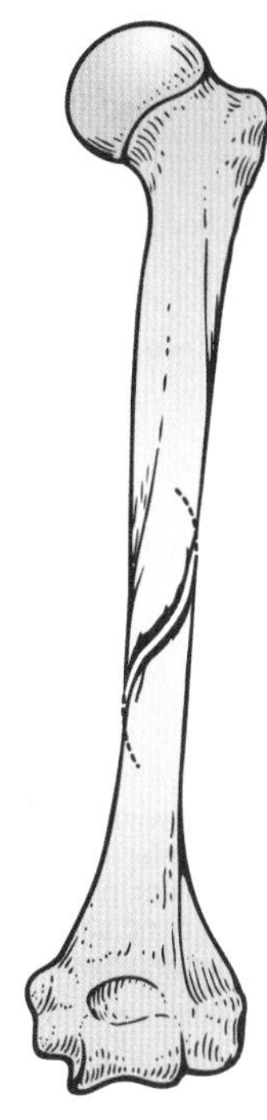

Impacted Fracture
The broken ends of the bones are forcefully jammed together.

Greenstick Fracture
The bone remains intact on one side, but broken on the other, in much the same way that a "green stick" bends; common in children, whose bones are more flexible than those of adults.

Transverse Fracture
The break occurs perpendicular to the long axis of the bone.

Oblique Fracture
The break occurs diagonally across the bone; generally the result of a twisting force.

Comminuted Fracture
The bone is splintered or shattered into three or more fragments; usually caused by an extremely traumatic direct force.

Spiral Fracture
The bone is broken into a spiral or S-shape; caused by a twisting force.

• **Fig. 15.7** Types of fractures. (From Niedzwiecki, B. (2022). Kinn's Medical Assisting Fundamentals [2nd ed.]. Elsevier.)

- Inflammatory response
- Blood supply blocked by pus, pus spreads into the blood vessels
- Decreased blood flow leads to bone necrosis
- There is a devascularized dead bone fragment (sequestrum)
- The new bone is formed around the dead bone (involucrum)

Symptoms of osteomyelitis are pain, fever and chills, malaise, redness and swelling, drainage, and dysfunctional movement. These manifestations can vary by age, risk factors, infection site, type of injury, and pathogen. Infections can be acute, subacute, or chronic. Osteomyelitis can be diagnosed by wound cultures, x-rays, bone scans, computed tomography (CT), and magnetic resonance imaging (MRI). It is typically treated with 4 to 6 weeks of intravenous (IV) antibiotic therapy, packing, and immobilization. Osteomyelitis can result in necrosis and amputation (Fig. 15.8).

Osteonecrosis

Osteonecrosis occurs due to lack of perfusion to the bone, or avascular necrosis. There is aseptic destruction of the bone from the lack of blood supply. This can occur from an embolism, vessel injury, steroid therapy, peripheral arterial disease, or ischemia from a fracture. The site of the lesion depends on the hypoperfused area and is very painful. It can be diagnosed by x-ray, CT, MRI, or bone scan and often requires a surgical repair. The affected area will need to be immobilized with limited weight-bearing during healing and anti-inflammatories would be used to treat pain. If left untreated, the disease will cause bone collapse and joint deterioration.

Osteoporosis

Osteoporosis is a progressive, metabolic bone disease. The equilibrium between osteoblasts and osteoclasts is disrupted. The structural integrity of the trabecular and cortical bone is impaired and bone mass starts to decrease.

Risk factors

- Age
- Genetics
- Hormonal and metabolic status
- Low physical activity

Pathogenesis

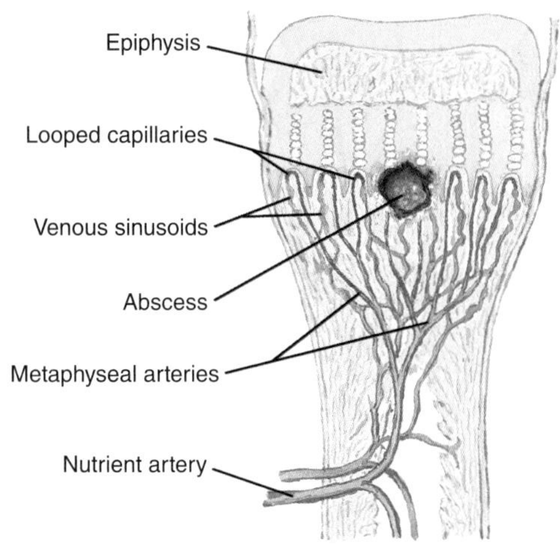

Terminal branches of metaphyseal arteries form loops at growth plate and enter irregular afferent venous sinusoids. Blood flow is slowed and turbulent, predisposing to bacterial seeding. In addition, lining cells have little or no phagocytic activity. Area is catch basin for bacteria, and abscess may form.

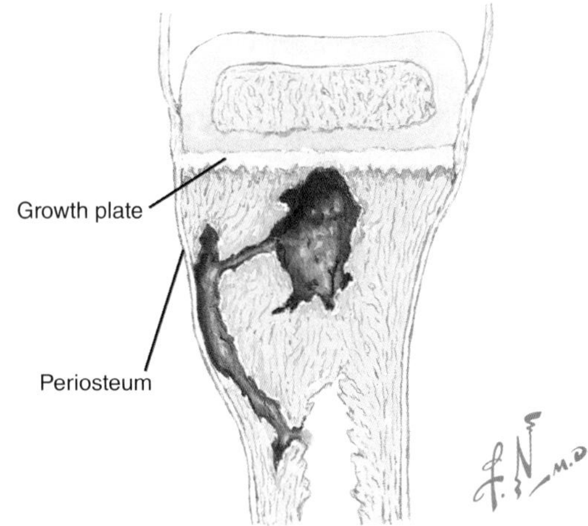

Abscess, limited by growth plate, spreads transversely along Volkmann canals and elevates periosteum; extends subperiosteally and may invade shaft. In infants under 1 year of age, some metaphyseal arterial branches pass through growth plate, and infection may invade epiphysis and joint.

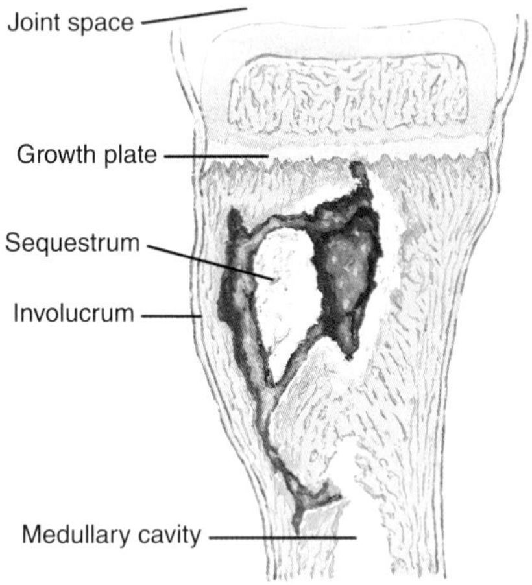

As abscess spreads, segment of devitalized bone (sequestrum) remains within it. Elevated periosteum may also lay down bone to form encasing shell (involucrum). Occasionally, abscess is walled off by fibrosis and bone sclerosis to form Brodie abscess.

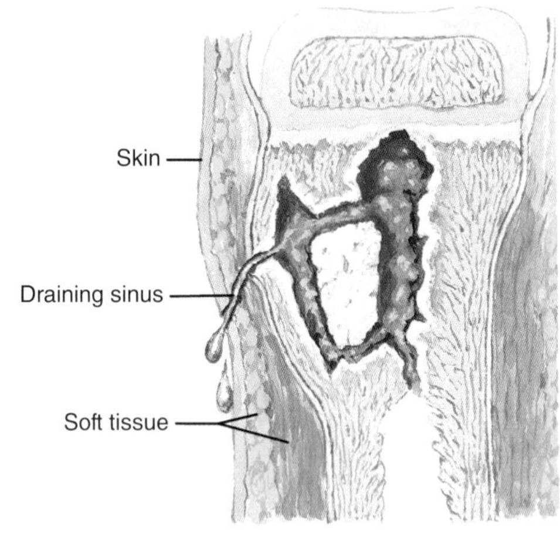

Infectious process may erode periosteum and form sinus through soft tissues and skin to drain externally. Process is influenced by virulence of organism, resistance of host, administration of antibiotics, and fibrotic and sclerotic responses.

• **Fig. 15.8** Pathogenesis of osteomyelitis. (From https://www.netterimages.com/pathogenesis-of-hematogenous-osteomyelitis-labeled-thompson-1e-orthopaedics-frank-h-netter-33648.html.)

- Comorbidities
- Medications
- Smoking
- Low body weight
- Red-S (assigned female at birth [AFAB] athletic triad)
  - Low energy/disordered eating
  - Menstrual disorders
  - Decreased bone density
- Early menopause

Diagnostics
- Labs—renal function, thyroid function, vitamin D, and calcium levels
- X-ray
- Dual x-ray absorptiometry (DEXA) scan

Clinical manifestations
- Pain
- Bone deformity
- Kyphosis
- Fractures
  - Colles' fractures—sudden due to fall, coughing
  - Diminished height—wedging and collapse of vertebrae
  - Impaired breathing
  - Impaired mobility
- Treatment
  - Weight-bearing exercise, exercise that improves balance
  - Calcium supplements with vitamin D
  - Alendronate (slows down osteoclasts); denosumab (RANKL inhibitor) (Fig. 15.9)

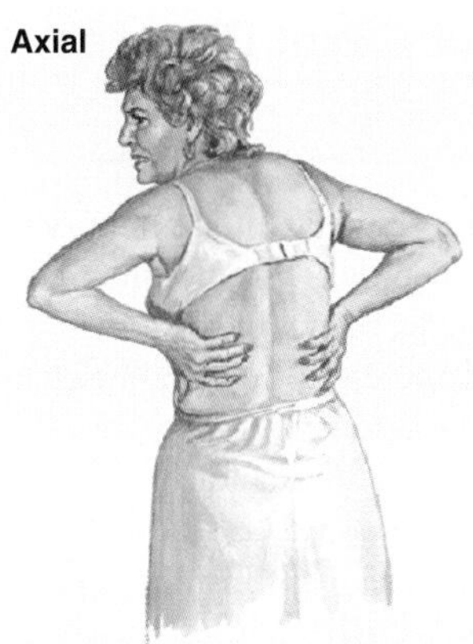

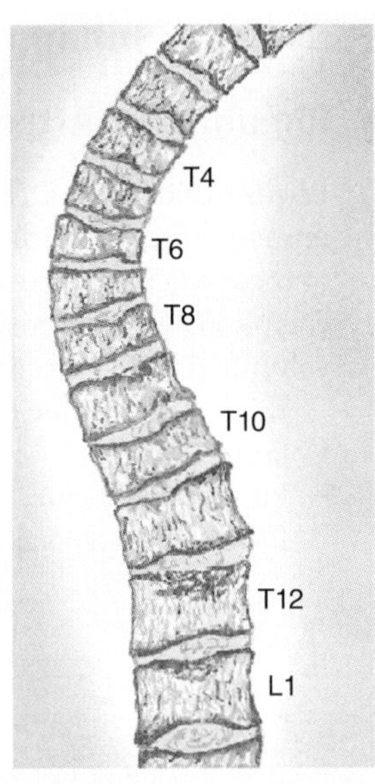

Characteristics of Osteoporosis	
Characteristic	**Description**
Etiology	Postmenopausal women, genetics, vitamin D synthesis deficiency, idiopathic
Risk factors	Family history, white female, increasing age, estrogen deficiency, vitamin D deficiency, low calcium intake, smoking, excessive alcohol use, inactive lifestyle
Complications	Vertebral compression fractures, fracture of proximal femur or humerus, ribs, and distal radius (Colles' fracture)

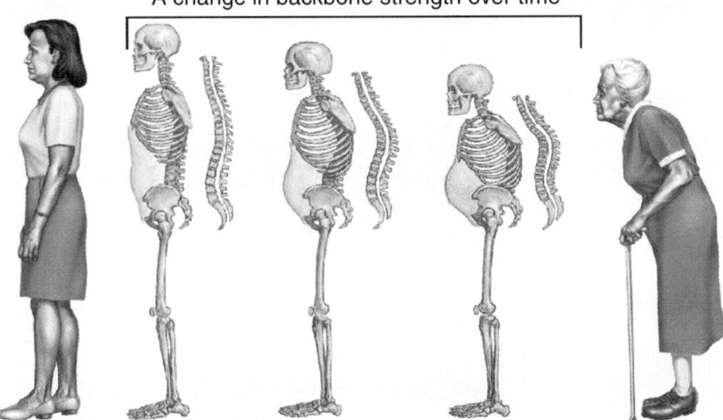

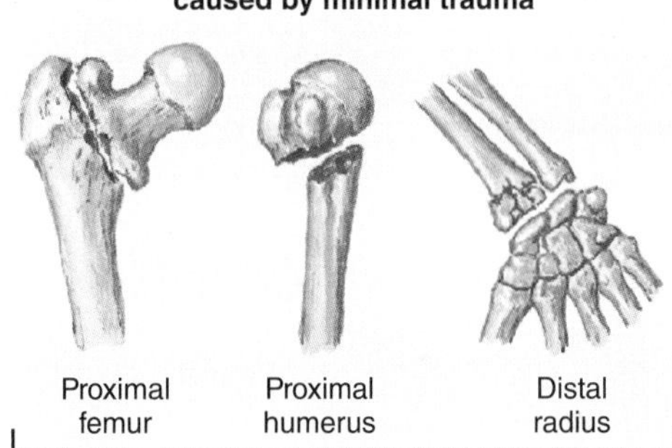

• **Fig. 15.9** Osteoporosis development. (From https://www.netterimages.com/osteoporosis-labeled-hansen-ca-2e-general-anatomy-carlos-frank-39978.html.)

Osteoarthritis

Osteoarthritis is a noninflammatory degenerative joint disease. It is the most common kind of arthritis and is preventable. Typically, osteoarthritis occurs in joints that are continually stressed, such as repetitive work injuries. There is a loss of articular cartilage, which is caused by protease enzymes and cytokines (tumor necrosis factor [TNF], interleukin [IL]) released during the inflammatory process.

- Articular cartilage develops fissures, thins, and pits and synovial fluid widens it
  - The synovium is the connective tissue that lines the inside of a joint capsule
- Subchondral bone thickening, exposure
- Fragments of bone and cartilage dislodged
- Bone becomes sclerotic
- Fluid leaks to form cysts; osteophytes (bony outgrowth) develop
- Joint capsule thickening, effusion
- Synovial inflammation

Clinical manifestations of osteoarthritis are typically localized and include:

- crepitus
- swelling
- misaligned joints
- Heberden and Bouchard nodes
- joint pain
- pain at night
- limited range of motion
- muscle wasting
- paresthesias
- stiffness
- joint enlargement

Osteoarthritis can be diagnosed by history and physical and x-rays.

Criteria include the following:
1. Pain worse with activity and better with rest
2. Pain worse in evening
3. Age greater than 45 years
4. Morning stiffness lasting more than 30 minutes
5. Bony joint enlargement
6. Limitation in range of motion

Treatment of osteoarthritis is largely symptom relief. Anti-inflammatory medications, physical therapy, weight reduction, assistive devices, and joint replacement surgeries are common treatment approaches (Fig. 15.10).

Systemic Inflammatory Joint Diseases

Rheumatoid Arthritis

Rheumatoid arthritis (RA) is a systemic, inflammatory, autoimmune disease. With RA, there is a chronic inflammation of the connective tissue. Synovial tissue (in the joint capsule) is typically affected first and there can be extra-articular involvement. RA is a progressive disease and incurable.

RA risk factors are epigenetic and include:
- familial history
- human leukocyte antigen class II histocompatilibity, D-related beta chain (HLA-DRB1) alleles

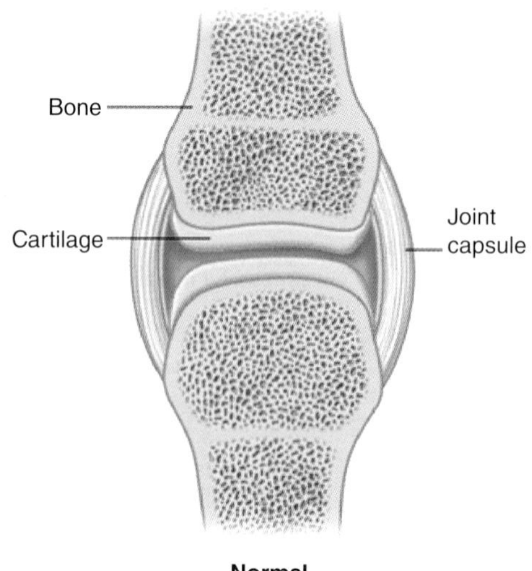

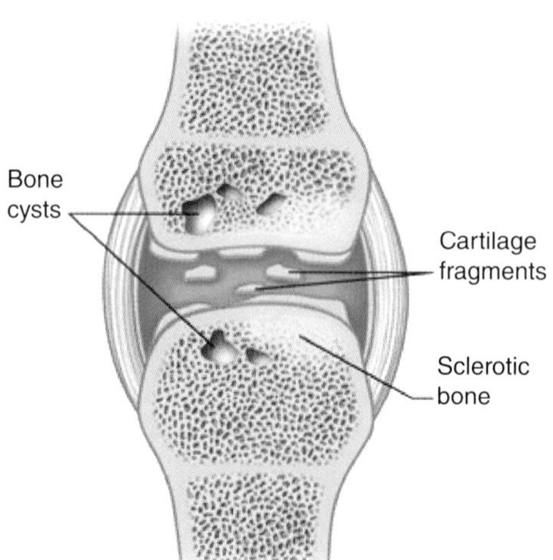

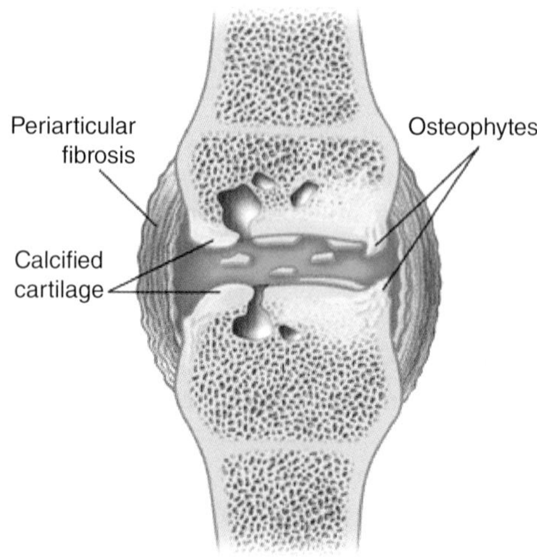

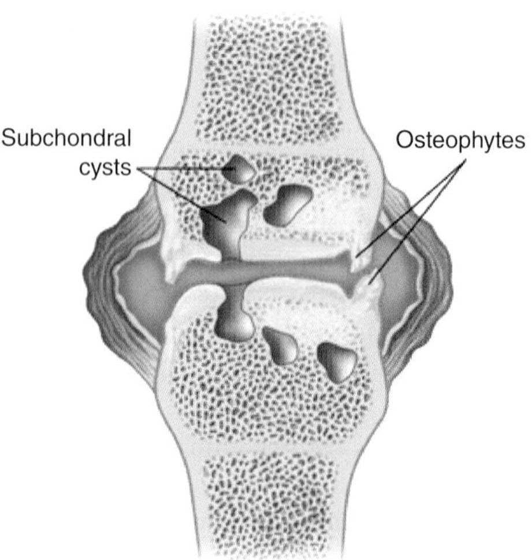

• **Fig. 15.10** Osteoarthritis. (From Paterson, K.L. et al. (2023) Foot and ankle biomechanics. Academic Press.)

- AFAB more than assigned male at birth (AMAB)
- smoking
- silica, asbestos, textile dust exposure
- gum infections
- dysfunctional gut microbiome
- obesity

RA is triggered by repeated environmental triggers and autoantibodies are formed against citrullinated proteins. This immune response can start in the lungs, gums, and gastrointestinal (GI) tract. These autoantibodies can be present for years before patients with RA actually become symptomatic. Some patients do not develop clinical disease. Once the inflammatory reaction begins in the synovium, angiogenesis (blood vessel growth) occurs. The synovium is infiltrated by inflammatory cells and autoantibodies begin to be produced in the synovium. Cytokines and chemokines are released by inflammatory cells, such as mast cells, and cause loss of cartilage. Chondrocytes secrete cytokines, damaging the cartilage. RANKL is released, activating osteoclasts causing bone erosion. The synovial membrane becomes swollen and projects into the joint space. This synovial swelling and cell proliferation is called a pannus.

RA typically starts in the distal, small, peripheral joints of hands and feet, progressing to proximal larger joints. A hallmark finding is joint stiffness and pain in the morning.

Clinical manifestations include the following:

- Localized manifestations:
  - Symmetric and bilateral
  - Affects hands and feet first (metacarpophalangeal [MCP], proximal interphalangeal [PIP])
  - Pain, worse in morning
  - Affects larger joints, such as wrists, elbows, knees, ankles later
  - Joint swelling
  - Rheumatic nodules
  - Joint deformities (boutonniere, swan neck, joint subluxation, hallux valgus)
  - Limited range of motion
- Systemic manifestations:
  - Sjögren syndrome (dry eyes, dry mouth)
  - Scleritis
  - Vasculitis
  - Nonhealing ulcers
  - Fatigue and weakness
  - Anorexia and weight loss

Diagnostics

- Testing for the presence of rheumatoid factor (RF) and anticitrullinated protein antibodies (ACPAs)
- Erythrocyte sedimentation rate (ESR) and C-reactive protein (CRP)
- Synovial fluid examination (high rates of leukocytes)
- X-rays and MRI

Diagnosing RA can be challenging. The American College of Rheumatology created diagnostic criteria. A total score of 6 or more indicates a diagnosis of RA.

Number and size of joints

- Inclusion of 2 to 10 affected large joints (1 point)
- Inclusion of 1 to 3 small joints (2 points)
- Inclusion of 4 to 10 small joints (3 points)
- Greater than 10 joints including at least 1 small joint (5 points)

Blood tests for RF or ACPA

- Low positive (2 points)
- High positive (3 points)

Blood tests for ESR or CRP

- Elevated (1 point)

Symptom duration

- Six weeks or more (1 point)

Treatments

Treatments to control RA inflammation are classified as disease-modifying antirheumatic drugs (DMARDs). These include methotrexate, hydroxychloroquine, and sulfasalazine. Corticosteroids are often used for RA flares. Pain is managed with nonsteroidal anti-inflammatory drugs (NSAIDs) (Fig. 15.11).

Gout

Gout is a chronic, inflammatory arthritis that affects typically one joint, but can affect more. In most cases, it is primary gout. Risk factors include age (40–50 years of age); AMAB; genetics; a diet high in meat, dairy and seafood; lack of exercise; alcohol; dieting; rapid weight loss; and metabolic syndrome. Gout occurs when there is an excess of uric acid, due to either overproduction or underexcretion by the kidneys. Urate crystals start to form, especially in the synovial fluid. The urate crystals cause an inflammatory response which causes swelling, redness, and tissue damage.

Typically, gout (or gouty arthritis) is episodic with exacerbations and remissions. The asymptomatic period in between gout exacerbations is called intercritical gout. Clinical manifestations are as follows:

- Abrupt onset
- Pain
- Redness and swelling
- Typically affects toes (can affect ankles, wrists, knees, hands, elbows)
- Gouty nephropathy
- Tophi
- Urate kidney stones

Gout is diagnosed by lab findings. Synovial fluid aspiration is the gold standard. Leukocytosis and high serum uric acid levels, as well as a 24-hour urine test for uric acid can aid in diagnosis. Treatment of gout is two-pronged—treatment of inflammation and reduction of uric acid. Colchicine and NSAIDs are first-line treatments for gout, with glucocorticoids for gout exacerbations. Allopurinol is the drug of choice when looking to reduce uric acid (Fig. 15.12A and B).

Study Guide for Chapter 15

Make sure that you have your class notes and textbooks on hand to answer these questions. A concept map is included to help you to diagram and link disease concepts together.

1. What are the components of the musculoskeletal system and how do they work together?

____

____

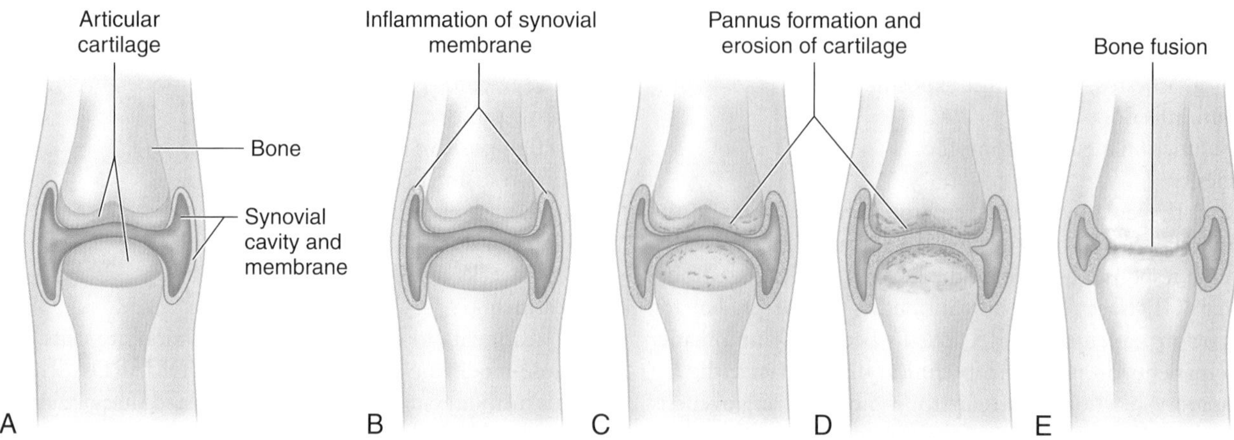

• **Fig. 15.11** Development and Progression of Rheumatoid Arthritis. (Linda Anne Silvestri: Saunders Comprehensive Review for the NCLEX-PN® Examination, 9, 9780443112874.)

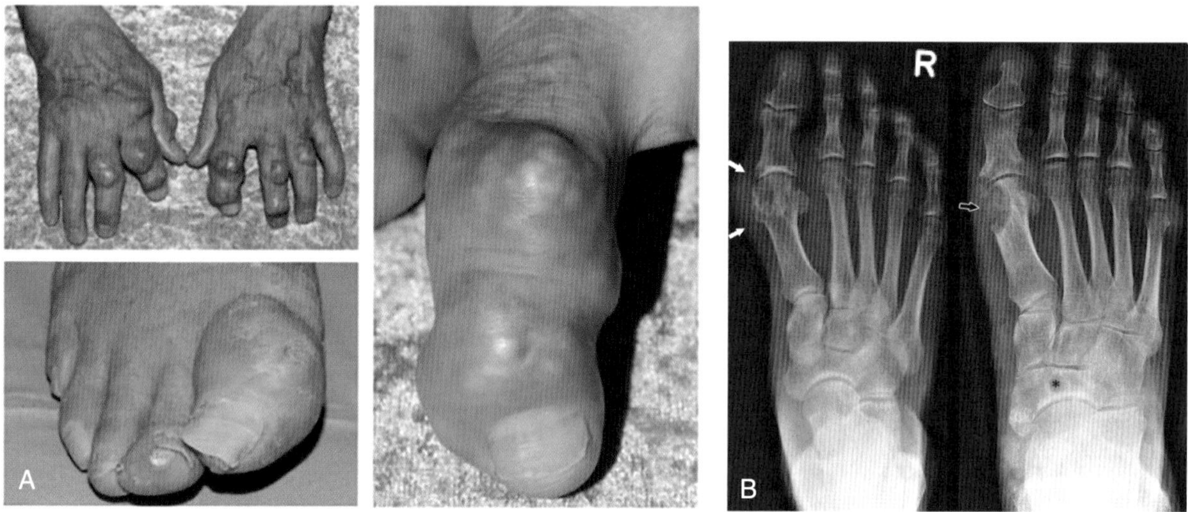

• **Fig. 15.12** (A and B) Manifestations of gout. (A. Image courtesy of Arthritis Research UK Primary Care Centre, Primary Care Sciences, Keele University, Keele, UK.)

2. Explain how the osteoblasts, osteoclasts, RANKL, calcitonin, PTH, etc. work together to keep skeletal processes in equilibrium.

3. What are the different types of musculoskeletal injuries?

4. Explain how the different types of fractures occur. How do they heal? How do we diagnose and treat it?

5. What are the complications associated with fractures? What is compartment syndrome and how do you treat it?

6. Compare and contrast the pathophysiology, diagnosis, symptoms, complications, and treatment for osteomyelitis and osteonecrosis.

7. What causes osteoporosis? How is it diagnosed and treated? What are the complications?

8. Compare and contrast the pathophysiology, symptoms, complications, diagnosis, and treatment for osteoarthritis and rheumatoid arthritis.

9. What is gout? Explain the pathophysiology.

10. How is gout diagnosed? What are the complications and treatments for gout?

Concept Map

Use this concept map to link each disease to its pathophysiology, diagnostics, causes, risk factors, complications, and clinical manifestations together. This way, you will be able to see the whole picture of the disease.

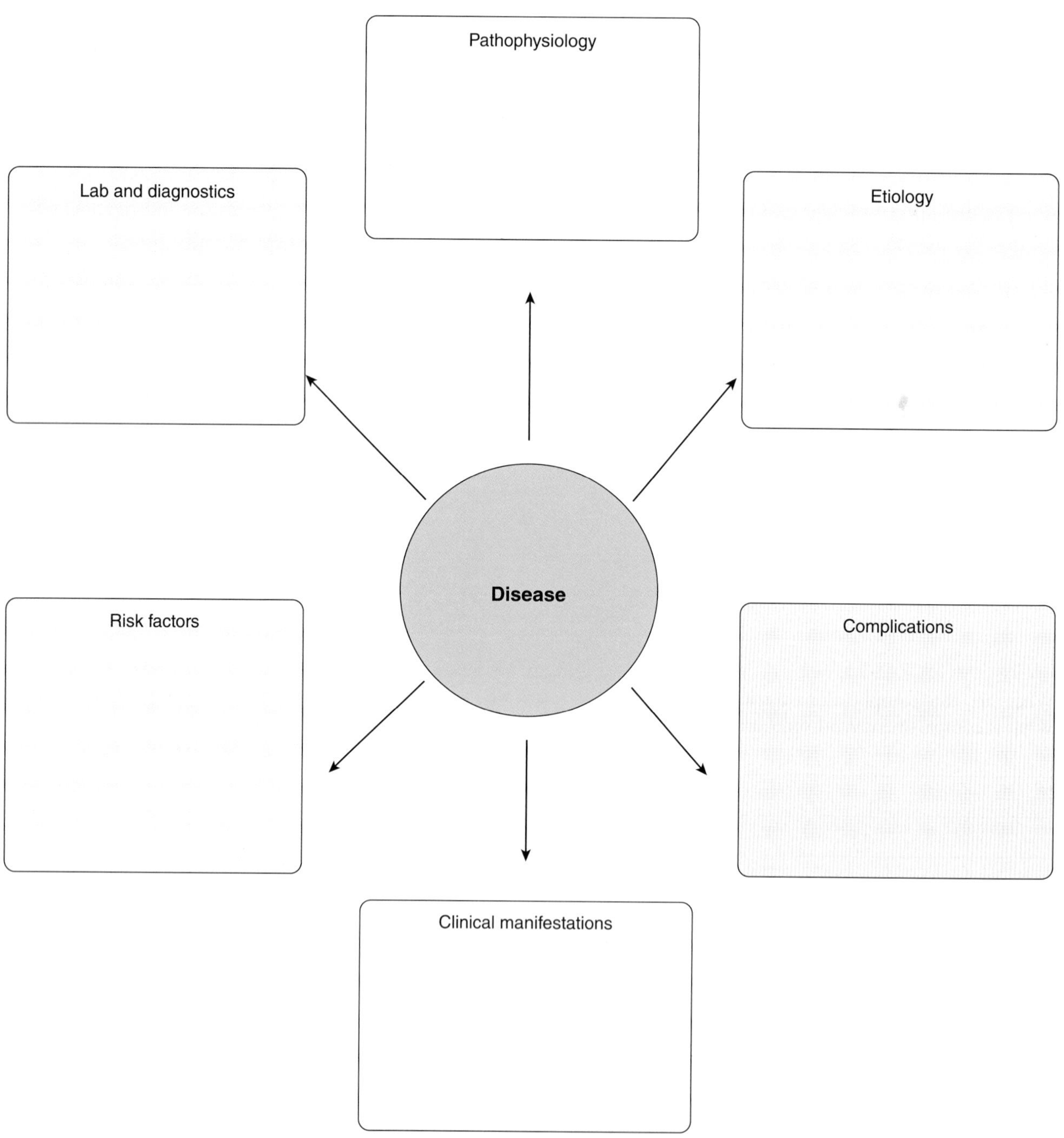

Case Studies for Chapter 15

Case Study 15.1

Shauna is a 65-year-old Black AFAB (she/her) who comes to the emergency room with acute pain and deformity in her right wrist after tripping over a rug. Shauna has a history of Crohn disease and osteoporosis. Currently, she is not taking any medications.

1. Explain the pathophysiological mechanisms behind osteoporosis.

2. What risk factors did Shauna have that caused her to develop osteoporosis? How would you treat her?

3. What measures can Shauna take to reduce the likelihood of fractures? What complications might she be at risk for?

AFAB, Assigned female at birth.

Case Study 15.2

Meera is a 50-year-old Southeast Asian AFAB (she/her) who presents to her provider with a deep puncture wound to her right foot from stepping on a nail 3 weeks ago. Meera's wife cleaned the wound and packed it, but the pain has now worsened. Meera has been taking ibuprofen for the pain. She has no significant past medical history and has no known drug allergies.

Vital Signs	Assessments
BP: 135/92 mm Hg HR: 88 beats per minute RR: 20 breaths/minute T: 101°F	Report of sharp, throbbing, constant pain in the right foot, radiating up the right lower leg; pulses intact Cannot bear weight on right leg Swelling and redness around the wound and extending up right foot to right ankle Feeling of malaise

1. What condition do you think that Meera would be at risk for? Why?

2. What role does the mechanism of injury play in the pathogenesis of this condition?

Diagnostics
WBC: 16,000/L ESR: high CRP: high Wound culture: +Staph infection X-ray: inflammation of periosteum; bone destruction in right foot and tissue swelling

The provider orders a CBC, wound culture, and x-rays of the right foot and lower leg.

3. What do these results mean? Explain. What other tests might be ordered?

4. What are the potential complications of Meera's condition?

5. What would Meera's treatment plan include?

AFAB, Assigned female at birth; *BP,* blood pressure; *CBC,* complete blood count; *CRP,* C-reactive protein; *ESR,* erythrocyte sedimentation rate; *HR,* heart rate; *RR,* respiratory rate; *T,* temperature; *WBC,* white blood cell.

Case Study 15.3

Rachel, a 35-year-old cis-female (she/her), presents to her provider with gradually increasing joint pain, swelling, and stiffness in the mornings, primarily in both hands. She states that the pain typically lasts for 2 hours and is accompanied by fatigue. Rachel has a past medical history of hypertension (well-controlled) and has an allergy to penicillin. She mentions that her mother has "arthritis."

1. Looking at Rachel's symptoms and history, what key clinical features would lead you to a diagnosis? What would your diagnosis be?

2. What are the genetic and environmental risk factors that contribute to this disease? Is this an autoimmune disease? Why or why not?

On exam Rachel has difficulty making a fist, and there is evidence of bilateral ulnar deviation and metacarpophalangeal (MCP) deformity. She says that she has a lot of difficulty gripping objects.

3. What labs would you expect the provider to order and what results do you expect to see to confirm the diagnosis?

4. What complications would you expect? How would you treat this disease?

Case Study 15.4

Marwan is a 45-year-old AMAB (he/him). He is seeking medical attention due to sudden-onset severe pain and swelling in his left big toe. He mentions a history of occasional joint pain but nothing as intense as his current episode. Gary has a family history of gout, and he admits to a diet high in meat and dairy products and has a glass of wine with dinner every night.

1. Given Marwan's symptoms and family history, what key clinical features would lead you to believe that he has gout?

2. How would you confirm that Marwan has gout?

3. What lifestyle changes would Marwan need to make? How would you treat gout?

AMAB, Assigned male at birth.

16

Putting It All Together—Looking at Real Patients With Multiple Comorbidities

Case Study 16.1

Julia is a 24-year-old trans-female (she/her) who has a 10-year history of eating disorders (anorexia and bulimia). The client had been in an eating disorders program and was doing well. Recently, due to external stressors, she stopped eating, started taking excessive amounts of laxatives, and lost 28 pounds in the last month. She came to the emergency room after having 3 days of severe vomiting and diarrhea.

Lab Test	Value (Interpretation)
pH	7.58
pCO_2	50 mm Hg
pO_2	80 mm Hg
HCO_3^-	34 mEq/L
Na	141 mEq/L
K	2.5 mEq/L
Ca	5.2 mg/dL
Creatinine	2.9 mg/dL
BUN	234 mg/dL
Glucose	72 mg/dL
Hgb	8.2 g/dL
Hct	22%
WBC	11,000/L
Plts	325,000 mm^3
ALT	469 units/L (high)
Serum osmolality	323 mOsm/kg

Body System	Assessment Findings
Vital signs	BP: 88/60 mm Hg; HR: 52 and irregular; RR: 24 breaths/minute; T: 97°F (oral); O_2 sat: 94% on room air Height: 5′7″; weight: 85 pounds
Neuro	Alert and oriented to person, place, and time; appears sleepy, extremely weak
Skin	Cool lower extremities; pale, poor skin turgor
Lungs	Diminished sounds in bilateral bases
Heart	Heart murmur: mitral valve regurgitation; abnormal ECG
Abdomen	Concave, + bowel sounds in all quadrants; hepatomegaly
Genitourinary	Oliguria; dark urine

On admission to the ED, labs and an arterial blood gas (ABG) were drawn.

1. Please interpret Julia's blood gas (pH, pCO_2, pO_2, and HCO_3).

____

____

____

____

2. Why does Julia have an ABG like this? What caused it?

____

____

____

____

After looking at the assessment and lab work, Julia is diagnosed with severe dehydration and slated for admission to the ICU.

3. The health care provider is worried about kidney damage. Is this a concern? Why?

____

____

____

____

4. What labs and assessment findings support this?

____

____

The health care provider reviewed Julia's lab results.

5. Would the provider find Julia's electrolyte levels to be normal? Which ones are abnormal and what led to the abnormality? Explain.

6. Would the provider be concerned about anemia? What kind of anemia? Explain the labs and pathophysiology that indicate this condition.

By day 3 of admission to the ICU, Julia's fluid and electrolyte levels have stabilized. However, she has several episodes of nausea and vomiting. The nurse does an abdominal assessment and finds that her bowel sounds are absent in the lower quadrants, but hyperactive in the upper quadrants. Abdominal distension is noted, and she is complaining of crampy 8/10 abdominal pain.

7. What would be a possible diagnosis for these new symptoms? Why?

On day 6, Julia's condition stabilized, and she seemed to be on the road to recovery. However, when the evening nurse came in to check on her, she was sitting up straight in bed, breathing fast, and looking anxious. On exam, Julia had crackles throughout both lung fields and tachypnea with an RR of 32 breaths/minute. When Julia started to cough, the nurse noticed pink frothy sputum.

8. What condition do you suspect that Julia has? Why?

9. Looking at her lab and assessment findings, which factors would have caused this new complication?

10. How can this diagnosis be confirmed?

ALT, Alanine transaminase; *BP,* blood pressure; *BUN,* blood urea nitrogen; *ECG,* electrocardiogram; *ED,* emergency department; *Hct,* hematocrit; *Hgb,* hemoglobin; *ICU,* intensive care unit; *O_2 sat,* oxygen saturation; *Plts,* platelets; *RR,* respiratory rate; *T,* temperature; *WBC,* white blood cell.

Case Study 16.2

Daniel is a 50-year-old Dominican American cis-male (he/him) who has not had regular health care since he was laid off 2 years ago. He has a history of smoking (20 years), hypertension, coronary artery disease, chronic bronchitis, type 2 diabetes mellitus, and stroke. He comes to the emergency room coughing and complaining of severe dyspnea. You are his emergency department nurse.

Lab Test	Value (Interpretation)
pH	7.30
pCO_2	50 mm Hg
pO_2	60 mm Hg
HCO_3^-	34 mEq/L
Na	140 mEq/L
K	5.7 mEq/L
Ca	9.5 mg/dL
Creatinine	3.8 mg/dL
BUN	400 mg/dL
Glucose	224 mg/dL
Hgb	17 g/dL
Hct	42%
WBC	10,000/L
Plts	170,000 mm^3
Troponin	0.2 ng/mL (normal)

Body System	Assessment Findings
Vital signs	BP: 173/98 mm Hg; P: 110 and irregular; RR 28 breaths/minute; T: 97.3°F (axillary); O_2 sat: 90% on room air Height: 5′3″; weight: 175 pounds
Neuro	Alert and oriented to person, place, and time; appears very anxious
Skin	Cool lower extremities; pale, 2+ edema to lower extremities
Lungs	Wheezing; diminished sounds bilaterally
Heart	Atrial fibrillation; abnormal ECG
Abdomen	Distended, hypoactive bowel sounds; hepatomegaly

1. What would your primary diagnosis be? Explain.

2. What risk factors could have contributed to his illness?

The health care provider reviewed Daniel's lab results.

3. Analyze Daniel's arterial blood gases. Are they normal? If not, explain what the cause would be.

4. What other lab results would the provider be concerned with? What might cause these issues? Explain the labs and pathophysiology.

After being treated for the condition above (Question 1), Daniel is slated for admission to the floor. While assessing him, the health care provider hears a heart murmur. The provider orders an echocardiogram, which shows that he has mitral valve regurgitation.

5. What implications might this finding have for Daniel? Explain.

6. What labs and assessment findings support this?

On day 3 of Daniel's admission, the nurse finds him flushed, sitting upright, and struggling to breathe. The pulse oximetry reading is 88% on 2 L of oxygen. When the nurse auscultates his lungs, diffuse crackles are heard throughout. The nurse notices 4+ edema in Daniel's lower extremities. The morning labs show that his BNP has increased to 8000 mg/dL.

7. What do you think has happened to Daniel? Why?

Daniel was transferred to the ICU. On day 5 of admission, the nurse notes that he has a distended abdomen. While the nurse is giving a bed bath to him, they notice that his eyes have a yellow tinge.

8. What would be a possible diagnosis for these new symptoms? Explain how this may be linked to Daniel's previous diagnoses and/or medical history.

On day 7 of admission, Daniel's condition has stabilized, and he seems to be on the road to recovery. When the evening shift nurse comes to assess him, they find that he is leaning to the right side, with right-sided facial droop. When the nurse assesses Daniel, the nurse finds that he cannot speak coherently.

9. What do you think has happened to Daniel?

10. Do you think that Daniel's condition has been caused by anything in his previous medical history, assessments, or labs? If so, explain the correlation.

BNP, B-type natriuretic peptide; *BP,* blood pressure; *BUN,* blood urea nitrogen; *Hct,* hematocrit; *Hgb,* hemoglobin; *ICU,* intensive care unit; O_2 *sat,* oxygen saturation; *Plts,* platelets; *RR,* respiratory rate; *T,* temperature; *WBC,* white blood cell.

Case Study 16.3

Davina is a 15-year-old Black AMAB (she/her) who states that she is exhausted, falling asleep in school, unable to concentrate, and losing weight, despite eating much more than normal. Her parents have brought her to the pediatric provider.

Vital Signs	Assessment	Labs
BP: 117/72 mm Hg HR: 88 beats per minute RR: 18 breaths/minute O_2 sat: 98% on room air T: 99°F	Tall, thin in appearance; skin is warm, dry; lips are cracked Has lost 10 pounds in 4 weeks; states that she is "always hungry and really thirsty"; states that she is urinating more than usual	Hct: 40% Hgb: 15 mg/dL K: 4.5 mg/dL Na: 150 mg/dL Creatinine: 1.0 mg/dL BUN: 20 mg/dL Glucose: 200 mg/dL

1. What do you think is happening to Davina? What evidence do you have?

2. How can you confirm this diagnosis?

3. Explain the pathophysiology of this disease.

Davina and her parents are referred to an endocrinologist and she is able to manage her condition well with a pump.

Five years later, Davina comes to see her provider for frequent abdominal pain and diarrhea. Her regular provider is not available, so she sees another provider that she is not familiar with. She reports that she has been having loose stool and diarrhea for the past few months, but it has gotten much worse in the past 3 weeks, with 6 to 8 episodes of nonbloody diarrhea. She states that she has been under stress recently, as she has just broken up with her partner. Her provider tells her that she probably has a gastrointestinal virus and to rest and keep up with her fluids. However, Davina's symptoms continue to get worse, and she comes back to see her regular provider the following week.

4. What do you think her diagnosis is and how is it related to the diagnosis in Question 1?

5. Describe the symptoms and complications of the disease. How could the disease be definitively diagnosed?

6. How do you treat this disease?

7. Do you feel that Davina's first provider treated her appropriately? Why or why not?

A few more years go by. Davina is now 28 years old and working as a software engineer. She is having palpitations and losing weight. Her blood sugars are well controlled, and she has been "pretty healthy." She tells her provider that she gets so hot and short of breath that she has had to stop exercising.

8. What do you suspect? Give your rationale.

9. What lab and diagnostic tests would you need to confirm a diagnosis?

AMAB, Assigned male at birth; *BP,* blood pressure; *BUN,* blood urea nitrogen; *Hct,* hematocrit; *Hgb,* hemoglobin; O_2 *sat,* oxygen saturation; *RR,* respiratory rate; *T,* temperature.

Appendix

Answers to Chapter 1 Case Studies

Case Study 1.1

1. In terms of inflammatory response, describe the vascular and cellular events.
   The initial phase of inflammation is the vascular phase. In this phase, Leah would see vasodilation and increased capillary permeability. Vasodilation would increase blood flow to the injured area; redness and warmth to the area would result. Chemical mediators (histamine, bradykinin, leukotrienes) would cause increased capillary permeability. This would cause exudate and proteins to escape into the tissues, which results in edema. The thick yellow exudate is pus, which is made up of dead neutrophils. Leah would see swelling, pain, and impaired function. Redness, warmth, swelling, pain, and loss of function are the cardinal signs of inflammation.
   The cellular phase refers to the migration of the leukocytes to the area of injury. Margination and tethering refer to the accumulation and adhesion of the leukocytes to the endothelium. The endothelial cells secrete selectin and integrin to help the cells adhere to and roll along the endothelium. Diapedesis is the transmigration of the leukocytes, or how they get into and out of the blood vessel. Finally, once the leukocytes reach the area of injury, chemotactica factors attract them to the right place. Phagocytosis then occurs, as the leukocytes move in to engulf pathogens and debris. Complement proteins help phagocytes recognize pathogens by coating their surfaces (opsonization).
2. Is this an acute or chronic inflammation? Is it systemic? Explain your answers.
   It would be classified as an acute inflammation. In this case, Leah's symptoms take place 2 days after the injury. Chronic inflammation is defined as an unsuccessful inflammatory response that has gone on for 2 weeks of longer. At this point, the inflammatory response is localized, without any known systemic effects such as fever.
3. What has caused Leah's worsening symptoms?
   Leah's symptoms have worsened and with the fever the inflammation has now become systemic. The redness, swelling, and pain have spread and become worse. She is also having generalized symptoms of fatigue and myalgia.
4. What lab work would you expect?
   The provider would likely order a complete blood count (CBC) to look for leukocytosis (increased white blood cell production), an erythrocyte sedimentation rate (ESR), and blood cultures to identify the pathogen. They may order C-reactive protein levels (CRP) as well.
5. How would you treat Leah's symptoms?
   Leah's symptoms suggest bacterial infection and would likely be treated with an intravenous infusion of antibiotics.

Case Study 1.2

1. What is the biopsy indicative of? Explain.
   The biopsy is indicative of a granuloma. A granuloma is composed of macrophages and lymphocytes. Giant cells are multinucleated cells formed by the fusion of macrophages.
2. Is this an acute inflammation or a chronic inflammation? Why?
   With Matt's long history of inflammatory bowel disease and finding of a granuloma, it would suggest that this is a chronic inflammation.
3. Explain why Matt is at a higher risk for cancer.
   Matt is at higher risk of a colorectal cancer because of the chronic nature of his inflammatory bowel disease. When tissue is constantly undergoing the inflammatory and healing process, the increased proliferation of cells could lead to cellular mutations, which could go on to result in cancer.
4. What would you say to Matt about the risk of getting cancer?
   "I understand your concern. While you are at increased risk of colorectal cancer because of your inflammatory bowel disease, this does not mean that you will definitely have a cancer diagnosis. You can try to prevent exacerbations by eating a healthy diet with a moderate level of fiber, drinking plenty of fluids, exercising, managing your stress levels, and not eating or drinking things that trigger exacerbations. There are also ways to prevent and catch any early signs of cancer, such as getting more frequent colonoscopies and being vigilant in looking for signs and symptoms of colorectal cancer, such as dark or bright red blood in stool, change in bowel habits, and pain during defecation."

Case Study 1.3

1. What stage of HIV infection is Kasey in? Describe the stage.
   HIV/AIDS occurs in three stages: acute HIV infection, chronic (latent) HIV infection, and overt AIDS. Kasey is in the acute HIV infection stage. This initial

phase has vague symptoms (sore throat, night sweats, nausea, vomiting, lymphadenopathy, fever, chills, and fatigue) that can be attributed to having a virus.

2. Do their symptoms fit with the HIV diagnosis?
   Yes, these symptoms fit with the diagnosis. Kasey reports having a sore throat and myalgias for 3 weeks, which are common symptoms of HIV.
3. What kind of HIV testing is done initially? Is just having one of those tests enough to confirm the diagnosis? Explain.
   Typically, antigen/antibody or antibody testing is done (enzyme immunoassay [EIA], enzyme-linked immunosorbent assay [ELISA], OraSure) first. These tests are screening tests (lab draws, finger sticks, oral swabs) that detect the presence of antibodies in the blood. If these tests show a positive result, then a confirmation test, such as the Western Blot, will need to be done before a positive diagnosis is made. There are also nucleic acid tests (NATs) that look for the presence of the virus in the blood. The NAT does not need a second confirming test.
4. How would you answer Kasey?
   "No, this does not mean a death sentence. HIV is now considered a chronic condition in many well-resourced countries. With a proper antiretroviral medication regimen, monitoring of viral load and helper T cells, many clients do not advance to AIDS."
5. What would you tell them?
   "Yes, it is possible to have a child as long as Kasey is taking antiretroviral medications and has an undetectable viral load. If the viral load is negligible, the chance of passing HIV to their partner is low. An HIV negative partner can also take the pre-exposure prophylaxis (PrEP) to protect themselves, though this may not be necessary in an undetectable viral load. Artificial insemination is an option as well."
6. How can they prevent the child from having HIV?
   If Kasey is taking antiretroviral medications and their viral load is undetectable, it is extremely unlikely that they will pass the HIV onto their child. However, Kasey must be receiving good prenatal care and their viral load and helper T cell levels must be carefully monitored.
7. Does this mean that the baby has HIV? Explain your answer.
   No, this does not mean that the child has HIV. Immunoglobulin G (IgG) is transmitted from the parent to the fetus, as IgG can cross the placenta. The child will have HIV antibodies because of this.
8. What would be the most definitive HIV test for a newborn?
   The definitive HIV test for the newborn would be a NAT test. Because of the HIV antibodies transmitted to the child from the parent, the only way to definitively diagnose HIV in the newborn would be to get a blood test that looks for the virus.

Answers to Chapter 2 Case Studies

Case Study 2.1

1. What disorder do you think that Mateo has? Why?
   Mateo has Marfan syndrome. Marfan syndrome is a genetic disorder that is autosomal dominant and typically familial. With this disease, there is a gene mutation that affects fibrillin-1 production (elastin) and causes connective tissue dysfunction. He has hallmark symptoms of Marfan syndrome: very tall, cardiac arrhythmias, and pectoris excavatum (concave) chest.
2. Explain the reason why Mateo may be short of breath, hypotensive, and tachycardic.
   People with Marfan syndrome often have cardiac issues—such as mitral valve prolapse, cardiac arrhythmias, aortic aneurysms, aortic dissection, heart failure, and sudden death. Due to his vigorous exercise, Mateo's heart went into ventricular tachycardia and his cardiac output decreased dramatically. The lack of cardiac output causes low blood volume, therefore low blood pressure. Because of the lack of oxygenated blood, his respiratory rate increases, and he is short of breath.
3. What would you say to Mateo about continuing his athletic activities?
   "Mateo, I know that you are a terrific athlete and love sports. However, because of your condition, you are at high risk of collapsing again if you participate in high impact activities. Marfan syndrome causes cardiac and blood vessel abnormalities, which may cause your heart to fail. This does not mean that you must stop exercising. You can still participate in low to moderate impact activities. I know this is hard to hear. I am here for you if you have questions."
4. What complications are associated with this disease and how can they be monitored?
   With Marfan syndrome, the ocular, skeletal, and cardiac systems need to be monitored. Individuals with the disorder may have ocular defects leading to myopia (nearsightedness) and retinal detachment. Skeletal abnormalities such as scoliosis and kyphosis are common. Finally, cardiac and vascular abnormalities can occur. Mateo should have yearly eye exams, exams for skeletal abnormalities and bone density testing, and a complete cardiac workup with an ECG.

Case Study 2.2

1. How would you answer Mia's spouse?
   "Tay-Sachs is an autosomal recessive genetic disease (chromosome 15) that causes lipid accumulation in the cells, affecting the brain and retinal neurons. Though Lana was normal at birth, the rapidly progressive nature of this disease has caused weakness, loss of muscle function, and loss of motor and mental functions. Unfortunately, there is no cure. Most of the care is supportive."

2. Explain how Mia could have a child with Tay-Sachs disease.

   Mia did not do anything wrong. She had a recessive gene for Tay-Sachs disease, which would not show any clinical symptoms. Unfortunately, the sperm donor also had a recessive gene for the disease. Lana has Tay-Sachs because she received both recessive genes. Mia could not have known this.

3. What is the prognosis for children with Tay-Sachs disease? Is there a way to find out if a child will be born with the disease? How?

   Lana will become very weak, and she may have seizures and lose her sight. Typically, children with this disease die around 4 or 5 years of age. Respiratory failure is a common cause of death. If Mia and her wife are considering having another child, they can ask the sperm donor to have genetic testing done to make sure that that they are not carrying the recessive gene for Tay-Sachs.

Case Study 2.3

1. Discuss any risk factors, including epigenetic risk factors, Patrick may have. What would be the next step in the assessment?

   Patrick has a history of type 2 diabetes mellitus, hypertension, and depression. These are all risk factors. He is also overweight, which is a risk factor as well. Multifactorial inheritance disorders are disorders that are both genetic and environmental in nature. This means that individuals with this disorder can be predisposed to certain diseases, but may be able to modify disease expression with environment and lifestyle. Hypertension, type 2 diabetes mellitus, depression, and obesity are all considered to be multifactorial inheritance disorders. As a nurse, the next step is to look at Patrick's environment and lifestyle.

2. How do the social determinants of health and health equity play a role in Patrick's health?

   The social determinants of health address the living conditions of both the individual and the community: safe housing, healthy food, jobs and income, education, health care, safe neighborhoods, and green spaces. The social determinants of equity address access to all of these conditions. From Patrick's comments, we can see that income is an issue. He cannot afford his medication, or the gym, and he does not have a place he can exercise. Patrick's diet is also affected, as he is forced to shop at a corner store, which may not have as many healthy options. Access to a good income, access to health care (medications), access to green spaces, and access to healthy food all seem to be out of reach for Patrick. This will impact his quality of life, overall health, and access to treatment. These are health inequities and must be noted and addressed by the health care team, as all individuals should have the opportunity to achieve good health and should not be disadvantaged from achieving this due to socioeconomic issues and lack of access.

3. How can the health clinic team help Patrick achieve his goal to become healthier?

   First, the team needs to find out what Patrick's goals are and details of what he is doing. Then, the team needs to help him reframe what exercise and healthy diet look like. An easy change may be for Patrick to start walking or biking to and from work for exercise, rather than taking public transportation or driving. If Patrick lives in an apartment building, climbing stairs could also be an option for exercise. To eat healthier, perhaps there are healthy options at the corner store. Many times, there are farmers' markets in the area. If Patrick is able to travel further, budgeting and planning meals for the week may be a good option. Finally, regarding medication, the clinic team should reevaluate his medications. Can he take generic medications or different medications that are just as effective at lower cost? Perhaps there is a better insurance plan or drug program to cover the cost.

Case Study 2.4

1. What would be the next step in properly diagnosing Leticia's condition?

   The next step would likely be a tissue biopsy. A biopsy is a sample of abnormal tissue that is taken so that it can be examined, and the condition can be diagnosed.

2. How would the social determinants of health and equity impact her diagnosis and treatment?

   Leticia does not have access to regular health care, specialized treatments, or medications because she does not have insurance. This lack of access impacts the length and quality of her life and signals a health inequity. Without further intervention, and access to free/low-cost mammography, she would not be able to have her condition diagnosed. If she is diagnosed with cancer, she would not have the insurance required to treat it.

3. What risk factors does Leticia have for breast cancer?

   Leticia has heart disease (atherosclerosis and hypertension) and is overweight. Hypertension has been found to be a risk factor in postmenopausal women. Atherosclerosis is a chronic inflammatory disease. Chronic inflammation can lead to cancer in postmenopausal women, including breast cancer. Chronic inflammation leads to increased cell proliferation during the injury and health process, which increases the chance of mutations. Atherosclerosis is often seen in conjunction with obesity, which is a risk factor because the adipose tissue produces inflammatory hormones. Obesity also leads to insulin resistance, causing increased insulin production and release. Insulin affects estrogen release, and greater levels of insulin lead to greater levels of estrogen. Too much estrogen may lead to cellular proliferation and cancer. Leticia also told her daughter that breast nodules were common occurrences in the family. This may mean that the family members are prone to having dense breast tissue, which is a risk factor for breast cancer. It may also mean that the family has a genetic mutation of the tumor suppressor genes BRCA1 and BRCA2, which is an indicator of high risk for breast and ovarian cancer. Leticia should receive genetic testing to find out if she has this mutation. If she does, immediate family members should also be tested. Treatment requires close monitoring and healthy diet and exercise. The most effective treatment if the client has BRCA 1 and 2 mutations is prophylactic mastectomy and bilateral salpingo-oophorectomy.

4. How advanced is Leticia's cancer?
   The breast cancer is advanced. The tumor is moderately large, greater than 5 cm across, it has spread to 1 or 2 lymph nodes, and there is distant metastasis.
5. Why is she scheduled for chemotherapy? Will surgery and chemotherapy get rid of all of the cancer cells? Why or why not?
   Surgery is done to remove most or all of the tumor; however, surgery may not be able to get rid of all of the tumor cells and will not be effective against metastatic cancer. Chemotherapy is used as an adjuvant systemic therapy that typically targets rapidly proliferating cells and is effective for metastatic cancer. The purpose of chemotherapy is not to kill all of the cancer cells, but to kill enough cancer cells so that the body's immune system can take over and destroy the remaining cancer cells.
6. What are three common side effects of chemotherapy? Explain the pathophysiology behind why these side effects occur.
   Most chemotherapy targets rapidly proliferating cells during cell division. However, it is not just cancer cells that proliferate rapidly. Cells in the gastrointestinal (GI) tract, bone marrow, skin, and hair are also rapidly dividing cells. This causes GI side effects such as stomatitis, mucositis, and diarrhea. Red blood cells, white blood cells, and platelets are destroyed in the bone marrow, causing anemia and fatigue, increased risk of infection, and bleeding. Chemotherapy affects skin and hair follicles and can cause dryness, itching, and redness to skin, as well as temporary hair loss during the course of the treatment. Finally, chemotherapy affects the medulla, stimulating the chemotherapy trigger zone and causing nausea and vomiting.
7. What could these symptoms be a result of?
   This could be a result of metastasis to the liver and the brain. The jaundice and ascites suggest spread to the liver and the confusion and agitation suggest metastasis to the brain.

Answers to Chapter 3 Case Studies

Case Study 3.1

1. Explain the pathophysiology behind the swelling and edema.
   Marcos has been on their feet, walking around in a warm climate. The fact that they have been on their feet more can lead to dependent edema. Gravity causes fluid to pool in the vessels of the lower legs and feet. This increases the hydrostatic or capillary filtration pressure. This increase in pressure causes fluid to move out of the blood vessels and into the tissues, causing edema.
2. What conditions may have led to this?
   The heat, the increase in activity (walking) in the hot climate, and the increased fluid intake may all have led to the swelling and edema that Marcos is experiencing.
3. Why did Nikhil ask this question? Why did he assess the lungs?
   Nikhil is asking to see if this is a case of fluid overload. Fluid overload can lead to increased hydrostatic pressure, causing edema. If there is high water intake, as in Marcos' case, fluid overload is likely. In severe fluid overload, the lungs will fill with fluid, called pulmonary congestion, causing dyspnea and respiratory issues. Nikhil wants to make sure that this is not happening to Marcos.
4. What does Marcos' response indicate? What condition do they have?
   Marcos' response indicates that they have fluid overload. Because they drank so much water to rehydrate, they likely have hypotonic hyponatremia. This means that they have drunk so much water that they have diluted out the sodium present in the blood. Remember that sodium is the major cation in the extracellular fluid. Symptoms of hyponatremia include: confusion, edema, lethargy, and decreased reflexes.
5. Does Marcos need to go to the hospital? How can their condition be treated?
   Unless there is fluid in their lungs, or they cannot keep fluid down due to vomiting, chances are that they do not need to go to the hospital. Instead of water, Marcos needs to drink fluids balanced with electrolytes and minerals, such as Pedialyte or Gatorade. This is likely not available in India, but oral rehydration therapy can be homemade, with six teaspoons of sugar and half a teaspoon of salt dissolved in a liter of water. They can also increase their salt intake.

Case Study 3.2

1. Does Sam have any electrolyte abnormalities? Which electrolytes?
   Yes, they do.

Potassium—6.5 mg/dL high
Magnesium—4 mg/dL high
Calcium—12 mg/dL high
Blood glucose—515 mg/dL high

2. How would you interpret Sam's arterial blood gas? If there is a disorder, how would the body compensate?

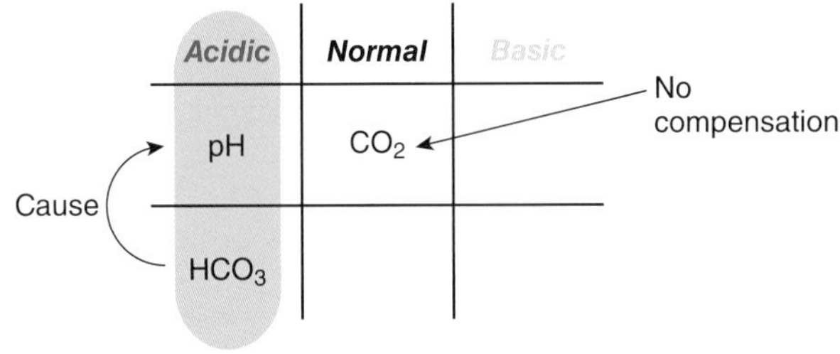

Looking at the tic-tac-toe diagram, the arterial blood gas (ABG) disorder is uncompensated metabolic acidosis. With metabolic acidosis, the chemical buffer automatically responds first. The lungs start compensating within minutes, with rapid, deep breaths to blow off CO_2. Finally, the kidneys respond last, taking hours to days, but compensate most thoroughly.

3. Are there any electrolyte imbalances that are common with Sam's condition? Explain.

Yes. Hyperkalemia, hypercalcemia, and hypermagnesemia are electrolyte imbalances that occur with metabolic acidosis. When the blood is acidic, proteins have decreased affinity for their substrates. Therefore, more ions are not bound to proteins. There are more free potassium, calcium, and magnesium ions, increasing their serum concentration.

4. How would you explain Sam's somnolence and respiratory rate? Explain the pathophysiology.

Acidemia causes decreased neuronal excitability and inhibition of metabolism. This initially leads to confusion, drowsiness, and lethargy, and can ultimately lead to somnolence and coma. Sam's increased respiratory rate is a compensatory response to the metabolic acidosis. The lungs are compensating with deeper and faster breaths to blow off the CO_2 and decrease acidity.

5. Why is Sam's face warm and flushed? What would cause their weak, rapid pulse?

Sam's face is warm and flushed due to arteriolar dilation. With acidemia, smooth muscles lose their tone, causing vasodilation. Vasodilation increases blood flow to the tissues, causing warmth and flushing.

Case Study 3.3

1. Based on the above information, which patient needs to be assessed first? Why?

Lei needs to be assessed first. All her electrolytes (K, Na, Ca, Mg) are out of normal range, more so than Kal or Jess. Lei's blood gas is also extremely high. Kal has mildly abnormal electrolytes. Finally, Jess has only one electrolyte out of normal range (Na).

2. Kal is complaining of numbness and tingling, especially around the mouth. Identify the electrolyte imbalance(s) this patient has that could be causing these symptoms.

Kal's potassium is mildly elevated (5.6 mg/dL), which causes neuromuscular excitability and paresthesias.

3. How would you interpret Kal's blood gas? What would cause this? What body system(s) will attempt to compensate?

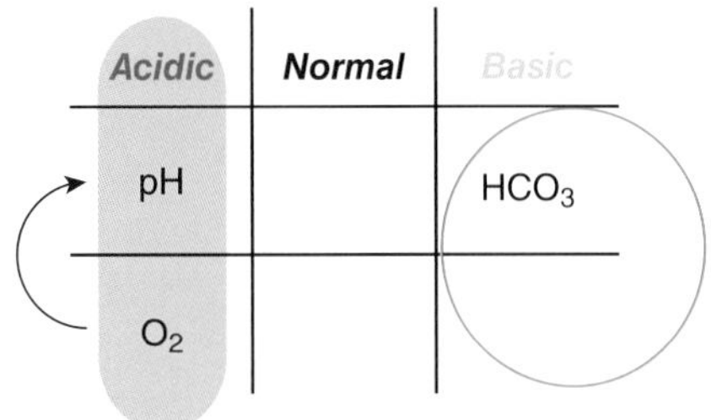

Kal has partially compensated respiratory acidosis. This is likely caused by poor oxygenation (hypoventilation) from pulmonary disease. The chemical buffer system will compensate first, then later, the kidneys. In this case, the lungs would not be able to adequately compensate, as lung disease is the issue.

4. Jess' blood pressure is 88/50 mm Hg and her heart rate is 116 beats/minute when lying down. When she attempts to sit up, she feels faint. What could be causing her symptoms?

Jess is hypernatremic and quite dehydrated. The decrease in blood volume causes the blood pressure and cardiac output to drop. The heart then beats faster to try and compensate for the decrease in cardiac output. The kidneys produce little to no urine to retain fluid. When Jess sits up, she experiences orthostatic hypotension, dizziness/syncope caused by the sudden drop in blood pressure (from the position change) and the corresponding increase in heart rate.

5. Would you treat Jess' sodium level? If yes, how?

Yes. Hypernatremia should be treated as noninvasively as possible. Jess does not have severe hypernatremia, so we would start with oral fluids. If she is unable to keep the fluids down, intravenous (IV) fluids, such as normal saline, would be started and infused slowly. Fast infusions or hypotonic solutions may cause cerebral edema and should be avoided unless the hypernatremia is severe.

6. What do Lei's blood gas results indicate? What condition does she have? What is an electrolyte disorder that often accompanies this condition?

Lei's blood gases indicate that she has uncompensated metabolic alkalosis, likely from the household cleaner. Electrolyte disorders that accompany this condition are hypokalemia, hypocalcemia, and hypomagnesemia. In an alkalotic situation, proteins bind more tightly to their substrates, binding up the electrolytes and leaving few free ions.

7. How would you account for her seizures and respiratory rate?
   Metabolic alkalosis causes increased neuronal excitability, which can lead to seizures. The decreased respiratory rate is caused by the lungs compensating for the alkalosis. By breathing less, CO_2 is retained, thereby increasing the acidity to neutralize the blood.
8. How would you explain Lei's heart rate and paresthesias?
   Along with Lei's alkalosis, which increases neuromuscular excitability, she has severe hypokalemia, hypomagnesemia, and hypocalcemia. All these electrolyte disorders affect the heart and can cause dysrhythmias. Severe hypocalcemia increases neuromuscular excitability and causes spasms, tetany, and paresthesia, as evidenced by Trousseau and Chvostek sign.

Answers to Chapter 4 Case Studies

Case Study 4.1

1. As the nurse, what would you notice about this client? How would you interpret this?
   As the nurse, you should note the age of the client, the fact that the client has dementia and is more confused than normal. The client is also sleeping more and the daughter reports foul-smelling urine.
2. What condition do you think that the client has? Does she show typical symptoms? Why or why not?
   The client's dementia may be progressing. However, dementia does not typically progress in 2 weeks, and it does not cause foul-smelling urine. A urinary tract infection (UTI) is the most likely diagnosis. Older adults tend to drink less and can be dehydrated. Hygiene can also be an issue with decreased mobility. Finally, confusion is typical with older adults as a symptom of a UTI, instead of nausea, dysuria, and abdominal pain.
3. Does the client's dementia play a role in this disorder? Why or why not?
   Yes, it does, especially in later stages of dementia. UTIs are commonly associated with dementia, due to hygiene and decreased intake of fluids.
4. What lab tests would you expect the provider to order?
   At this point, the provider would probably order a urine analysis and urine culture. It is important to order both. The client would be started on a broad-spectrum antibiotic. Depending on the results of the urine culture, the antibiotics may be changed to better target the pathogen. Typically, the bacteria is *Escherichia coli*, which suggests fecal contamination.
5. How has the client's condition progressed? Explain the pathophysiology.
   With the increased severity in symptoms, it seems that the client's condition has progressed to become pyelonephritis. When a UTI is not treated, or not completely resolved, bacteria from the urethra travel up the ureter and can cause a renal infection. Generally, one kidney is infected, though both can be infected. The flank pain is a hallmark sign of pyelonephritis. Fever, lethargy, and nausea are also common.
6. What lab results would you expect to see?
   The urinalysis would show white blood cells and bacteria. There would be pyuria (pus) and microscopic hematuria. The urine culture may come back positive for bacteria. However, if the client has been taking antibiotics, it may impact the urine culture.
7. How would this condition be treated?
   This condition is typically treated with intravenous (IV) antibiotics and the client is often hospitalized. Renal imaging may be done to see if there is any obstruction or hydronephrosis.
8. Why type of acute kidney injury (AKI) would the client most likely have? Explain the pathophysiology and complications.
   Pyelonephritis happens within the kidney and affects the structure of the kidney. It can cause an intrarenal AKI. This could lead to acute tubular necrosis, due to sepsis and inflammatory response, which decreases the amount of oxygen to the kidneys, decreases the glomerular filtration rate (GFR), and ultimately may cause renal failure.

Case Study 4.2

1. As the nurse, what would you notice about the client's symptom history and vital signs?
   The client has periorbital edema, leg edema, and is seeing blood in his urine. The client's blood pressure is quite high for his age as well.
2. What disorder might this client have? Explain what may have caused this issue and what symptoms support your diagnosis.
   The client likely has nephritic syndrome. Nephritic syndrome is an inflammatory response that typically occurs with bacterial infection (streptococcus, staphylococcus) and autoimmune disease and causes damage to the glomerular filtration barrier. There are three layers to the barrier—the endothelium, the glomerular basement membrane, and the podocyte layer. Due to the inflammatory response, capillary permeability increases and there is a huge loss of albumin from the blood, causing fluid to move into tissues, which leads to edema. The renin-angiotensin-aldosterone system (RAAS) tries to compensate for intravascular fluid loss by increasing sodium retention, which leads to fluid retention and hypertension. White blood cells and red blood cells are also lost and filtered through the kidneys which is why blood (hematuria) and pus (pyuria) are seen in the urine.
   This differs from nephrotic syndrome. Nephrotic syndrome is also caused by an inflammatory process and involves the deposition of immune complexes in the glomerulus with increased capillary permeability. The inflammatory process causes clots, scarring, and damage

to the glomerulus. This results in massive proteinuria and generalized edema. To make up for this, the liver makes more lipoproteins. This leads to hyperlipidemia and eventually, as lipoproteins are excreted through the urine, lipiduria. With nephrotic syndrome, gross hematuria and pyuria are not typically seen, though microscopic amounts of blood can be seen.

3. What role, if any, would social determinants of health play in this case?
   Health care access may be an issue, as the client has not been to a provider recently and lives in a rural community. Untreated or undertreated streptococcal and staphylococcus infections may progress to glomerulonephritis and result in nephritic syndrome. The lack of access to health care, living in a rural area, would contribute to the client's renal issues.
4. What do you notice about the labs? How do these values support your diagnosis?
   Much of the lab work is abnormal. The creatinine is slightly high (normal 1.2 mg/dL) and the BUN is high (normal 6–21 mg/dL). Serum sodium is normal and serum potassium is slightly above normal (3.5–5 mg/dL). LDL levels are also normal, though on the higher side. However, albumin levels are quite low, which is seen in third spacing and edema. Hemoglobin levels are low, which would make sense, as the client is losing blood in his urine. The client's white blood cell level is high due to inflammation, and his urine shows hematuria, pyuria, and proteinuria. These results confirm nephritic syndrome, as there are blood, white blood cells, and protein in the urine. Loss of protein in the urine would cause edema. If it was nephrotic syndrome, the client would be oliguric, have hyperlipidemia and lipiduria, and would not have hematuria or pyuria.
5. How would you treat someone with this disorder?
   The underlying cause of nephritic syndrome would need to be treated. This client likely had untreated streptococcal or staphylococcal infection. This would be treated with antibiotics. Inflammatory and autoimmune disease would be treated with corticosteroids or immunosuppressive drugs. Resulting hypertension and edema would be treated with antihypertensives and diuretics.

Case Study 4.3

1. What do you notice about Josie's condition? How would you interpret these findings and make a diagnosis?
   Josie has not urinated in 8 hours, which is a medical emergency and suggests an obstruction and urinary retention. Nausea and vomiting are common symptoms of urinary retention. Their abdomen is distended and painful due to the full bladder. When the catheter was placed, it was difficult to place, which often happens with benign prostatic hyperplasia (BPH). The urine could be dark due to bleeding. Josie's diagnosis is urinary retention and obstruction due to BPH.
2. Did the nurse respond appropriately? How could the nurse have made Josie more comfortable?
   No, the nurse did not respond appropriately. The nurse's response made Josie uncomfortable. When assessing a client, the nurse could have asked them how they would like to be addressed and explained the procedure prior to catheterizing them. The nurse also should have made sure they were comfortable with the procedure and asked if they had any questions or concerns.
3. How would this condition lead to acute kidney injury (AKI)? What type of AKI would this lead to?
   Because the obstruction is postrenal and below the ureterovesicular junction, it will affect both kidneys. The obstruction will cause the urine to back up into the ureters and both kidneys, which may cause hydronephrosis and hydroureter. If not treated, this would result in a postrenal AKI.
4. Do the labs support a diagnosis of AKI? Why or why not?
   Yes, they do. Josie's GFR has decreased below 60 mL/minute/1.73m^2, which indicates kidney injury. Their creatinine is elevated, as is their BUN. These are all indicators of the progression to postrenal AKI. Josie's blood osmolality is also slightly elevated, but that could be an indicator of mild dehydration due to nausea and vomiting.
5. What complication(s) may arise in Josie's case?
   Josie now has a catheter placed. Blood in his urine indicates that there was likely some trauma with the catheter placement. Josie is at high risk of a catheter-associated urinary tract infection.

Case Study 4.4

1. How is diabetes related to chronic renal failure?
   Diabetes and the associated hyperglycemia cause a thickening of the glomeruli capillary basement membrane. This increase in cells causes a decrease in the diameter of the capillary lumen, which in turn leads to decreased glomerular filtration rate (GFR).
2. Which lab tests would indicate that Maria was in the beginning stages of renal failure?
   One of the first indicators of renal failure is microalbuminuria, or excretion of albumin in the urine. Increasing hyperglycemia and hypertension also causes damage to the capillaries.
3. The provider tells Maria that she needs to eat healthier and suggests limiting salt, meat, beans, and rice. Maria is dismayed as these are staples of her diet. She asks you, "Do I have to get rid of these foods? What will I eat?" How would you answer her?
   It is important for the nurse to let Maria make changes to her diet without getting rid of all her foods she normally eats. It is important to consider the culture of each individual and not assume that what works for one client will work for another. It is crucial to get a sense of Maria's normal diet, what spices and oils she uses. It is essential to meet Maria where she is. Portion

control may be a way that Maria can continue to eat familiar foods as well. Referring her to a nutritionist or dietician may help as well.

4. Explain the pathophysiology behind her symptoms.
   As Maria's renal failure has progressed to end-stage renal failure, her kidneys are no longer functioning. The kidneys act as a filter to remove nitrogenous wastes, such as urea and creatinine. In renal failure, the kidneys are unable to remove these wastes. They accumulate and are toxic to the brain, causing confusion and behavior changes. The kidneys normally secrete erythropoietin, which stimulates the production of red blood cells. As the kidneys fail, erythropoietin production falls. This leads to less erythropoietin production and anemia. Finally, the kidneys activate vitamin D. Without vitamin D, calcium cannot be absorbed from the gut. The kidneys cannot retain calcium as they normally do. With the decrease in serum calcium levels, the parathyroid glands go into overdrive and secrete parathyroid hormone (PTH) to restore serum calcium levels. However, the only place that calcium can be accessed is from the bone. Remember that the kidneys and the intestines cannot absorb or retain calcium because of renal failure. So PTH causes the release of calcium from bone. Bone breakdown results and fractures due to osteoporosis are a common occurrence for clients with renal failure.
5. During her hospitalization, the provider tells Maria and her family that her heart is failing. Her partner asks, "I don't understand why her heart is failing. She has issues with her kidneys." How would you reply?
   I would let the partner know that all our organ systems are connected. Because the kidney cannot filter and excrete fluid, fluid is retained causing fluid volume excess. This causes the heart to work harder, due to the extra blood volume. The heart can compensate, but eventually it will fail. The other issue is that the kidneys play a major role in electrolyte balance. In renal failure, potassium is retained, and causes hyperkalemia. This leads to arrhythmias and possible heart failure.

Answers to Chapter 5 Case Studies

Case Study 5.1

1. As the nurse, what would you notice about Leo's assessment?
   Leo's main symptoms are weakness, dizziness, and syncope. He has a low blood pressure, mild tachycardia, irregular heartbeat, has fatigue and dyspnea, and a grayish cast to his skin. He is also anxious, with a loss of appetite and dark stools.
2. How would you interpret the assessment? What do you think is the specific cause of Leo's weakness and dizziness?
   Leo's weakness, dizziness, and syncope are related to the low blood pressure, tachycardia, fatigue, loss of appetite, and dyspnea. His skin also has a grayish cast, which can be indicative of pallor in melanated individuals. Low blood volume and lack of oxygenation would lead to all these symptoms. Low blood volume/hypoxia would cause the heart to compensate by beating faster and would also cause increased rates of breathing and dyspnea. Leo has all the hallmark signs of anemia.
3. What orders would you anticipate from the provider? (Labs)
   The provider would likely order a complete blood count, which includes hematocrit, hemoglobin, platelets, red blood cell (RBC) and white blood cell counts, and mean corpuscular volumes. RBC indices (size, shape, and physical characteristics of RBCs) may also be ordered.
4. What is Leo's specific diagnosis? Support your answer with the lab results.
   Leo's Hgb and Hct are both quite low, and his MCV is low also. This suggests iron-deficiency anemia (microcytic). His reticulocytes are slightly elevated, which means that immature RBCs are being produced at a higher rate than normal to compensate for the low Hct/Hgb levels. Note that Leo's PT is high, meaning that it takes longer for his blood to clot. As Leo is on anticoagulants, this is expected.
5. Leo tells the nurse, "I eat lots of protein. Why do I have this condition?" How can the nurse respond?
   Iron-deficiency anemia occurs for different reasons. A low iron intake is just one of the reasons. This is probably not the issue, as Leo has stated that he eats a lot of protein. Blood loss and intestinal malabsorption are other reasons that iron-deficiency anemia can occur. Further testing is needed to determine the exact cause of the anemia.
6. The provider orders an endoscopy and a colonoscopy. Why would these be ordered?
   A common cause of iron-deficiency anemia is gastrointestinal (GI) bleeding. Leo is on an anticoagulant, which increases chances of bleeding. He has also reported a loss of appetite and dark stools, which could be indicative of bleeding. Melena, dark and tarry stool, is a sign of GI bleeding. The provider has ordered the endoscopy and colonoscopy to see if Leo has upper or lower GI bleeding, as well as any malabsorption issues.
7. How would Leo's condition be treated?
   It depends on the cause of the anemia. If Leo has GI bleeding, it will have to be addressed. Anticoagulants may need to be discontinued or changed. With a severe loss of blood, oxygen and transfusions would need to be initiated. If it is an issue with iron intake or malabsorption, supplemental iron would be administered, either orally or intravenously.

Case Study 5.2

1. Looking at Krishna's past medical history and her symptoms, what might be some reasons for her confusion?
   Krishna has a history of urinary tract infections, which can cause confusion in the elderly. She also has

hyperlipidemia, hypertension, and is prediabetic (type 2 diabetes). These conditions can lead to changes in blood vessels and hypoperfusion, leading to dementia. Krishna is also hard of hearing and has a language barrier, which increases the risk of dementia.

2. Looking at the results, what do you think the diagnosis of the patient is? Support your answer with the lab results.

   Krishna looks to have anemia. Her hematocrit and hemoglobin are both low and her mean corpuscular volume is high. Her urine results look to be within normal limits and her head CT and chest x-ray are normal. It looks as if Krishna has megaloblastic anemia, specifically cobalamin (B_{12}) deficiency. This is because with cobalamin deficiency, there are neurological changes, such as confusion and paresthesia.

3. Soma is surprised by the results and says to the nurse, "I really don't understand how my mom has this disorder. She has never had this before. What could this come from?" What are three questions the nurse can ask to find out possible causes of this disorder?
   - Does your mother's plant-based diet contain any dairy or forms of animal or fish protein? Please describe her diet.
   - Has your mother been diagnosed with any gastrointestinal issues, specifically anything that has caused destruction to the stomach lining? If so, please give more details.
   - Has your mother ever had any abdominal surgeries? If so, please specify.

4. Krishna wants to know more about her condition and how to treat it. As the nurse, how would you explain things so that Krishna is able to understand?

   "Krishna, because of the change in your diet, you are no longer getting an important vitamin, vitamin B_{12}. This is what is causing your confusion, fatigue, and the tingling and numbness. To fix this, you have some options.
   - You can start eating meat, fish, and poultry products again.
   - You can supplement with oral B_{12}.
   - You can receive B_{12} shots.

   It is important to take care of this because the confusion and numbness and tingling can get worse and become permanent."

Case Study 5.3

1. As the interpreter translates, Bella's father starts to cry. He tells the interpreter that he and her mother don't have the disease and does not understand how Bella has this disease. He asks how she got sickle cell disease (SCD) and says that this disease only happened to people of African descent. How would you address his question?

   You would explain that SCD is an autosomal recessive genetic disease. Bella's parents are carriers, meaning that they only have one copy of the recessive gene. However, they both passed on the recessive gene to Bella, so she has the disease.

   SCD occurs in regions where malaria is endemic. Because the cell is sickled, it prevents malaria. Brazil is a country where malaria is endemic.

2. Explain the pathophysiology behind SCD and the conditions that would cause red blood cells to change shape.

   The mutation in SCD causes abnormal hemoglobin production (HbS). This causes the red blood cell to "sickle" or to stiffen and elongate. The sickling episodes are triggered by stressors. Emotional stress, pain, infection/illness, dehydration, and lack of oxygen are all stressors that would cause sickling.

3. Is sickling permanent? Which symptoms occur with sickling episodes?

   Initially, sickling is not permanent. Once the stressors are addressed (hydrating, treating pain, decreasing stress, treating illness, or giving oxygen), the red blood cells resume their normal shape. However, over time, with repeated sickling episodes, red blood cells will assume the sickled shape permanently.

   Symptoms occur because the sickled red blood cells cause occlusions within the blood vessel. These occlusions lead to tissue hypoxia, which causes severe pain. These occlusions can occur in any part of the body and can cause pain, swelling, fever, pallor, jaundice, and shortness of breath. Note: Bella would also have all the symptoms of anemia because the sickled red blood cells do not have a long lifespan and are destroyed prematurely. Complications of SCD are stroke, myocardial infarction, heart failure, acute chest syndrome, and an enlarged spleen (spleen destroys red blood cells).

4. How is this disease treated?

   Preventing sickling episodes is key. Getting vaccinations, prophylactic antibiotics prior to medical/dental procedures, keeping hydrated, and reducing stress are all important. For some patients, hydroxyurea is a medication that prevents sickling. Stem cell transplants can be effective in curing SCD. Unfortunately, this is not a possibility for a large number of patients with SCD.

5. Bella's parents tell the nurse (through the translator) that they recently moved from Brazil, they do not have family or friends locally, and that they do not have a lot of resources. How can this impact Bella's care? How can the nurse intervene?

   Bella needs consistent follow-up due to her SCD. She needs preventative care (vaccines, antibiotics) and medical care during any sickling episodes. She also needs access to antisickling medications. A healthy environment, good diet, and exercise are important. However, with housing insecurity, this may be difficult. Social determinants of health (housing, safety, education, etc.) are key in maintaining Bella's health. The nurse should refer Bella's parents to a social worker/case manager, who will check in and help them navigate the different services Bella may need.

Case Study 5.4

1. What do you notice about Vicky's symptoms and how they correspond to her labs?
   Vicky has a normal hematocrit and hemoglobin, so does not have anemia. However, she has low platelets and her clotting time is slower than normal. This leads us to believe that Vicky has thrombocytopenia.
2. The provider orders an antiplatelet antibody test, which comes back as abnormal. What diagnosis would you infer from these data? Explain the pathophysiology.
   Vicky looks to have immune thrombocytopenic purpura (ITP). In adults, ITP is triggered by a viral illness. This causes autoantibodies to develop against platelets, which then destroys the platelets, lowering platelet levels and potentially causing bleeding and hemorrhaging.
3. Would you treat this disorder? Why or why not?
   No. At this time, the client should not receive platelets, as to do so would increase clotting risk. Infusion of platelets should be done only when platelets are under 20,000 or at risk of spontaneous bleeding. Taking preventative measures to reduce risk of bleeding would be advised.
4. Is this an acute or chronic issue? What complications could result?
   This could become a chronic issue in adults. In children, ITP is typically an acute response to a viral illness. Some complications would be brain hemorrhages, anemia, fatigue, internal bleeding (such as urinary and gastrointestinal bleeding).

Answers to Chapter 6 Case Studies

Case Study 6.1

1. Looking at Myra's history and assessment, what are you concerned about?
   I would be most concerned with her high blood pressure, her worsening headache, and blurry vision. I would also be concerned about her weight and nonadherence to medications.
2. What do you think Myra's diagnosis is? What could have caused this?
   Myra's diagnosis would be hypertensive crisis, specifically, hypertensive emergency. Her blood pressure is above 180 systolically and above 120 diastolically. This indicates a hypertensive crisis. Her headache and blurry vision suggest target organ damage to the brain, hypertensive encephalopathy. The cause would most likely be her medication nonadherence, as that is one of the most common causes of hypertensive crisis.
3. What complications could result from this?
   Further damage to target organs could result. She could have a hemorrhagic or ischemic stroke, vascular dementia, renal failure, retinal damage, and blindness.
4. What would you want to discuss with Myra? What may some of her barriers be?
   I would first want to discuss her blood pressure and a treatment plan to reduce her blood pressure gradually. I would then want to discuss her medication nonadherence. Many times, the social determinants of health and equity play a role in medications and nonpharmacological treatments. I would look at access to health care, healthy food, safe and clean spaces, and health literacy. I would want to ask her about her barriers with hypertensive and hyperlipidemia medications, as well any barriers to a healthy diet and exercise. I will discuss the health risks she may face if her condition goes unchecked. I would also ask about her weight, but sensitively, as many clients feel that they are being judged or that weight is not a priority for them. Blaming patients or making them feel guilty leads to poor health outcomes. It is better to take patient priorities into consideration when making a care plan.
5. What do you think Myra's condition has evolved into? How would you relate this to Question 2? Explain the pathophysiology.
   Chronic hypertension causes endothelial damage. She already has hyperlipidemia. This can lead to atherosclerotic plaque formation. This plaque is partially obstructing a coronary artery, causing chronic ischemic heart disease, with stable angina. Stable angina resolves with nitroglycerin and rest.
6. What tests would you run to confirm the diagnosis?
   I would perform an ECG, stress tests, and possibly an arteriogram.
7. What would you diagnose her with now? How is this different from Question 5?
   Myra's condition has progressed to acute coronary syndrome, most likely ST elevation myocardial infarction. The plaque has progressed and is now completely obstructing the coronary artery, causing these symptoms. The hypoxia causes myocyte cell death and tissue necrosis.
8. What lab tests would confirm this?
   An ECG should be done, and serum biomarkers (creatinine kinase-MB, troponin) should be run. The ECG may show ST elevation, a Q wave, or an ST depression and inverted T wave. The serum biomarkers will be elevated.
9. What is the priority?
   The priority is to reperfuse the heart as quickly as possible. This means performing a cardiac catheterization, ideally within 90 minutes of symptom onset. This means unblocking the coronary artery with a stent or a "clot busting" medication. The faster the reperfusion, the less damage and necrotic tissue.
10. What complications would you see?
    Arrhythmias are a common complication—anytime the structure of the heart changes, the electrical pathway changes. Heart failure from cardiac dysfunction and

stroke from thromboemboli are also common symptoms. Pericarditis may also result from tissue necrosis and healing, inflammation, and immune response (Dressler syndrome). In severe cases, cardiogenic shock may result.

Case Study 6.2

1. What do you think is happening to the patient? Explain your diagnosis.
   This could potentially be a ruptured aortic aneurysm or an aortic dissection. The sudden ripping pain suggests that it is an aortic dissection. The severity of the pain coupled with the unequal blood pressures in both arms would point to a dissection.
2. Why are the blood pressures in both arms different? Why are the extremities cool to touch?
   This is due to compression or blockage of the left aortic artery. Because the rupture is an emergent and catastrophic event, cardiac output is decreasing, and blood is shunted away from the periphery to the brain, heart, and lungs.
3. Why do you think these symptoms are occurring?
   As cardiac output drops, perfusion decreases, and tissues start to get ischemic. The brain does not receive enough oxygenated blood. Carbon dioxide levels in the brain go up and the brain vessels vasodilate. The client will be increasingly confused, lethargic, and somnolent and go into circulatory shock.
4. How would you treat this condition?
   This is a surgical emergency. To treat the symptoms, blood transfusions or plasma volume expanders can be used.

Case Study 6.3

1. What may have caused the DVT to occur? Explain the pathophysiology.
   Long periods of immobility cause venous stasis. According to Virchow triad, venous stasis, hypercoagulability, and venous injury put clients at high risk for DVTs. The client spent 10 hours sitting on a flight, which may have induced the clot to form.
2. Could the DVT have been prevented? How?
   Yes. The client could have gotten up during the flight, stretched and walked periodically.
3. How would you explain the condition and treatment to the client?
   I would tell them that the long flight and remaining immobile for 10 hours caused the blood to pool in their lower extremity and form a clot. In order not to dislodge the clot, the client now needs to be immobile and take blood thinners to help break down the clot and keep more clots from forming. It the clot does not break down, it will have to be removed surgically. I would also advise taking walks and stretching if on long flights.
4. What do you think the client's diagnosis is now? Explain.
   The client's DVT likely became dislodged and moved to the lungs, becoming pulmonary emboli. Dyspnea, anxiety, and tachycardia are hallmarks of pulmonary emboli.

Case Study 6.4

1. What would you diagnose the patient with? Explain the pathophysiology.
   I would diagnose the client with peripheral arterial disease. The client likely has atherosclerosis. Atherosclerosis can occur in all arterial vessels, including peripheral vessels. The atherosclerotic lesions occluded the peripheral arterial vessels, causing pain with exertion. Gravity helps the oxygenated blood move down into the legs, causing dependent rubor. Clients need to dangle their legs to get any circulation in their lower extremities. Due to having no circulation, the legs are thin with muscle atrophy, shiny, and hairless.
2. What are some risk factors causing this condition?
   Family history, hyperlipidemia, hypertension, atherosclerosis, diabetes, and smoking.
3. What complications could you expect with this client?
   If the peripheral arterial vessels are occluded, small dark extremely painful ulcers (lateral ankle and toes), gangrene, and tissue necrosis would set in, resulting in amputation.

Case Study 6.5

1. How would you assess the mass? What findings would you expect?
   You would very gently palpate the mass and auscultate it. You would likely feel a thrill and hear a bruit.
2. What would you diagnose this client with? Is this an emergent condition? Why?
   The client has an abdominal aortic aneurysm. If there is a palpable abdominal mass, it is a large aneurysm (>5 cm) and an emergent condition needing surgery. The surgery is done to repair the aortic artery. If surgery is not done, the aneurysm may rupture, and the client may hemorrhage.

Answers to Chapter 7 Case Studies

Case Study 7.1

1. What condition/disease do you think Jess has?
   Jess may have rheumatic heart disease (RHD).
2. How did Jess get this condition/disease? Explain the pathophysiology.
   RHD is caused by untreated strep throat infections. The bacteria then travel to other parts of the body through the blood and the disease becomes systemic. Bacterial vegetations may form on the heart valves and cause permanent valvular damage, leading to stenosis or regurgitation. With a systolic murmur, it is likely that Jess has mitral valve stenosis.

3. What complications would you be worried about? Why?
   One complication would be the formation of emboli. The bacterial vegetations can break off and cause pulmonary emboli or strokes. Also, as the valve gets progressively more damaged, blood will accumulate in the left atrium, and the left atrium will dilate. Eventually, blood will start to backflow into the lungs through the pulmonary vein. The left ventricle will contract harder to preserve cardiac output, causing left ventricular concentric hypertrophy. Ultimately, this will lead to heart failure.
4. How do the social determinants of health and equity affect Jess' case?
   Because Jess is unhoused, he may have difficulty with stable access to care. He needs to be followed and treated; however, having to keep moving may make this impossible. He may lack money to pay to see a provider or buy medications and a safe living environment, which would contribute to the worsening of his condition.

Case Study 7.2

1. Why might Nevil be experiencing palpitations and have a murmur? Explain the pathophysiology.
   Nevil has Marfan syndrome, which is a connective tissue disorder affecting blood vessels and the heart. One of the symptoms of Marfan syndrome is mitral valve prolapse. With mitral valve prolapse, the mitral valve is mucinous and can degenerate, leading to mitral valve regurgitation. Accompanying the mitral valve prolapse is dysregulation of the autonomic nervous system. The sympathetic nervous system is dysfunctional and triggers when it should not, which would cause the palpitations and dizziness. The murmur occurs when the ventricles contract, so it is a systolic murmur.
2. What would be some things Nevil can do to avoid these symptoms?
   Nevil should avoid caffeine and other stimulants to keep from having palpitations and anxiety.
3. Has Nevil's condition progressed? What would his diagnosis be? Explain the pathophysiology behind Nevil's symptoms.
   Nevil's condition has progressed to mitral valve regurgitation. The shortness of breath and paroxysmal nocturnal dyspnea are because blood is backflowing from the left atrium into the lungs. With mitral valve regurgitation, there is volume overload and eccentric hypertrophy, decreasing cardiac output, and causing fatigue. Finally, atrial fibrillation is a common dysrhythmia with left atrial dilation and would feel like fluttering.
4. Explain why Nevil's condition could progress to heart failure.
   Eccentric hypertrophy causes elongation and thinning of the left ventricle. This makes it harder for the left ventricle to contract and the oxygen demand is higher. Eventually the left ventricle will fail, and Nevil's cardiac output will decrease. A valve replacement or other surgical interventions would be necessary to maintain cardiac output. Nevil is also from the Cherokee Nation. Studies have shown that Black, indigenous, and people of color (BIPOC) individuals do not receive the same level of care for heart failure as do White assigned males at birth.

Case Study 7.3

1. Why would the school require a cardiac exam and ECG?
   Hypertrophic cardiomyopathy and arrhythmogenic right ventricular dysplasia are the two most common causes of death in young athletes. Schools and colleges now require ECGs and cardiac exams for all athletes for this reason.
2. What would you say to Mia?
   I would explain that with hypertrophic cardiomyopathy, it is possible that she may have serious cardiac dysfunction with extreme activity. The left ventricle, which is typically muscle, has defective proteins that cause it not to contract properly, and causes decreased cardiac output. I would tell her that she can participate in low to moderate impact activities, but unfortunately, she will probably not be able to participate in lacrosse, as it may cause too much of a demand on the heart.

Case Study 7.4

1. What do you think caused the code? Explain the pathophysiology.
   COVID-19 can cause a systemic inflammatory response leading to pericarditis and pericardial effusions. The sharp chest pain, fever, cough, and shortness of breath point to pericarditis. The muffled heart sounds and jugular vein distension are indicators of cardiac tamponade, as suggested by Beck triad (muffled heart sounds, hypotension, and jugular vein distension).
2. What type of shock did the client experience? Explain.
   Cardiac tamponade would be an example of obstructive shock. Obstructive shock occurs when cardiac output drops drastically due to a cause outside of the heart. In this case, it is due to the rapid accumulation of pericardial fluid in the pericardial sac. Tension pneumothorax and tumors compressing the heart are also causes of obstructive shock.

Answers to Chapter 8 Case Studies

Case Study 8.1

1. Should Kai wait to seek treatment? Why or why not?
   No, Kai should not wait to seek treatment. Thinking back to early and late-phase asthma, Kai was wheezing and coughing, and the rescue inhaler was not working. The inflammatory response with asthma gets worse with

late-stage asthma, with the airway becoming hyperresponsive and narrowing with airway edema and mucus. Late-stage asthma can lead to respiratory failure.

2. How might climate change and social determinants of health cause increased prevalence of asthma?

Climate change can cause and exacerbate asthma attacks. With climate change, air pollutants have increased, irritating the lungs. The temperature has gone up globally, which adds heat stress to the mix, another factor which can exacerbate asthma. Wildfires are much more common and much larger than before. The smoke adds pollutants to the air, making it hard for clients with asthma to breathe. Also, living in an environment polluted by factories, chemicals, and landfill will also exacerbate asthma. Social determinants of health and equity must also be looked at. Access to care, a healthy living and working environment, access to a job with a healthy work environment, education, and good food are all factors to look at. Marginalized communities may not have access to these determinants of health, or have limited access, which can cause their asthma to get worse.

3. Explain the pathophysiology behind early and late-stage asthma.

Early-stage asthma encompasses the vascular phase of inflammation. Mast cells release histamine, vasodilation and bronchoconstriction occur, and goblet cells start to secrete mucus. If medications are not taken and inflammation is not controlled, it continues to progress. Mast cells produce prostaglandins and leukotrienes, which function similar to histamine, but are much longer acting. The airway becomes hyperresponsive and even more mucus is produced and released, occluding the airway further.

4. What are the symptoms of severe asthma?

With severe asthma, the airway is so occluded it is difficult to move air. Breath sounds are more distant; wheezing is on inspiration and expiration on auscultation. The client is extremely dyspneic, tachypneic, typically tachycardic. The client is no longer able to cough up mucus, has difficulty saying more than two to three words at a time, and is using accessory muscles to breathe.

Case Study 8.2

1. Looking at the data, do you think that Rhea has chronic bronchitis or emphysema? Provide evidence.

Rhea has signs of both chronic bronchitis and emphysema. Signs of chronic bronchitis that Rhea has are a productive cough, right lower extremity edema, and CO_2 retention. Signs of emphysema are an O_2 saturation above 90%, tachypnea, tachycardia, and a lower-than-normal alpha-1 antitrypsin level.

2. The provider, after assessing Rhea, asks, "Are you sure you've never smoked?" Rhea denies smoking. For what other reasons could she have developed lung disease?

There is a stigma associated with chronic obstructive pulmonary disease (COPD) and smoking. Smokers are often uncomfortable seeking treatment for COPD because they feel that they are to blame, or that society blames them for smoking. However, there are other reasons that COPD occurs. Rhea grew up in a house where the cooking was done over a charcoal fire. The smoke from the cooking fires can damage the lungs. It is estimated that over 75% of Indian assigned female at birth (AFAB) have COPD because of cooking fires. Also, she grew up in a home where secondhand smoke was an issue for 18 years. This history could explain why Rhea has COPD. Providers should not assume people are always smokers.

3. Outline the major differences between emphysema and chronic bronchitis.

Emphysema is a disease of the alveoli. The lack of alpha-1 antitrypsin causes elastase to accumulate and break down the elastic fibers in the lungs. The alveolar walls are destroyed, and air can go in, but there is no elastic recoil, so air cannot be expired. This causes hyperinflation of the lungs. The symptoms of emphysema are dyspnea, tachypnea, barrel chest, and thin physique. Chronic bronchitis is a disease of the airways. Irritants, such as smoking and pollution, can cause chronic bronchitis. This causes an increase in goblet cells and mucus glands, and there is a hypersecretion of mucus. There is an inflammatory response in the bronchi and bronchioles, and chronic irritation, which results in bronchospasm, chronic cough, narrowing, and recurrent infection. Symptoms include cyanosis, wheezing, shortness of breath, edema, and secondary polycythemia.

Case Study 8.3

1. Jon's parents are very upset. They ask, "We thought he was tested at birth for this. Why is this showing up now?" What would you say to them?

Cystic fibrosis (CF) is a genetic disorder, a mutation of the CFTR gene. This causes defective protein channels to form. These channels absorb chloride ions. The genetic defect can lead to a partial deficiency in normal proteins, rather than a complete deficiency. It is possible that Jon had enough normal protein channels to compensate when he was a baby and now the deficiency is now more pronounced.

2. As a clinician, how would you explain the progression of the disease? What treatments will Jon potentially need?

This deficiency causes defective chloride channels, which lead to chloride not being able to be reabsorbed. With that, less water and sodium are reabsorbed, making the mucus thick and sticky. With sweat glands, the opposite happens. Chloride, along with water and sodium, is excessively excreted. The thick mucus causes breathing difficultics, chronic cough, frequent infections, chronic inflammation with interleukin, oxidant, and elastase release. Bronchioles get dilated and have pockets where mucus accumulates, and bacteria can thrive. Semen and vaginal secretions are also affected resulting in infertility. Pancreatic enzyme release and bile release are also affected, and steatorrhea, malnutrition, and diabetes can result.

3. What is the prognosis of an individual with cystic fibrosis?
   Typically, individuals with CF live until their 20s or 30s, sometimes 40s. It is not a curable disease. Supportive treatments such as oxygen, antibiotics, chest physiotherapy, bronchodilators, mucolytics, and pancreatic enzymes should be given.

Case Study 8.4

1. What do you think Abena has? What would cause this to happen?
   Abena has pulmonary emboli. The COVID virus causes a systemic inflammatory response and activates bradykinin, which causes increased clotting. This increase in clotting likely caused pulmonary emboli.
2. What are the hallmark symptoms of this disease? How can you diagnose this?
   Hallmark symptoms are tachycardia, tachypnea, lower O_2 saturations, a low-grade fever, and a cough with blood-tinged sputum. You can diagnose this with an elevated D-dimer and a chest computed tomography (CT) scan.
3. What would this condition do to the V/Q ratio?
   Pulmonary emboli block the pulmonary artery. This would result in a decrease in perfusion, but unchanged ventilation, at least initially. This would be a high V/Q ratio.

Answers to Chapter 9 Case Studies

Case Study 9.1

1. Explain the pathophysiology of the disease. Is this a definitive diagnosis? Why or why not?
   Indrani appears to have COVID-19. A home test has varying degrees of accuracy. A polymerase chain reaction (PCR) test for COVID would be the definitive test.
2. What precautions should she take?
   She should isolate for 10 days and wear an N-95 mask when she is around people either outdoors or indoors. Other precautions are getting the COVID vaccines, boosters, and bivalent vaccine.
3. What is causing these symptoms? Should she go to the emergency room right away? Explain.
   Initially, the virus binds to angiotensin-converting enzyme-2 (ACE-2) receptors in the nose, pharynx, stomach, and kidneys. This causes the initial cough, runny nose, and diarrhea symptoms. However, as COVID progresses and viral replication continues, the virus infiltrates the lungs. This causes inflammation, increased mucus and edema, and hyaluronic acid to accumulate, making it very difficult to breathe. This can result in acute respiratory distress and respiratory failure.
4. Could her post discharge symptoms be linked to COVID? Explain.
   Yes. The virus causes systemic inflammation and an upregulation of bradykinin, or bradykinin storm. These increase clotting and damage to vessels and organs. It is very likely that the virus caused the stroke and caused small vessel damage in the brain. Long COVID, due to inflammatory changes and clotting, is a syndrome resulting in many COVID patients and brain fog is one of the common symptoms.

Case Study 9.2

1. Looking at the vitals and assessment, what diagnosis would you expect for Sam? Why?
   I would expect that Sam has croup. The barking cough, tachypnea, stridor, and retractions all suggest croup.
2. What is causing the stridor, retractions, and cough? Explain the pathophysiology.
   The swollen, narrowed airways are causing the stridor and barking cough.
3. Why would these medications be ordered?
   The airway is extremely inflamed and there is bronchoconstriction. Epinephrine is a catecholamine that causes bronchodilation. Steroids decrease inflammatory response, decreasing the edema and swelling in the airways.

Case Study 9.3

1. Looking at the assessment, what is Dave's diagnosis? Are his symptoms typical?
   Dave has influenza B. Prodromal symptoms for viral infections are rigors, high fever, myalgia, headache, and nausea, so Dave does have typical symptoms.
2. What would you expect the treatment to be?
   Antibiotics cannot be taken for viral infections. Rest, fluids, antipyretics, and nonsteroidal anti-inflammatories can be taken. Within 48 hours of symptom onset, Tamiflu may be effective as well.
3. Why has Dave's illness progressed?
   Dave has developed sinusitis and pneumonia. These are secondary complications of influenza. The influenza virus infiltrates and damages the lining of your nasal/sinus passages, as well as your respiratory tract, allowing bacteria to colonize and thrive.
4. Is this a bacterial or viral disease? How do you know?
   This is a bacterial pneumonia. On the x-rays, you can see consolidation. This happens in bacterial pneumonia because of the alveolar exudate. Dave also has a productive cough with brownish sputum, which also suggests bacterial infection. If it was a viral infection, there would be inflammation of the alveolar septum and lung interstitium, with no exudate. Viral infections do not consolidate and are often not seen on x-ray.
5. On auscultation, what lung sounds would you expect to hear?
   As there is exudate you could hear crackles, rhonchi, and diminished breath sounds in the right lower lobe.

Case Study 9.4

1. Does this mean that Gina has tuberculosis? Why or why not?
   No. This does not definitively mean that Gina has tuberculosis (TB). Gina could have gotten a BCG vaccine, which would show a false positive. She could also have latent TB, which would show up as positive on the tuberculin test. A chest x-ray for latent TB would need to be done. The gold standard for diagnosis is sputum cultures.
2. Describe the course of tuberculosis in a healthy individual.
   Tuberculosis is an airborne bacterium (*Mycobacterium tuberculosis*). When a healthy individual is exposed, the bacteria can enter the body through the airway and invade the lung tissue. The alveolar macrophages try to kill the bacteria but cannot. Granulomas, called Ghon foci, then form to seal off the bacteria within the lung or other affected organs.
3. What is the difference between primary and secondary tuberculosis infection?
   Primary tuberculosis is the initial infection, which typically results in latent infection, but can result in active or miliary infection in those who are immunocompromised. Secondary TB is a reinfection from someone previously exposed or reactivated latent TB. In immunocompromised individuals, this can progress to clinical symptoms, such as low-grade fever, blood-tinged sputum, cough, fatigue, anorexia, dyspnea, and weight loss.
4. What risk factors caused Gina to develop primary tuberculosis?
   Autoimmune disease and type 2 diabetes mellitus would cause immunocompromise.
5. What complication(s) might Gina's experience as a result?
   This can lead to antibiotic resistance. It becomes more difficult to treat once TB is resistant, leading to chronic disease.

Answers to Chapter 10 Case Studies

Case Study 10.1

1. What condition do you think she has? What indicates this?
   Allison has Graves disease. Her T4 and TSH levels as well as her symptoms (jitters, diaphoresis, weight loss, palpitations, and hair loss) indicate this. High glucose levels can occur, as she has both type 1 diabetes mellitus (DM) and Graves disease and she is likely dehydrated, so her BUN may be high as well.
2. How did she get this condition? Explain the pathophysiology.
   Type 1 DM is an autoimmune disease. Once you have one autoimmune disease, you are more likely to get another. With Graves disease, antibodies bind to the TSH receptors on the thyroid glands, blocking the receptor from binding with TSH. The antibodies then stimulate the thyroid gland to produce more T3 and T4. Graves disease is triggered and exacerbated by stressors, and there are exacerbations and remissions.
3. What are some of the severe complications of this condition?
   With Graves disease ophthalmopathy (bulging eyes), goiter, and thyroid storm are some of the more severe complications. Thyroid storm occurs with severe hyperthyroidism and causes high fevers, palpitations, chest pain, anxiety, and dyspnea. Often, clients in thyroid storm feel as if they are having a myocardial infarction. This is a medical emergency and treatment needs to be swift.
4. How would you explain Allison's condition now?
   Allison had her thyroid removed and now is dependent on medication to replace her thyroid hormones. It may be possible that she is not getting enough of the hormone replacement and now has signs of hypothyroidism. She may need to have her medication level adjusted.
5. How could you verify this?
   You should verify this by checking her labs. Free T4, TSH, and low glucose would be indicators. Her symptoms (weight gain, lethargy, hypothermia) suggest that she has hypothyroidism.
6. What are the complications of this condition?
   Severe hypothyroidism can lead to myxedema coma. With myxedema coma, you will see lethargy, confusion and depression, hypothermia, hypoglycemia, and fluid retention. Without treatment, this will lead to a coma and death.

Case Study 10.2

1. What diagnostic tests might the provider run to help diagnose Tara?
   The provider should do a complete blood count, a basal metabolic panel, and a urine test. They should also check Tara's blood sugar.
2. What would you diagnose Tara with? Explain the pathophysiology of the disease.
   I would diagnose Tara with Addison disease. Tara already has one autoimmune disease, which makes her more susceptible to having another autoimmune disease, which Addison disease is. They have the hallmark symptoms of hypoglycemia, hypotension, vomiting, and diarrhea.
3. What tests would verify this?
   Adrenal gland stimulation tests, blood and urine cortisol levels, and serum adrenocorticotrophic hormone (ACTH) levels could verify this.
4. How would this condition be treated?
   Tara would need to supplement with glucocorticoids.

Case Study 10.3

1. What condition would you diagnose Kalyani with? Why?
   Kalyani has Cushing syndrome caused by the oral steroids. She has the hallmark signs: moon face, visceral weight gain, and bruising. She is also hyperglycemic.

2. Is this a primary, secondary, or tertiary condition?
   This is iatrogenic Cushing syndrome and is a primary condition. This is the most common cause of Cushing syndrome.
3. As her nurse, what teaching would you do regarding her antirejection medication?
   You should advise Kalyani not to stop her steroid suddenly, as it would cause adrenal insufficiency. She needs to taper her steroids if she is reducing the dose.

Case Study 10.4

1. What do you suspect is happening to Dario? Explain.
   With his symptoms of nausea, vomiting, confusion, fruity breath, and hot skin, he may have diabetic ketoacidosis (DKA). He also denies drinking alcohol. With the extreme hyperglycemia in DKA, Dario's blood would be concentrated with glucose, and he would be extremely dehydrated, and his skin would be hot to touch. The ketoacidosis would cause his breath to smell like acetone. Nausea, vomiting, and obtundation are also hallmark signs of DKA.
2. Why would the police think that Dario had been drinking alcohol?
   Dario appears inebriated, as he is unsteady, confused, and has fruity breath. It is common to mistake DKA for alcohol use.
3. What lab findings would you expect with this condition?
   Serum glucose: 250 to 800 mg/dL
   Arterial blood gas (ABG): pH 6.9 to 7.3
   Metabolic panel: hyperkalemia >5 mg/dL
   Bicarbonate <15 mEq/L
   Serum osmolality: >300 mOsm/kg
   Urine: + urine ketones, +glucose
4. Is this a medical emergency? Why or why not? How would this be treated?
   DKA is a medical emergency, as hyperglycemia, acidosis, and electrolyte and fluid imbalances cannot be reversed without intensive medical intervention. Intravenous (IV) fluids, IV bicarbonate, IV insulin drip, and telemetry and monitoring of electrolytes are required.

Case Study 10.5

1. The provider looks at the report and has some concerns. What do you think that the provider is concerned about?
   Trevor has high blood pressure and is symptomatic with headaches and dizziness. Trevor also has high serum glucose levels and his HbA1c is elevated. Finally, he has high triglycerides and low HDL.
2. What might be a potential diagnosis for Trevor? Explain using the results above.
   Trevor looks to be prediabetic, hypertensive, and has hyperlipidemia. His glucose levels and blood pressure were elevated, and his triglycerides were elevated.
3. What would you diagnose Trevor with? Provide rationale(s).
   Trevor's consistently elevated glucose levels and HgA1c indicate that he has type 2 diabetes mellitus (T2DM). He also has hyperlipidemia, with high triglycerides.
4. The provider talks to Trevor about a condition called metabolic syndrome. When the provider leaves, Trevor turns to you, his nurse. He is visibly upset. He says, "I work hard to be healthy, to provide a safe and loving home for my family, and now I have this syndrome? I don't even understand what it is and what it has to do with my diagnosis!" What would you say to Trevor?
   Trevor's triglycerides are very high, he is extremely hypertensive, and has hyperglycemia (insulin resistance). This fits the criteria for metabolic syndrome. Metabolic syndrome is an indicator of cardiovascular disease, combining symptoms to assess for cardiovascular risk, instead of just looking at T2DM in isolation.
5. What are the complications that could result from Trevor's condition?
   With metabolic syndrome, Trevor has a higher risk of stroke, myocardial infarction, coronary artery disease, pulmonary emboli, peripheral artery disease, and T2DM.

Answers to Chapter 11 Case Studies

Case Study 11.1

1. What is the reason behind Doreen's pain?
   Nonsteroidal anti-inflammatory drugs (NSAIDs) inhibit prostaglandin production and release. Prostaglandin is needed to produce the mucus that lines and protects the stomach mucosal layer from pepsin and hydrochloric acid.
2. What would you diagnose her with?
   Acute gastritis from ibuprofen ingestion.
3. How can she treat the pain?
   Doreen can treat the pain with antacids, H2 receptor blockers, and proton pump inhibitors to reduce the amount of acid. She should avoid ibuprofen and other NSAIDs.
4. Has her condition progressed? Why or why not?
   Yes, the severe cramping abdominal pain and the fact that it improves with food indicate that Doreen's gastritis has advanced to become a peptic ulcer, specifically a duodenal ulcer.
5. What are the risks with this condition?
   If the duodenal ulcer perforates, it can cause gastrointestinal bleeding and peritonitis.
6. What has happened to Doreen? Explain the pathophysiology.
   It appears that Doreen's ulcer has perforated, and the gastric contents will go into the peritoneum and cause peritonitis. The hallmark signs of peritonitis are rigid, painful abdomen, fever, and paralytic ileus, which is why the nurse could not hear bowel sounds.

Case Study 11.2

1 What condition/disease does Ryan have? Explain the pathophysiology.
   Ryan has appendicitis. Appendicitis is when a fecalith is trapped within the appendix, causing inflammation, edema, lack of perfusion, gangrene, and ulceration. If the appendix ruptures, it can result in peritonitis.
2. What are the hallmark symptoms of this condition/disease?
   Low-grade fever, right lower quadrant (RLQ) pain (McBurney point), guarding, and leukocytosis.
3. Is this the right decision? Why or why not?
   Ryan should not leave. The relief he feels is his appendix rupturing. The relief will be temporary as he will start having severe pain once peritonitis sets in.

Case Study 11.3

1. Krishna is worried and asks, "Is this serious? How did I get this?" What would you tell her?
   This is a very common disease. It is caused by a lack of fiber and fluid in the diet and the constipation that results. The straining causes partial herniations to occur in the sigmoid colon. These are painless and typically asymptomatic.
2. What is the difference between diverticulosis and diverticulitis?
   Diverticulosis consists of partial herniations and is typically asymptomatic. Diverticulitis is when the diverticula get inflamed and infected. With the lower left quadrant pain, it shows that Krishna has diverticulitis.
3. Krishna asks if she can try to eat more fiber. What would you tell her?
   With diverticulitis, adding fiber to the diet would exacerbate the pain and infection. When the diverticulitis resolves, adding fluid and fiber to her diet would help.
4. What is the treatment for diverticulitis?
   I would tell her that when she has diverticulitis, she needs to be NPO, rest her bowel. Intravenous (IV) antibiotics, IV fluids, and pain medications are needed.

Case Study 11.4

1. What labs would you expect to be ordered to find out the cause of these symptoms?
   Complete blood count, basal metabolic panel, thyroid panel, blood cultures, and stool specimens would be some of the labs ordered.
2. What are two differential diagnoses?
   Inflammatory bowel disease and gastroenteritis (inflammation of stomach lining) would be two diagnoses.
3. What do these findings indicate?
   Rose has severe abdominal pain, nausea, vomiting, and diarrhea. These findings indicate that Rose has inflammatory bowel disease, specifically Crohn disease. The skip lesions would indicate Crohn disease rather than ulcerative colitis. Lesions would also look like cobblestones with Crohn disease.
4. What complications would you be worried about?
   With Crohn disease, complications would be fistulas, perforations, hemorrhaging, strictures, peritonitis, and nutritional deficiencies.
5. Is this condition curable? What can be done?
   Crohn disease is not curable. There are exacerbations and remissions that are triggered by stressors. Reducing stress, pain medications, anti-inflammatories, steroids, immunosuppressants, and surgery are measures that may be helpful.

Case Study 11.5

1. Does this mean that Raquel is constipated?
   It does not mean that Raquel is constipated. They still have bowel sounds in all quadrants. Also, people have different bowel patterns. The end-stage cancer may affect their bowel movements.
2. What suggestions would you make to Raquel?
   I would tell Raquel that they should increase fluid and fiber in her diet, if possible. They do have end-stage cancer, so they may not be able to tolerate fiber and fluid.
3. Why is the nurse concerned about obstruction? What would cause this?
   At this point, Raquel is constipated. As the fecal obstruction gets larger, it will obstruct the colon. Being bedridden or not ambulating as much, having weak abdominal and pelvic muscles, not being able to take in fiber and fluid, and taking opiates can cause severe constipation, impaction, and obstruction. Also, with abdominal cancers, tumors can obstruct the colon.
4. Would increasing fluids and fiber help at this stage? Why or why not?
   Fluid and fiber do not relieve constipation, they prevent constipation. Adding fluid and fiber once someone is constipated is just worsening the obstruction. At this stage, the client would need laxatives, suppositories, and possibly an enema.

Case Study 11.6

1. What five questions would you ask Rawan's parents to find out what the cause of her illness is?
   - How long has she been ill?
   - When did the symptoms start?
   - What did she eat and drink in the last week?
   - How much weight has she lost?
   - Were there any others around her who were sick with the same symptoms?
2. What do you think Rawan's diagnosis may be? Why?
   Rawan's diagnosis may be cholera or dysentery. Damascus has been bombed repeatedly and there is a lack of clean water and food. Damage to sewage systems has left sewage overflowing inside and outside of homes. This is the perfect breeding ground for cholera. Because of being watery diarrhea, with lack of clean water, it is likely cholera.

3. What would you be most concerned about? Why?
   Cholera causes profound dehydration, due to vomiting and diarrhea. That would also create pH and electrolyte imbalances, especially sodium and potassium imbalances. Rawan is tachycardic and tachypneic. Also, she may be hypoglycemic, as she is not able to keep anything down. She is listless with a weak cry, a neurological concern.
4. Rawan's parents are very upset. They feel that they caused her illness. What would you tell them?
   I would tell them that it is not their fault, and they did the best they could do under the circumstances. The lack of clean water, lack of food, and sewage issues are all a condition created by war.
5. How would you treat this illness?
   Rawan needs cardiac monitoring and oxygen. Intravenous (IV) fluid resuscitation with glucose should be started, with careful monitoring to avoid cerebral edema. She also needs IV antibiotics to treat the cholera. Finally, pH and electrolyte imbalances must be monitored and corrected.

Answers to Chapter 12 Case Studies

Case Study 12.1

1. Joe is extremely upset. He says, "I haven't touched drugs in 35 years! I've been faithful to my wife! How did I get this?" How would you answer him?
   Hepatitis C is a chronic disease that is transmitted by needles and blood products, not sex. Joe could have contracted hepatitis C from blood products or intravenous (IV) needles over 35 years ago and hepatitis C could have been latent or in remission.
2. Joe states that he does not want to take medication for something that has no symptoms and is not affecting his lifestyle. Is this the right decision? Explain.
   Hepatitis C is a chronic disease that has exacerbations and remissions. With chronic inflammation, scarring and fibrosis occurs, eventually causing liver cirrhosis, failure, and possible liver cancer. Even though Joe does not have symptoms currently, the damage over time will build up and could cause death. Treatment is Joe's decision, but Joe needs to be fully informed about the progression of the disease.
3. Are Joe's symptoms indicative of hepatitis C? Explain the pathophysiology of these symptoms.
   Yes, they are. With liver disease, bile production and release are affected, which is needed for fat digestion. Without it, digestive issues, malabsorption, and weight loss may occur. Also, with liver inflammation, hepatomegaly and liver tenderness occur. Finally, with liver disease, the liver is not able to conjugate bilirubin to make bile. The bilirubin builds up in the blood, causing jaundice.
4. Is hepatitis C treatable? How?
   Yes, it is. It is treatable with antivirals. It may take 12 to 24 weeks to treat, but once cured, the client can contract hepatitis C again.

Case Study 12.2

1. What do you think is happening to Milo? What may have led to this condition?
   COVID causes systemic inflammation and microemboli to form. This could lead to liver injury.
2. What is causing Milo's confusion and distended abdomen?
   Hepatic encephalopathy can occur with liver disease, as ammonia and other toxins build up in the blood. These toxins disrupt neurotransmitters and cause confusion and disruption in neural impulses. The distended abdomen comes from a lack of protein (decreased oncotic pressure) and increased fluid in the mesenteric vessels (increased hydrostatic pressure). There is also an increase in aldosterone (Na and water retention), as the liver is not able to make the enzymes to break down the hormone.
3. Why would Milo's condition cause diarrhea and jaundice?
   A healthy liver conjugates bilirubin and makes bile, which is recycled to help emulsify fats and is excreted in the feces. A diseased liver would not make bile, which would cause fats to be undigested and be excreted as fatty foul-smelling diarrhea. Jaundice is due to the bilirubin building up in the blood, as the liver cannot conjugate it.
4. Are there other labs that are abnormal? Explain why.
   Liver function tests are elevated, BUN and creatinine are elevated indicating acute renal failure, bilirubin is elevated because the liver cannot create bile, and albumin is low as the liver cannot produce proteins. Anemia may be occurring because of the renal failure, as the kidney may not be able to produce erythropoietin.
5. Why has Milo's condition changed?
   The COVID infection may have caused acute fulminant hepatitis. This is a rapid acceleration of liver injury to liver failure.
6. Use the labs to explain the pathophysiology of Milo's symptoms.
   Milo's ammonia level is quite high, which causes confusion and drowsiness, due to hepatic encephalopathy. Milos' bilirubin is very high, which would lead to jaundice. Finally, Milo has hepatorenal syndrome, with acute kidney failure, apparent in the high creatinine and BUN values and oliguria.
7. Why would Milo start to bleed?
   The liver is not making clotting proteins and clotting factors, and not storing vitamin K, all of which will increase clotting time.

Case Study 12.3

1. What would you suspect as a diagnosis? Why?
   Champane's symptoms demonstrate the Charcot triad—right upper quadrant (RUQ) pain, jaundice, and fever. This is indicative of cholangitis, biliary obstruction, and inflammation.

2. Was the nurse correct in asking Champane to wait for pain medications? Why or why not?
   No. You cannot assess someone in severe pain properly. Champane is getting anxious and complaining of severe pain. Something to consider—often clinicians and providers are biased when it comes to care and pain medications. The fact that Champane is Black may be affecting her care. A common myth is that Black individuals do not feel pain. The nurse should have advocated for pain management first, before continuing with the assessment.
3. Why would Champane's condition be considered a medical emergency?
   Champane has significant hypotension, tachycardia, fever, and decreased oxygen saturation, as well as agitation and delirium. These are signs of septic shock, which is a medical emergency.
4. What diagnosis would you give Champane? How would this be treated?
   Champane has the all the signs and symptoms of Reynolds Pentad (hypotension, confusion, jaundice, fever, and Right upper quadrant [RUQ] pain), which indicates acute suppurative cholangitis, with pus in the bile ducts, which is a surgical emergency. An ERCP would be done, emergency decompression and bile stent may be placed, intravenous (IV) antibiotics would be given, and the bile ducts would need to be cleaned out.

Case Study 12.4

1. Looking at the assessment data, what would you suspect Blue's diagnosis is? Why?
   I would suspect that Blue has acute pancreatitis secondary to cystic fibrosis, with her sudden left upper quadrant (LUQ) pain, fever, and nausea. She has high WBC (leukocytosis), elevated CRP (inflammation), and elevated serum amylase and lipase, which are common in acute pancreatitis.
2. How can you diagnose Blue's condition?
   You could perform an abdominal ultrasound, computed tomography (CT) scan, or endoscopic retrograde cholangiopancreatography (ERCP).
3. Is this connected to Blue's cystic fibrosis diagnosis? If so, explain the connection.
   Yes, it is related. With cystic fibrosis, chloride channels are affected by a genetic mutation, causing mucus to become thick and sticky. With pancreatic enzymes, mucus secretions are important in carrying them through the pancreatic duct and into the small intestine. Due to the thick mucus, pancreatic enzymes cannot travel to the small intestine, and activate prematurely in the pancreas, destroying the pancreatic tissue.
4. What complications would you be concerned about?
   I would be concerned about it developing into systemic inflammation and sepsis, perforation → peritonitis, chronic pancreatitis, secondary diabetes mellitus, malabsorption syndrome, and pancreatic cancer.

Answers to Chapter 13 Case Studies

Case Study 13.1

1. Why can't Rosa feel her legs? What other symptoms of this condition would you look for?
   Rosa has spinal shock. It is the body's immediate response to spinal trauma. There is paralysis and loss of reflexes. There is loss of bowel and bladder function and sensation below the level of injury. There is also a vascular, or neurogenic, response. The sympathetic nervous system (SNS) is inhibited within the smooth muscle, causing vasodilation (hypotension) and bradycardia above the level of injury, as the parasympathetic nervous system (PNS) is unopposed.
2. Is this condition permanent?
   No, it is not. It typically lasts 2 to 3 days but can last longer. The true damage and symptoms of the spinal cord injury will not be able to be determined until the spinal shock resolves.
3. With a C6 spinal injury, what complication(s) would you be most worried about?
   The primary injury is to C6. However, the inflammation and edema can lead to further damage both above and below C6, called the secondary injury. There can be vascular damage, ischemia, and demyelination of neurons. I would worry most about respiratory failure, as the C4 phrenic nerve enervates the diaphragm and controls breathing. I would worry that secondary injury may cause damage to C4.
4. What is happening to Rosa?
   Rosa is experiencing autonomic dysreflexia.
5. What symptoms justify your answer?
   Rosa has a high blood pressure and a low heart rate. This shows the SNS response above the level of injury with the exaggerated PNS response of bradycardia. Vasodilation (PNS) causes the sweating and flushing.

Case Study 13.2

1. What would you suspect? Is this an emergency? Why or why not?
   Yes, this is a medical emergency. Geo likely has an epidural hematoma. This is an arterial bleed between the skull and dura mater. With this type of injury there is a brief loss of consciousness, followed by a lucid period, then loss of consciousness, and coma.
2. Explain the pathophysiology of the diagnosis. What complication would you be worried about?
   The arterial bleeding compresses the brain and increases the intracranial pressure. According to the Monro-Kellie doctrine, if one component of the intracranial pressure (ICP) (blood, brain tissue, cerebrospinal fluid) increases, the other components must decrease. Here bleeding has increased, so the complication to look for is brain herniation.

Case Study 13.3

1. Was this the right decision? Why or why not?
   No, it was not. Secondary impact syndrome is when there is a second concussion before the symptoms from the first concussion have subsided. This causes rapid swelling and edema of the brain and is often fatal. Studies have shown that Black athletes are put back into the game with concussions at a higher rate than White athletes, often due to access to care issues.
2. Lee asks, "Can I go back to playing football next week? We have a big game!" What would you say?
   I would say that it typically takes 1 to 2 weeks to heal, sometimes longer. Lee needs to be symptom-free before going back to playing football, otherwise he is at risk of second impact syndrome.
3. Lee tells you that he is having difficulty focusing in class and getting through assignments. Are these normal symptoms of concussion?
   Yes, they are. Blunt force trauma causes the brain, suspended in cerebrospinal fluid (CSF), to hit the skull. This can damage the tissues, vessels, and nerves, causing a diffuse transient brain injury called a concussion. Common symptoms are loss of concentration, headaches, irritability, and insomnia.

Case Study 13.4

1. If you were the triage nurse, what would you do next? Why?
   I would institute droplet precautions and bring Lizzie back to a room and isolate her, as she has symptoms of meningitis and would need to be ruled out for bacterial meningitis. Lizzie has fever, photophobia, neck pain, vomiting, and +Kernig sign, all symptoms of meningitis. I would also make sure that the room was dark, as she has photophobia.
2. Why is a head CT scan done prior to the lumbar puncture?
   If intracranial pressure (ICP) is increased, a lumbar puncture would relieve the pressure, causing cerebrospinal fluid (CSF) to flow out quickly and causing the brain to herniate through the foramen magnum.
3. What do Lizzie's lab results and assessments tell you? Explain the pathophysiology.
   Lizzie's WBC is high, signifying ongoing infection. D-dimer is also high, which means that there is systemic infection and clotting. Platelets are low, which is concerning, as increased clotting is part of disseminated intravascular coagulation (DIC). Once clotting factors and platelets run out, then hemorrhaging will begin. The long clotting time is also an indicator of DIC. Finally, the CSF is cloudy, which is an indicator of bacterial meningitis.

Answers to Chapter 14 Case Studies

Case Study 14.1

1. Looking at these results, what would you suspect is causing Cassandra's symptoms? Which results support your diagnosis?
   Cassandra's WBC is slightly elevated, her ESR and CRP are both high, which suggest systemic inflammation. The numbness and diplopia occurred after a viral illness. With the initial viral illness, numbness and tingling and double vision, differential diagnoses would be stroke, myasthenia gravis, and multiple sclerosis.
2. Does Cassandra have risk factors for a stroke? If so, what are they?
   Cassandra's only risk factors are that she smokes. She is fit, her LDL and HDL are both in a healthy range, and she exercises. The fact that she is Black has no bearing on her risk factors, as race is not genetic. Cassandra is at fairly low risk for a stroke.
3. What does the MRI suggest that Cassandra has?
   The MRI shows lesions in the brain stem and left brain. She also has progressive fatigue and loss of balance. This appears to be multiple sclerosis. Multiple sclerosis (MS) is a diagnosis of exclusion. The next step would be a lumbar puncture.
4. Cassandra tells the nurse that she does not want a lumbar puncture because she is afraid that she will be paralyzed. What would you say to her? Why is a lumbar puncture important?
   Ultimately, the decision is Cassandra's. The benefit of the lumbar puncture is that it may show antimyelin antibodies specific to MS. There is always risk associated with any procedure, but there is almost no risk of paralysis with lumbar puncture, as performed by a trained provider.
5. Have these findings confirmed your diagnosis? Explain the pathophysiology of the diagnosis.
   MS cannot be definitively diagnosed until death, and it is a diagnosis of exclusion. MS is an epigenetic disease. Cassandra was genetically predisposed to MS. A viral trigger caused an inflammatory and immune reaction. Autoreactive T and B cells cross the blood-brain barrier and attack and destroy myelin sheaths and oligodendrocytes. Over time, with the destruction of myelin sheaths and of the oligodendrocytes, neuronal conduction stops and there is neuronal death. This causes brain atrophy and affects both white and gray matter.
6. How would you respond?
   I would empathize with Cassandra about her misdiagnosis. I would let her know that neuromuscular diseases are often difficult to diagnose, and the diagnosis is one of exclusion. The other issue is that MS is wrongly thought to be a disease that exclusively affects White individuals. The reality is that MS is often

misdiagnosed and undertreated in people of color. This contributes to a late diagnosis with worse symptoms and prognosis.

Case Study 14.2

1. What diagnosis do Tony's symptoms suggest? What findings might confirm this?
   The recent viral illness, ptosis, facial droop, and autoimmune disease all point to myasthenia gravis (MG). It is more likely to occur if there is history of autoimmune disease already. Tony has Addison disease, so they are more likely to have MG.
2. Explain the pathophysiology of the disease. What may have triggered it?
   MG is an acquired autoimmune disease. The autoantibodies bind to acetylcholine receptors in the neuromuscular junction and block the receptors from binding to acetylcholine. Over time, the receptors are destroyed by these autoantibodies. Acetylcholine is an excitatory neurotransmitter. Without acetylcholine, there is decreased transmission of nerve impulses which results in muscle weakness. MG typically has exacerbations and remissions, set off by triggers such as stress and illness. Tony's viral illness probably triggered this.
3. The provider orders a chest CT. Why would the provider order this?
   Often the cause of MG is a thymoma. A thymoma is a tumor (often malignant) that grows slowly within the thymus gland. The thymoma can cause the development of autoreactive T cells. It can be detected in a chest CT and removal often results in remission of the disease.
4. Can this disease be cured? Why or why not?
   Unfortunately, MG cannot be cured. It is a chronic, autoimmune disease. However, symptoms can be treated, and the disease can go into remission, either temporarily or permanently.

Case Study 14.3

1. Shyam tells the nurse that no one in the family has a history of Parkinson disease. He asks how Radhika could have gotten the disease. What can the visiting nurse say?
   Parkinson disease (PD) is an epigenetic disease but is rarely inherited. The exact cause of the disease is unknown. Parkinsonian symptoms can also be caused by medications and other toxins.
2. What is the pathophysiology behind Parkinson disease? Explain the mechanism.
   With PD, the cause is unknown. It is thought that oxidative stress and mitochondrial dysfunction are part of the reason it that occurs. With PD, there is a loss of dopamine producing neurons in the basal ganglia. Dopamine is an inhibitory neurotransmitter, which means that muscles stay contracted and cannot relax. With PD, there can also be a mutation of the alpha synuclein protein in the neurons. This mutation causes the protein to accumulate, forming Lewy bodies and causing Lewy body dementia.
3. Explain the reason for her falls and confusion.
   With PD, there are muscle rigidity, slowness of movement, and tremors. As the disease progresses, balance is affected and individuals stoop forward, throwing off their balance. This is likely causing Radhika's falls. The confusion may result from accumulation of alpha synuclein proteins, causing Lewy body dementia.
4. What can be done for Parkinson disease? Is it curable?
   Unfortunately, PD is progressive and not curable. Symptoms can be treated. Levodopa-carbidopa is a medication that can alleviate symptoms. It is composed of synthetic dopamine. Symptoms such as pain, spasms, depression, anxiety, sleep, skin, bowel, and bladder issues can all be addressed with medication or nonpharmaceutical approaches, such as meditation. An interdisciplinary approach is most beneficial for clients with PD.

Case Study 14.4

1. On arrival, Rose had a fingerstick glucose done and IV placed before being rushed off to get a head CT scan. What is the rationale for these actions?
   Hypoglycemia symptoms can mimic stroke symptoms. That is why a blood sugar is always taken when clients are brought in with stroke symptoms. A head CT needs to be done emergently to determine whether the stroke is hemorrhagic or ischemic.
2. What may have caused Rose's stroke? Explain how Rose's risk factors may have contributed.
   Rose had hypertension, type 2 diabetes mellitus (T2DM), and hyperlipidemia. All of these would suggest metabolic syndrome. With these conditions, Rose has a high probability of atherosclerosis and cardiovascular disease. With atherosclerosis, a thrombus can occlude a cerebral artery and cause a stroke. The two transient ischemic attacks (TIAs) that Rose had are also indications that Rose was likely have a stroke.
3. Does this mean that Rose did not have a stroke? Explain.
   No. This tells you that the stroke is not hemorrhagic. Damage from ischemic stroke does not show up right away and would not be visible on a head CT. It is important to determine if the stroke is hemorrhagic or ischemic prior to treatment with fibrinolytics.
4. What is the priority in treating a client with a stroke? Explain.
   The priority is reperfusion, the same as it is with a myocardial infarction. With a stroke, the infarcted area is called the core. The core becomes necrotic and is permanently damaged. However, the surrounding area, the penumbra, is hypoxic and damage can be reversed. That's why reperfusion and oxygenation must occur quickly, to limit the damage.

5. Will Rose fully recover function? Why or why not?
   It depends on the level of injury and the function. The necrotic area will become scarred and will not be able to conduct neural impulses. However, there is neural plasticity, which means that the neural networks can grow, change, and rewire itself to perform functions that were previously performed in other areas of the brain. Depending on the severity of the stroke, Rose will likely regain full or partial function.
6. Is this Alzheimer disease? What are the structural changes associated with Alzheimer disease? Explain the pathophysiology.
   Rose has a history of Alzheimer disease in her family. There is a genetic association, so this may likely be Alzheimer disease. With Alzheimer disease, there are mutations in chromosomes 19 and 17. The mutations in chromosome 19 causes the misfolding of beta-amyloid proteins. This causes them to accumulate outside the neurons and form neuritic plaques. The mutation of chromosome 17 causes the tau proteins to build up inside the neurons, causing neurofibrillary tangles. The plaques and tangles disrupt neuronal transmission and cause neuronal death.
7. Could these cognitive changes be due to her stroke? Explain.
   Yes. Vascular dementia is caused by atherosclerosis and hypoperfusion of the brain. In Rose's case, she may have mixed dementia, both Alzheimer and vascular dementia.

Answers to Chapter 15 Case Studies

Case Study 15.1

1. Explain the pathophysiological mechanisms behind osteoporosis.
   Osteoporosis is characterized by a reduction in bone density, leading to increased bone fragility and susceptibility to fractures. The balance between bone resorption and bone formation is disrupted, and osteoclasts break down more bone than osteoblasts form. The structural integrity of the bone is impaired and the bone "thins."
2. What risk factors did Shauna have that caused her to develop osteoporosis? How would you treat her?
   Osteoporosis has many risk factors, such as older age, postmenopausal AFAB (due to lack of estrogen), lack of calcium and vitamin D, smoking, medications (steroids), and immobility. Initially, Shauna would be treated with RICE (rest, ice, compression, and elevation). Pain should be treated with nonsteroidal anti-inflammatory drugs (NSAIDs), unless the patient has contraindications, such as bleeding. The wrist should be splinted until the swelling goes down and then casted if needed. Circulation, sensation, and movement should be checked regularly.
3. What measures can Shauna take to reduce the likelihood of fractures? What complications might she be at risk for?
   Shauna should be advised to follow-up with her provider and consider supplementing her calcium and vitamin D. Low-impact, weight-bearing exercises can also reduce the risk of fracture. Medications such as alendronate, which slows down osteoclast activity, and denosumab, which inhibits the receptor activator of nuclear factor kappa beta ligand (RANKL), can also prevent the progression of osteoporosis and reduce the risk of fracture. Complications that could result are Colles fractures (sudden fractures with coughing or a fall), vertebral compression fractures, kyphosis, difficulty breathing (due to less compliance), impaired mobility, and pain.

Case Study 15.2

1. What condition do you think that Meera would be at risk for? Why?
   Meera would be at risk for osteomyelitis or infection of the bone. The penetrating injury that Meera has sustained by stepping on a nail would be the cause of this. Meera's symptoms—fever, throbbing pain in right foot and lower leg, redness and swelling, inability to bear weight on the right leg, and malaise—all point to osteomyelitis as the diagnosis.
2. What role does the mechanism of injury play in the pathogenesis of this condition?
   Meera appears to have acute pyogenic osteomyelitis, most likely a *Staphylococcus aureus* infection from the penetrating injury.
   - Invasion of pathogen
   - Inflammatory response
   - Blood supply blocked by pus, pus spreads into the blood vessels
   - Decreased blood flow leads to bone necrosis
   - There is a devascularized dead bone fragment (sequestrum)
   - The new bone is formed around the dead bone (involucrum)
3. What do these results mean? Explain. What other tests might be ordered?
   These results serve to confirm the diagnosis of osteomyelitis. With this condition, there are leukocytosis and inflammation, which cause elevated white blood cell counts, ESR, and CRP. The wound culture indicates a staphylococcus infection, which is a common cause of osteomyelitis. I would expect the provider to consider ordering a magnetic resonance imaging (MRI) of the right lower extremity.
4. What are the potential complications of Meera's condition?
   If left untreated, the wound could progress to become necrotic and gangrenous, which would mean that the right foot would need to be amputated. The infection could also spread to the blood and cause sepsis and shock.

5. What would Meera's treatment plan include?
   Meera would need to be on an intravenous (IV) antibiotic regimen for 4 to 6 weeks. The antibiotic medication depends on bacterial sensitivity and resistance. Pain management would typically be achieved with nonsteroidal anti-inflammatory drugs (NSAIDs). The wound should be packed and dressed, and the limb should be splinted and immobilized.

Case Study 15.3

1. Looking at Rachel's symptoms and history, what key clinical features would lead you to a diagnosis? What would your diagnosis be?
   Rachel has bilateral pain in the small joints of her hands, swelling and stiffness in the mornings. This pain lasts over an hour and is accompanied by fatigue, which is a systemic symptom. All of this indicates rheumatoid arthritis (RA).
2. What are the genetic and environmental risk factors that contribute to this disease? Is this an autoimmune disease? Why or why not?
   RA risk factors are epigenetic and include:
   - familial history
   - human leukocyte antigen class II histocompatibility, D related beta chain (HLA-DRB1) alleles
   - assigned female at birth (AFAB) > assigned male at birth (AMAB)
   - smoking
   - silica, asbestos, textile dust
   - gum infections
   - dysfunctional gut microbiome
   - obesity

   RA is triggered by repeated environmental triggers, which causes autoantibodies to be formed against citrullinated proteins. This immune response often starts in the lungs, gums, and gastrointestinal (GI) tract. These autoantibodies can be present for years before patients with RA actually become symptomatic. Once the inflammatory reaction begins in the synovium, angiogenesis (blood vessel growth) occurs. The synovium is infiltrated by inflammatory cells and autoantibodies begin to be produced in the synovium. Cytokines and chemokines are released by inflammatory cells, such as mast cells, and cause loss of cartilage. Chondrocytes secrete cytokines, damaging the cartilage. The receptor activator of nuclear factor kappa beta ligand (RANKL) is released, activating osteoclasts and bone erosions. The synovial membrane becomes swollen and projects into the joint space, causing a pannus to form.
3. What labs would you expect the provider to order and what results do you expect to see to confirm the diagnosis?
   I would expect the provider to order a complete blood count (CBC), erythrocyte sedimentation rate (ESR), C-reactive protein (CRP), rheumatoid factor (RF), and anti-cyclic citrullinated peptide (CCP) antibody levels. In RA, white blood cell (WBC), ESR, and CRP levels would be elevated. RF and CCP antibodies would also be present. Aspiration of the synovium would show high levels of leukocytes.
4. What complications would you expect? How would you treat this disease?
   RA could progress to larger joints and cause deformities, loss of function, and immobility. Systemic autoimmune symptoms such as Sjögren syndrome (dry eyes, dry mouth), scleritis, vasculitis, fatigue, weakness, and weight loss. RA is managed with disease-modifying antirheumatic drugs (DMARDs), such as methotrexate. For exacerbations, steroids are prescribed. Pain is generally treated with nonsteroidal anti-inflammatory drugs (NSAIDS).

Case Study 15.4

1. Given Marwan's symptoms and family history, what key clinical features would lead you to believe that he has gout?
   Gout, or gouty arthritis, occurs because of excess uric acid (urate). The urate forms crystals, which then collect in the joint synovium, causing inflammation. Pain, redness, and swelling are hallmark signs of inflammation. Marwan also states that he has a family history of gout, he eats a lot of meat and dairy products, and drinks alcohol. All of this can lead to high uric acid concentrations.
2. How would you confirm that Marwan has gout?
   Lab tests, such as white blood cell (WBC), erythrocyte sedimentation rate (ESR), and C-reactive protein (CRP), would be run to detect leukocytosis and inflammation. I would expect all of these labs to be high. The gold standard is aspiration of the synovial fluid. If there are urate crystals in the synovial fluid, it is a confirmation of gout.
3. What lifestyle changes would Marwan need to make? How would you treat gout?
   Marwan should consider changing his diet so that he is not eating as much meat or dairy. He should also consider cutting down his alcohol intake. Treatment would consist of colchicine and nonsteroidal anti-inflammatory drugs (NSAIDs) for inflammation and allopurinol to decrease the amount of uric acid.

Answers to Chapter 16 Case Studies

Case Study 16.1

1. Please interpret Julia's blood gas (pH, pCO_2, pO_2, and HCO_3).
   Julia's blood gases indicate partially compensated metabolic alkalosis.
2. Why does Julia have an ABG like this? What caused it?
   Julia has severe vomiting and diarrhea, which likely caused her alkalosis. As she has an eating disorder where she is vomiting often, she would be vomiting acid, so she

would be alkalotic. The fact that she has an eating disorder and has taken laxatives means that the cause is metabolic. The pH is 7.58 which is basic, the HCO_3 is high which means metabolic alkalosis. CO_2 is higher; therefore, it is compensating. Because pH is not back to the normal range it is only partially compensated.

3. The health care provider is worried about kidney damage. Is this a concern? Why?
   Yes, it is a big concern. Julia's labs show that she has elevated BUN and creatinine. She also has oliguria, which means that the glomerular filtration rate (GFR) is decreased. If there is a decreased GFR the blood is not being filtered through the kidney.
4. What labs and assessment findings support this?
   Julia's BUN and creatinine are both high, and she has oliguria and dark urine. All of these are indications of renal injury. Julia's liver enzymes are also elevated (ALT). If she has liver disease (cirrhosis), it can lead to hepatorenal syndrome, which would cause the kidneys to fail. Finally, Julia is extremely dehydrated, which can lead to prerenal kidney failure.
5. Would the provider find Julia's electrolyte levels to be normal? Which ones are abnormal and what led to the abnormality? Explain.
   Metabolic alkalosis can lead to Julia's hypokalemia, hypocalcemia, and hypomagnesemia. In alkalotic conditions, proteins hang on to their substrates. This means that there are less free ions in the blood. The body is trying to compensate the alkalosis and therefore the H^+/K pump is activated. This would cause the H^+ to be pumped outside of the cell in exchange the potassium into the cell. This would cause hypokalemia in this case. Her eating disorder could also cause malnutrition leading to hypomagnesemia, which can lead to hypoparathyroidism. Remember that the parathyroid glands need magnesium to function! Hypoparathyroidism leads to hypocalcemia.
6. Would the provider be concerned about anemia? What kind of anemia? Explain the labs and pathophysiology that indicate this condition.
   Yes. Julia has low hemoglobin and hematocrit which could result from iron-deficiency anemia. That would also explain why she is extremely weak. She is likely not eating enough so therefore there is malabsorption of iron from her diet leading to iron-deficiency anemia. Julia also has kidney injury. Kidneys produce erythropoietin, which stimulates red blood cell production. When kidneys are failing, they may not be able to produce red blood cells. This would be anemia of chronic disease.
7. What would be a possible diagnosis for these new symptoms? Why?
   She is suffering from a mechanical small bowel obstruction. She exhibits the symptoms of borborygmi (hyperactive bowel sounds above the obstruction site, hypoactive below the obstruction site), nausea and vomiting (N/V), abdominal pain, and distention. Her pain is crampy (noncontinuous) so it would be a mechanical obstruction instead of a nonmechanical obstruction.
8. What condition do you suspect that Julia has? Why?
   Julia may be suffering from a pulmonary embolism. This could be an embolus from a deep vein thrombosis caused by immobility or from clotting caused by the mitral valve regurgitation. She has the hallmark findings of a pulmonary embolism—the anxiety, tachycardia, low-grade fever, dyspnea, and pink frothy sputum.
9. Looking at her lab and assessment findings, which factors would have caused this new complication?
   There are many factors leading to clotting and pulmonary embolism. On admission, Julia was extremely dehydrated, which leads to hypercoagulable conditions and clotting (Virchow triad). Julia's mitral valve regurgitation (MVR) would lead to left atrial dilation, which may cause atrial arrhythmias and clots, which may have traveled to her pulmonary arteries. Immobility may have led to a deep vein thrombosis, which could have broken off and traveled to her lungs.
10. How can a diagnosis of pulmonary embolism be confirmed?
   A D-dimer measures clotting fragments. A high D-dimer indicates that you may have a clotting issue, a pulmonary embolus. To confirm, a chest CT must be done.

Case Study 16.2

1. What would your primary diagnosis be? Explain.
   Daniel's primary diagnosis appears to be an exacerbation of his chronic obstructive pulmonary disease (COPD), specifically chronic bronchitis. He is wheezing, has a low oxygen saturation, diminished lung sounds, peripheral edema, and cool extremities. The wheezing, cough, and low O_2 saturation would point to COPD as the diagnosis. The edema and ascites point to cor-pulmonale, right-sided heart failure caused by lung disease. A myocardial infarction can be ruled out because the troponin level is normal.
2. What risk factors could have contributed to his illness?
   Daniel has multiple risk factors that would lead to COPD and heart failure. Daniel has a history of smoking, hypertension, and obesity. He also has coronary artery disease, chronic bronchitis, and type 2 diabetes mellitus. All these factors contribute to a diagnosis of metabolic syndrome. Having metabolic syndrome leads to a high-risk cardiovascular disease. Finally, we must take the social determinants of health and equity into consideration. He was laid off 2 years ago and likely has financial stressors, as well as a lack of access to medical care. He may also have issues with housing and getting healthy food to eat. Psychosocially, he may be stressed, anxious, and depressed, which would exacerbate his disease progression and toxic stress.

3. Analyze Daniel's arterial blood gases. Are they normal? If not, explain what the cause would be.
   Daniel's arterial blood gas (ABG) is not normal. He has partially compensated respiratory acidosis. His acidic pH, high CO_2, and an increase in HCO_3 indicate partial compensation. Daniel's acidosis is caused by his chronic lung disease, as he has low levels of oxygen and high levels of retained carbon dioxide.
4. What other lab results would the provider be concerned with? What might cause these issues? Explain the labs and pathophysiology.
   Daniel's potassium level is high, which would be a big concern. As Daniel is in acidosis, the kidneys are getting rid of H^+ to correct acidosis and retaining potassium in exchange, causing hyperkalemia. The buffer system would push the H^+ into the cells, causing the potassium to be pushed out into the blood. Daniel's glucose levels are also quite high, indicating poorly managed type 2 diabetes mellitus. His BUN and creatinine are also high, indicating poor kidney function. This may be because heart failure and diabetes are closely related to kidney failure. Diabetes causes microangiopathy, damaging kidney vessels. Heart failure decreases perfusion to kidneys, causing hypoxic damage.
5. What implications might this finding have for Daniel? Explain.
   The aortic stenosis causes concentric hypertrophy of the left ventricle to push the blood into the aorta. Eventually, due to the high oxygen demand, the left ventricle will start to fail and the blood will back up into the left atrium, causing dilation and arrhythmias such as atrial fibrillation. The blood will then back up into the lungs, contributing to pulmonary congestion and hypoxia, eventually leading to heart failure.
6. What labs and assessment findings support this?
   Daniel has an abnormal ECG, showing atrial fibrillation, an echocardiogram finding of aortic stenosis, respiratory acidosis, and a low O_2 saturation.
7. What do you think has happened to Daniel? Why?
   Daniel is experiencing acute pulmonary edema due to heart failure. Daniel's oxygen saturation is only 88% on 2 liters of O_2, and there are crackles throughout his lungs, indicating that his lungs are filled with fluid, causing dyspnea hypoxia, and increasing edema. His BNP is very high as well. BNP is the best indicator of heart failure, as a high BNP is the body's attempt to correct fluid overload.
8. What would be a possible diagnosis for these new symptoms? Explain how this may be linked to Daniel's previous diagnoses and/or medical history.
   Posthepatic portal hypertension from heart failure. Daniel has jaundice, as evidenced by yellowing of conjunctiva. This is caused by bilirubin not being able to be conjugated by the liver. The unconjugated bilirubin then builds up in the blood and causes the yellow coloring. With liver disease, Daniel's liver would not be able to make protein and he would have hypoalbuminemia. The distention is from a decrease in colloidal osmotic pressure (lack of protein) and increase in hydrostatic pressure which results in fluid shunting to peritoneum. This is consistent with her hepatomegaly and distended abdomen from when he first presented to the hospital.
9. What do you think has happened to Daniel?
   Daniel is having a left-brain stroke. This is evident from the right-sided facial droop and paralysis. He also has difficulty speaking, which is a function of the left brain.
10. Do you think that Daniel's condition has been caused by anything in his previous medical history, assessments, or labs? If so, explain the correlation.
   Daniel has metabolic syndrome, which indicates high risk for cardiovascular events such as stroke. Type 2 diabetes mellitus is also associated with macroangiopathy and cardiac disease. He has coronary artery disease and hypertension, which lead to atherosclerosis and formation of thrombi and emboli. Finally, his ECG shows atrial fibrillation. This can lead to clots in the left atrium, which can then travel to the brain, causing a stroke.

Case Study 16.3

1. What do you think is happening to Davina? What evidence do you have?
   Davina appears to have type 1 diabetes mellitus (T1DM). Her clinical manifestations are the "3 Ps," polyuria, polydipsia, and polyphagia. She appears dehydrated and has lost a significant amount of weight in a short period of time. Looking at her labs, the serum glucose is very high.
2. How can you confirm this diagnosis?
   T1DM is an autoimmune disease. Circulating pancreatic autoantibodies to islet cells and insulin may be present and should be tested for to distinguish it from type 2 DM. Repeat fasting glucose should be done.
3. Explain the pathophysiology of this disease.
   T1DM is an autoimmune disease that is predisposed by genetic mutations on multiple genes (i.e., chromosome 6). T1DM is thought to be triggered by epigenetic stressors, such as viral illness (Coxsackie, rotavirus, mumps, rubella, influenza B, and COVID-19). Viral illnesses are thought to trigger autoantibody destruction of the beta cells, rendering the patient insulinopenic.
4. What do you think her diagnosis is and how is it related to the diagnosis in Question 1?
   Davina may have inflammatory bowel disease, most likely Crohn disease, given the nonbloody diarrhea. This is an epigenetic and autoimmune disease thought to be caused by dysfunctional intestinal microbiome, intestinal epithelial cell dysfunction, and genetic mutations. It is related to Davina's previous diagnosis of T1DM because both are epigenetic and autoimmune diseases. When an individual has one autoimmune

illness, there is a high risk of having other autoimmune disorders.

5. Describe the symptoms and complications of the disease. How could the disease be definitively diagnosed?

   Crohn disease causes chronic bowel inflammation and partial-to full-thickness ulcerations throughout the gastrointestinal (GI) tract, from the mouth to the anus. The initial lesions are superficial, but progress to all layers of the GI tract, and ultimately cause scarring. These areas of inflammation cause granulomas that look like "cobblestones" and are often called skip lesion because they do not progress in an orderly fashion and can "skip" around the GI tract. Symptoms consist of diarrhea 6 to 8 times a day, abdominal pain, and urgency. The disease has exacerbations and remissions and is often triggered by stressors such as illness and emotional stress. Complications are malabsorption, malnutrition, strictures, fistulas, and weight loss. The disease can be definitively diagnosed by capsule endoscopy, colonoscopy, and magnetic resonance imaging (MRI).

6. How do you treat this disease?

   The treatments for this would be anti-inflammatory medications, such as mesalamine, steroids, and immunosuppressants, such as methotrexates. For severe disease, biologic monoclonal antibodies, such as infliximab, can be used.

7. Do you feel that Davina's first provider treated her appropriately? Why or why not?

   Davina's provider should have looked more deeply into her symptoms and history. Historically, inflammatory bowel diseases (IBDs) are underdiagnosed in the Black population. In fact, IBD was thought to be a disease of "White people." Although the prevalence of IBD is increasing, many providers still wrongly diagnose the disease, even when it presents with hallmark symptoms, as in Davina's case. I would say that there was provider bias and also lack of knowledge of current practice on the provider's part.

8. What do you suspect? Give your rationale.

   I would suspect a thyroid disorder, specifically hyperthyroidism. Both Graves disease and Hashimoto disease are autoimmune diseases. As Davina has T1DM and Crohn disease already, she would be more prone to an autoimmune thyroid disorder. She has the symptoms of hyperthyroidism—palpitations, weight loss, shortness of breath, and heat intolerance. Both Hashimoto and Graves disease show signs of hyperthyroidism initially. With Hashimoto disease, hyperthyroidism evolves into hypothyroidism as the thyroid gland is destroyed. Further information is needed to distinguish the specific disease process.

9. What lab and diagnostic tests would you need to confirm a diagnosis?

   An ultrasound would confirm thyroid enlargement. For specific diagnosis, I would want to see thyroid stimulating hormone (TSH) and thyroxine (T4) levels, also thyroid autoantibody levels. You would see antithyroid antibodies with Hashimoto disease and thyroid receptor antibodies with Graves disease.

Index